ESSENTIALS OF THYROID
CANCER MANAGEMENT

ESSENTIALS OF THYROID
CANCER MANAGEMENT

Edited by
ROBERT J. AMDUR, MD
Professor, Department of Radiation Oncology
University of Florida College of Medicine
Gainesville, Florida USA

ERNEST L. MAZZAFERRI, MD, MACP
Professor, Department of Medicine
University of Florida College of Medicine
Gainesville, Florida USA
Emeritus Professor and Chairman of Internal Medicine
Ohio State University
Columbus, Ohio USA

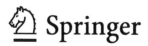 Springer

Robert J. Amdur, MD
Department of Radiation Oncology
University of Florida College of Medicine
2000 S.W. Archer Road
Gainesville, FL 32610-0385
USA

Ernest L. Mazzaferri, MD, MACP
Department of Medicine
University of Florida College of Medicine
2000 S.W. Archer Road
Gainesville, FL 32610-0385
USA

ESSENTIALS OF THYROID CANCER MANAGEMENT

Library of Congress Cataloging-in-Publication Data

A C.I.P. Catalogue record for this book is available
from the Library of Congress.

ISBN-10: 0-387-25713-6   e-ISBN: 0-387-25714-4   Printed on acid-free paper.
ISBN-13: 978-0387-25713-6

Printed in the United States of America.

9 8 7 6 5 4 3 2 1   SPIN 11054801

springeronline.com

CONTENTS

CONTRIBUTING AUTHORS

Robert J. Amdur, MD
Professor
Department of Radiation Oncology
University of Florida
College of Medicine

Heather M. Brown, MD
Assistant Professor
Department of Pathology,
Immunology and Laboratory Medicine
University of Florida
College of Medicine

Jonathan Gang Li, PhD
Assistant Professor
Department of Radiation Oncology
University of Florida
College of Medicine

Siyong Kim, PhD
Assistant Professor
Department of Radiation Oncology
University of Florida
College of Medicine

Chiray Liu, PhD
Associate Professor
Department of Radiation Oncology
University of Florida
College of Medicine

Nicole A. Massoll, MD
Assistant Professor
Department of Pathology, Immunology
and Laboratory Medicine
University of Florida
College of Medicine

Ernest L. Mazzaferri, MD, MACP
Professor
Department of Medicine
University of Florida
College of Medicine,
and Emeritus Professor and
Chairman of Internal Medicine
Ohio State University

William M. Mendenhall, MD
Professor
Department of Radiation Oncology
University of Florida
College of Medicine

Pamela L. Sandow, DMD
Clinical Associate Professor
Department of Oral and Maxillofacial
Surgery and Diagnostic Sciences
University of Florida
College of Dentistry

Illona M. Schmallfuss, MD
Assistant Professor
Department of Radiology
University of Florida
College of Medicine

George Snyder
Radiation Safety Officer
Shands Hospital, Gainesville, Florida

Douglas B. Villaret, MD
Assistant Professor
Department of Otolaryngology
University of Florida
College of Medicine

ACKNOWLEDGEMENT

We thank Chris Morris for helping us get permission to use figures from other publications and Jessica Kirwan for preparing the manuscript.

PREFACE

The goal of this book is to provide Endocrinologists, Surgeons, Nuclear Medicine Physicians, and Radiation Oncologists with practical advice about managing patients with thyroid cancer. This book will not replace the excellent publications that focus on a highly specific topic or provide an exhaustive review of major subjects from the perspective of a particular specialty. These kinds of publications will always be an important source of information for both students and experienced practitioners. The void that we see is the lack of a single, concise, up-to-date reference that is applicable to all of the specialists who make clinical decisions about thyroid cancer patients. *Essentials of Thyroid Cancer Management* will fill this void in a manner that is both user-friendly and technically comprehensive.

For reading efficiency, this book contains the minimum of text required to explain how to make sound clinical decisions in specific situations. We rely heavily on tables, diagrams, graphs, photographs, and other figures to convey this information. Subjects are addressed in a large number of chapters that each focus on a relatively narrow topic. In some cases, there is overlap between the information in multiple different chapters so the reader does not have to page back and forth between different sections of the book.

As occurs in every area of medicine, there is controversy about important issues in the management of thyroid cancer. We think explanations are most effective when they are concise and definitive. For this reason, we present our opinions and recommendations and simply note when others have divergent views. In most chapters, this book describes only one way of managing thyroid cancer patients. Reasonable people will disagree with some of the recommendations in this book and we respect the alternative viewpoints of our colleagues.

Robert J. Amdur and Ernest L. Mazzaferri

PART 1. INTRODUCTION

1.1. BASIC THYROID ANATOMY

ROBERT J. AMDUR, MD AND ERNEST L. MAZZAFERRI, MD, MACP

The normal thyroid gland is located in the anterior neck at the level of the thoracic inlet (Fig. 1). The majority of the gland consists of two lateral lobes connected anteriorly by the isthmus. Approximately 50% of people have a pyramidal lobe, which is a remnant of the distal end of the thyroglossal duct. There is variability in the superior extent of the pyramidal lobe between the thyroid and hyoid bone. The pyramidal lobe is usually located just to the left of midline.

In adults the average thyroid gland weighs 10 to 20 grams and measures approximately 5 × 5 cm in the superior–inferior and medial–lateral dimensions (Pankow 1985). Superiorly the lateral lobes of the thyroid usually extend to level of the middle of the thyroid cartilage. Inferiorly the thyroid usually extends to the level of the sixth tracheal ring. Laterally the thyroid lies just medial to the common carotid arteries. The thyroid wraps around 75% of the circumference of the trachea and the most posterior aspects of the lateral lobes may touch the esophagus (Fig. 2). The anterior surface of the thyroid is just deep to the strap muscles of the neck.

The location of the thyroid gland relative to important structures in the neck explains the presenting symptoms of locally advanced thyroid cancer, potential surgical complications, and the complexity of planning external beam radiotherapy. The main structures of interest are the recurrent laryngeal nerve, the trachea, the esophagus, the sympathetic trunk, the vagus and phrenic nerves and the carotid arteries. Figure 2 does not show the parathyroid glands and spinal cord. The parathyroid glands lie close to the posterior surface of the thyroid and vary in number and exact location. The parathyroid glands are discussed in more detail in a later chapter that focuses on the thyroidectomy procedure.

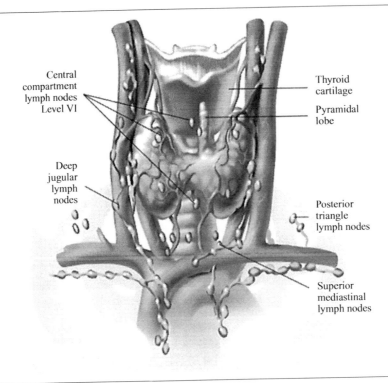

Figure 1. Anatomic location of the thyroid gland relative to the larynx, major vessles and draining lymphatics. (Reproduced with permission from MedImmune, Inc 2002.)

The spinal cord is located in the midline, approximately 4 cm posterior to the thyroid gland. This distance, and the intervening muscles of the floor of the neck and bone of the vertebral column, makes it so that tumor rarely spreads directly from the thyroid area to the spinal canal. The proximity of the thyroid gland to the spinal cord is a major factor when planning external beam radiotherapy.

LYMPHATIC DRAINAGE

The thyroid gland has a dense lymphatic network characterized by interconnections that drain each area of the gland in multiple different directions. The concept of a stepwise progression of nodal metastasis from one nodal station to another determines the extent of the neck dissection for thyroid cancers and the extent of the irradiated volume in patients who receive external beam radiotherapy (Qubnain 2002).

According to the sixth edition of the Cancer Staging Handbook organized by the American Joint Commission on Cancer, the first echelon nodal metastases from thyroid cancer are the nodes of the central compartment of the neck, the nodes of the superior

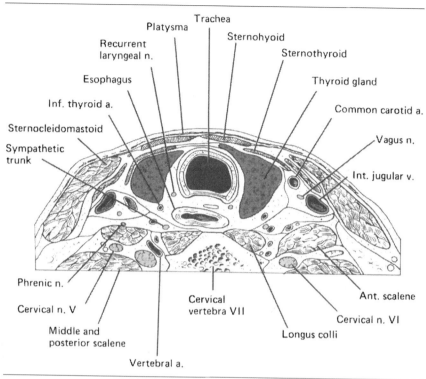

Figure 2. Axial section through the neck at the level of the C-7. (Redrawn from Eycleshymer AC, Schoemaker DM: A cross-section anatomy. New York, D. Appleton-Century, 1938:55.)

mediastinum, and the lateral cervical nodes (AJCC 2002). Figure 3 is a diagram of the boundaries of level I-VII nodal stations. The central compartment nodes are level VI, which is bounded by the hyoid bone superiorly, the suprasternal notch inferiorly, and the carotid arteries laterally. The specific nodal groups that drain the thyroid in the level VI compartment are the paralaryngeal, paratracheal, and prelaryngeal (Delphian) nodes. The level VII nodes are those of the superior mediastinum that lie superior to the innominate vein. The lateral cervical nodes include nodes in both level III and IV: Bilateral metastases are common.

THE PAROTID DUCT (STENSEN'S DUCT)

Stensen's duct, named after a Danish physician anatomist Niels Stensen (1638–1686), is the excretory duct of the parotid gland. About 7 cm long, it courses anteriorly over the masseter muscle and buccal fat pad, and then bends medially to pierce the buccinator muscle, ending intraorally at the level of the second maxillary molar (Netter 1965). Stensen's duct may develop sialadenitis or obstruction following I-131 therapy.

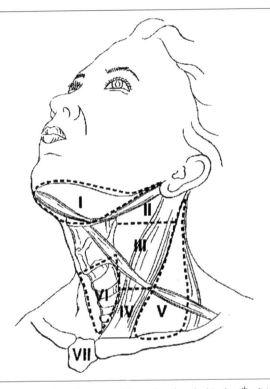

Figure 3. Schematic of the lymph node stations of the neck as described in the 6th edition of the AJCC staging manual.

REFERENCES

American Joint Committee on Cancer. 2002. AJCC Cancer Staging Manual, 6th edn. New York: Springer **22:**29 (nodal stations) and 90–97 (nodal drainage).

Netter, FH (ed). 1965. Anatomy of the Thyroid and Parathyroid Glands. The CIBA Collection of Medical Illustrations. Endocrine System and Selected Metabolic Diseases. New York: CIBA **4:**41–42.

Pankow, BG, J Michalak, and MK McGee. 1985. Adult human thyroid weight. Health Phys **49:**1097–1103.

Qubnain, SW, et al. 2002. Distribution of lymph node micrometastases in PN0 well differentiated thyroid carcinoma. Surgery **131:**249.

1.2. THYROID AND PARATHYROID PHYSIOLOGY

ERNEST L. MAZZAFERRI, MD, MACP AND ROBERT J. AMDUR, MD

The purpose of this chapter is to review the details of thyroid anatomy and physiology that facilitate an understanding of thyroid cancer management.

EMBRYOLOGY

The thyroid is embryologically derived from the primitive foregut and neural crest cells. The gland is comprised of two types of secretory cells: follicular cells that arise from the embryonic foregut and C cells that are derived from the neural crest (Santisteban 2005). These two cell types, respectively, synthesize thyroid hormone and calcitonin, the two main classes of hormones in the gland. The functional subunits of the thyroid are sphere-shaped follicles that contain an intra-luminal pool of colloid. Cuboidal follicular cells that synthesize and secrete thyroid hormones make up the lining of each follicle (Fig. 1). A thin layer of connective tissue containing a dense network of capillary and lymphatic vessels separates the follicles from each other. Within the interfollicular connective tissue, and interspersed among the follicular cells, are the thyroidal C cells that synthesize calcitonin.

THYROID HORMONE

The thyroid gland produces two biologically active forms of thyroid hormone: thyroxine (3, 5, 3', 5' iodothyronine or T_4) and triiodothyronine (3, 5, 3' iodothyronine or T3) (Engler 1984). Both contain an outer phenyl ring and an inner tyrosine ring attached by an ether linkage (Fig. 2). Conceptually it is useful to think of T4 as the

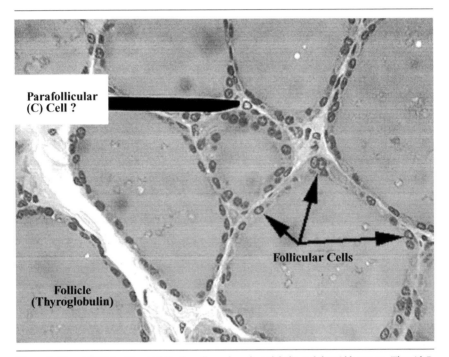

Figure 1. Thyroid follicle. Thyroid follicular cells produce thyroglobulin and thyroid hormone. Thyroid C cells, synthesize and secrete calcitonin.

storage and transport form of thyroid hormone and T3 as the metabolically active form. Most (~80%) thyroid hormone in the thyroid gland and plasma is T4, which is rapidly converted to T3 in skeletal muscle, liver, brain and other tissues by removal of an outer ring 5' iodine molecule. T3, and to a much smaller extent T4 (which acts mainly as a prohormone), are bound to specific nuclear receptors in peripheral cells that interact with regulatory regions of genes, influencing their expression. The tissue concentration of T3 almost completely determines the biologic effect of thyroid hormone. Levothyroxine (T4) alone is effective thyroid hormone replacement therapy because T3 is almost exclusively derived from T4.

IODINE AND THYROID FUNCTION

Iodine is essential for normal thyroid function (Fig. 2). The minimum daily intake necessary to prevent iodine deficiency goiter is 50 µg and the recommended daily intake is 150 µg. Urinary iodine is a reflection of iodine intake. Urinary iodine level was about 600 to 700 µg/L per day in the U.S. a few years ago but has been falling in recent years and now averages only about 150 µg/L (Hollowell 1998; Hollowell 2002).

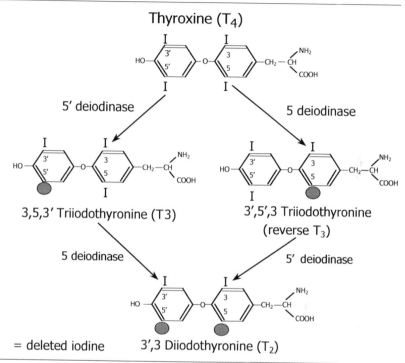

Thyroxine (T₄)

5′ deiodinase

5 deiodinase

3,5,3′ Triiodothyronine (T3)

3′,5′,3 Triiodothyronine (reverse T₃)

5 deiodinase

5′ deiodinase

● = deleted iodine   3′,3 Diiodothyronine (T₂)

Figure 2. The normal thyroid produces 80 to 100 µg of T_4 per day. About 10% of T_4 is degraded each day and about 80% is deiodinated, 40% to form T_3 and 40% to form rT_3 and the remaining 20% is conjugated with glucuronide and sulfate, deaminated and decarboxylated to form tetraiodothyroacetic acid (tetrac) or the two rings are cleaved. About 80% of the T_3 is formed by 5'-deiodination (outer ring) of T_4 in extrathyroidal tissue. This reaction is catalyzed by 5'deiodinase which occurs in abundance in the liver and kidney, but some deiodination occurs in most other tissues. There are two types of 5'-deiodinase (types I and II). Type I is the predominant form in the liver, kidney and thyroid, and deiodinates in the following order: $rT_3 > T_4 > T_3$. Type II is the predominant deiodinating enzyme in the brain, pituitary and skin and deiodinates $T_4 > rT_3$. Most T_3 (~80%) is produced by extrathyroidal deiodination of T_4 and the rest by the thyroid gland. Total T_3 production is 30 to 40 µg per day. Its degradation, mostly by deiodination, is much more rapid than that of T_4, reaching about 75% each day. The production rate of rT_3 is 30 to 40 µg per day, nearly all of which is extrathyroidal Degradation of rT3 is mostly by deiodination, and is even more rapid than that of T_3.

Ingested iodine is rapidly absorbed and distributed in the extracellular iodine pool, which it leaves via transport into the thyroid gland or by renal excretion. Expansion of the extracellular iodine pool is caused by iodine-containing drugs such as amiodarone or radiographic contrast materials such as Telepaque® or Oragrafin®. When this occurs, administered I-131 is so diluted within the expanded iodine pool that only a small fraction of I-131 is captured by the thyroid. This is why it is necessary to measure urine iodine levels when there is any question that a patient being prepared for I-131 therapy may have been exposed to pharmacologic doses of iodine. It also underscores

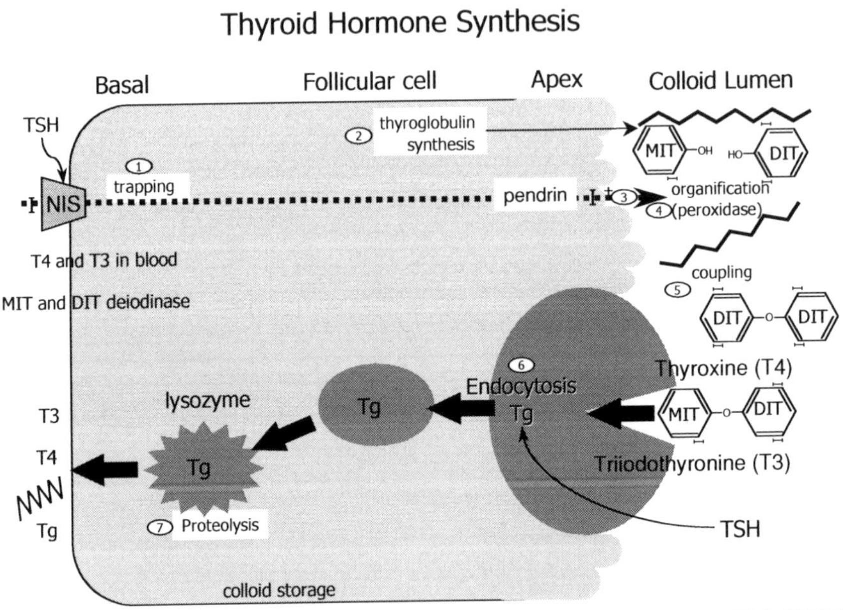

Thyroid Hormone Synthesis

Figure 3. Thyroid hormone synthesis. Thyroid hormones are synthesized in the thyroid gland via the following steps: (1) thyroid iodide transport (trapping), a TSH-stimulated process mediated by sodium-iodide symporters at the basolateral membranes of the cell; (2) synthesis of thyroglobulin, a 660 kilodalton protein composed of two non-covalently linked subunits that contain tyrosyl residues; thyroglobulin is synthesized and glycosylated in the rough endoplastic reticulum and then incorporated into the exocytotic vesicles that fuse with the apical cell membrane, only then are tyrosine residues iodinated; (3) iodide is transported by pendrin, a membrane iodide-chloride transporter, to exocytotic vesicles fused with the apical cell membrane; (4) oxidation of iodide is catalyzed by thyroid peroxidase, which produces iodination (organification) of about 10% of the tyrosine residues in thyroglobulin; (5) coupling of tyrosine residues produces T_4 by coupling two diiodotyrosine residues and T_3 by coupling one monoiodotyrosine and one diiodotyrosine within a thyroglobulin molecule; coupling is not a random process, instead T_4 and T_3 are formed at regions of the thyroglobulin molecule with unique amino acid sequences; (6) to liberate T_4 and T_3, thyroglobulin is reabsorbed into the thyroid follicular cells in the form of colloid droplets (endocytosis); (7) the colloid droplets fuse with lysosomes in which thyroglobulin is hydrolyzed to T_4, T_3 and the thyroid hormones and about 100 μg of thyroglobulin is released from the thyroid each day, a tiny fraction of the 25 mg that must be hydrolyzed to yield the 100 μg of T_4 that is secreted each day.

the necessity of a two-week low iodine-diet in preparation for I-131 therapy, even in patients who have not been exposed to iodine-containing drugs.

THYROIDAL IODINE TRANSPORT

Iodine is transported into thyroid follicular cells against an electrochemical gradient (Fig. 3). Its transmembrane transport is linked to that of sodium, and is energy-dependent and saturable, and requires oxidative metabolism. It is transported via the sodium–iodine symporter (NIS), a transmembrane protein located in the basolateral membrane of follicular cells, which responds to thyrotropin stimulation (thyroid stimulating hormone, TSH) (Smanik 1996). Functional NIS is also present in the malignant follicular cells of papillary, follicular and Hürthle cell cancers that concentrate I-131 after intense TSH stimulation (Shen 2001). In some thyroid cancers, however, NIS is not responsive to TSH, or is absent, which causes them not to take up I-131. NIS is also present in a variety of nonthyroidal tissues such as the parotid glands, breast tissues, gastric mucosa and nasolacrimal ducts, explaining why they may sustain injury from I-131 therapy.

A phenomenon termed the Wolff–Chaikoff effect is an acute decrease in thyroid hormone production and release that occurs when large amounts of iodine accumulate in the thyroid follicular cell in response to the administration of pharmacologic doses of iodine. However, after about 2 days there is an adaptation to this effect that spontaneously decreases the transport of iodine into the follicular cell, even in the presence of continued high plasma iodide concentrations. This lowers intrathyroidal iodine concentration below a critical inhibitory threshold thus allowing thyroid hormone synthesis and secretion to resume. Escape from the Wolff-Chaikoff effect is caused by an iodine-induced decrease in NIS that blocks iodide transport into the follicular cell (Eng 1999).

THYROID HORMONE SYNTHESIS, STORAGE AND RELEASE

Iodine, after entering into and rapidly diffusing through the thyroid follicular cell, is transported through the apical membrane of the cell by pendrin, a membrane-bound iodide–chloride transporter (Fig. 3). It is here that the first process of thyroid hormone synthesis begins with the rapid oxidation of iodine to iodide molecules that then bind to tyrosyl residues (organification) of thyroglobulin, a 660 kilodalton glycoprotein synthesized by follicle cells (Van Herle 1979). Iodinated thyroglobulin rapidly moves into intra-luminal colloid stores, becoming their main component. Thyroid hormones (T_3 and T_4) are synthesized by the coupling of iodinated tyrosine molecules and remain attached to the thyroglobulin stored in colloid until leaving the gland. Under normal circumstances the thyroid gland stores enough thyroid hormone to maintain T_3 and T_4 within physiologic levels for about 2 weeks. Thus, serum thyroid hormone levels fall over several weeks after total thyroidectomy has been performed for differentiated thyroid carcinoma.

In response to TSH stimulation, colloid droplets are taken from the lumen into the follicular cell by a process termed endocytosis in which they are hydrolyzed, releasing into the circulation each day about 80 to 100 μg of T_4 and only a small amount ($\sim$10 μg) of T_3, along with about 100 μg of thyroglobulin. This process also occurs to some extent in differentiated malignant follicular cells, thus providing a unique means of monitoring a patient's status postoperatively by measuring serum thyroglobulin (Tg) levels (Van Herle 1975).

The process of thyroid hormone synthesis and secretion is regulated by a feedback loop in which thyrotropin-releasing hormone (TRH) increases the secretion of TSH, which stimulates the synthesis and secretion of T3 and T4 by the thyroid gland, and both hormones in turn inhibit TRH release and TSH secretion (Fig. 4).

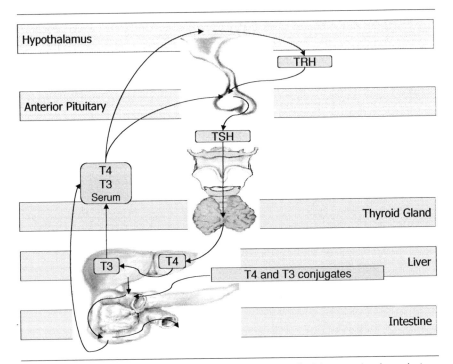

Figure 4. Regulation of thyroid hormone synthesis and secretion. Feedback loops regulate the synthesis and secretion of thyroid hormones (thyroxine [T4] and triiodothyronine [T3]). Regulation of thyroid secretion involves signals from the hypothalamus (thyrotropin-releasing hormone [TRH]) which in turn regulates the secretion of thyrotropin (thyroid stimulating hormone, [TSH]). Thyroidal synthesis and secretion of thyroid hormone is regulated by TSH. Type I deiodinase converts T4 to T3, and also converts T3 to reverse T3. The liver deiodinases converts T4 to T3 and then to mono- and diiodotyrosine.

Once released into the blood, 99.95% of T4 and 99.5% of T3 are bound to several serum proteins, termed thyroxine-binding globulin (TBG), transthyretin (TTR, formerly termed thyroxine-binding prealbumin) albumin and lipoproteins. Thyroid hormone bound to these proteins is in equilibrium with the unbound (free) thyroid hormone- the biologically active component of circulating T4 and T3 (Engler 1984). The serum half-life of T3 and T4 is determined by their binding affinities to carrier proteins. The T3-carrier protein bond is relatively weak, resulting in a short serum half-life of about 12 hours, whereas T4 is bound more tightly and thus has a longer serum half-life of about 7 days. This is why T3 is often substituted for T4 before withdrawing thyroid hormone for I-131 therapy.

Most (~80%) T4 is converted to T3 in the liver and many other tissues by the action of T4 monodeiodinases, while the rest is conjugated with sulfate and glucuronide in the liver, excreted in the bile and partially hydrolyzed in the bowel (Fig. 4). This is why diffuse hepatic uptake of I-131 is seen on a whole body scan when radiolabeled T4 is released into the circulation from normal thyroid tissues or differentiated thyroid cancers that have taken up and been treated by I-131.

Thyroid hormone, mainly in the form of T3, has critical actions on virtually all cells in the body; however, there are especially important effects of thyroid hormone on the heart and bone that occur with deliberate levothyroxine over-treatment, which can cause serious loss of bone mineral density in post-menopausal women, and atrial fibrillation and measurable cardiac dysfunction in both sexes.

CALCITONIN

Calcitonin is a 32-amino acid polypeptide. In pharmacologic doses it inhibits osteoclastic bone resorption, but the physiologic role of calcitonin is minimal in the adult skeleton where its effects are transient, probably because of calcitonin receptor downregulation. The effects of calcitonin deficiency are unknown, mainly because studies have been unable to separate the effects of calcitonin deficiency from hypothyroidism. Calcitonin is produced by, and is the main tumor marker for, medullary thyroid carcinoma (Machens 2005). Tumor secretion of calcitonin that occurs in medullary thyroid carcinoma may cause diarrhea or facial flushing in patients with advanced tumor stage.

PARATHYROID HORMONE (PTH)

PTH is one of two major hormones controlling calcium and phosphate metabolism. Its secretion is regulated by serum ionized calcium acting via an exquisitely sensitive calcium-sensing receptor on the surface of the parathyroid cells. Within seconds of the induction of hypocalcemia, PTH is released as the biologically active form of the hormone, an 84-amino acid polypeptide with a 2 to 4 minute half-life in plasma. The immediate effect of PTH is to rapidly mobilize the readily available skeletal stores of calcium that are in equilibrium with the extracellular fluid (Felsenfeld 1999). Later, it stimulates the release of calcium (and phosphate) by activating bone reabsorption. PTH thus maintains ionized serum calcium concentrations within a narrow range. The hormone also stimulates renal tubular calcium reabsorption and inhibits renal tubular phosphate reabsorption, thereby further raising both the serum calcium and phosphate concentrations.

VITAMIN D

The other major hormonal control of calcium and phosphate metabolism is mediated by vitamin D, a fat soluble vitamin that is readily absorbed from the intestine or synthesized in the skin in response to ultraviolet light. Vitamin D travels to the liver where it, and endogenously synthesized vitamin D3, are metabolized to 25-hydroxyvitamin D (calcidiol) (Compston 2000). PTH and hypophosphatemia both stimulate the renal enzyme $1,\alpha$-hydroxylase, which converts calcidiol to 1,25-dihydrovitamin D (calcitriol, Rocaltrol®), a form of vitamin D that is 100-fold more potent than its precursor. The most important biological action of calcitriol is to promote intestinal calcium absorption. These physiologic responses to hypocalcemia explain why calcium replacement alone is insufficient therapy for hypoparathyroidism: calcitriol synthesis is impaired by the

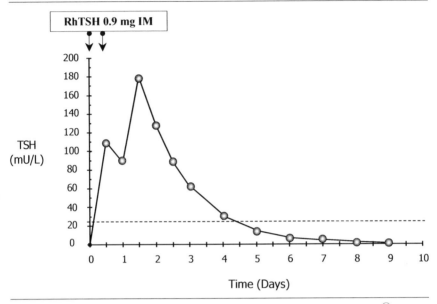

Figure 5. Serum TSH levels after two injections of recombinant human TSH-alpha (Thyrogen®) used to stimulate I-131 uptake and serum thyroglobulin levels. Fig. supplied by the Genzyme Corporation Cambridge, Massachusetts, U.S.A.

low serum PTH levels and oral calcium is simply not sufficiently absorbed without calcitriol.

PHARMACEUTICAL NAMES OF TSH, T3 AND T4 AND VITAMIN D PREPARATIONS

To practitioners that do not routinely manage patients with thyroid disease, it is useful to have a reference that lists the commercial trade names of TSH, T3 and T4:

- **Thyrotropin (TSH):** Recombinant Human Thyroid Stimulating Hormone (rhTSH) THYROGEN®
  - **Activity and pharmacodynamics:** TSH levels peak about 3 to 24 hours after injection, with a serum half-life of about 24 hours (Fig. 5). This varies according to the patient's body weight. It is not necessary to measure serum TSH levels after Thyrogen® injection.
  - **Thyroid cancer in adults:** Usual adult dose is 0.9 mg IM on two consecutive days, 24 hours apart.
    - For radioiodine imaging or use with FDG-PET scanning the isotope should be given 24 hours following the final Thyrogen® injection.
    - For serum Tg testing, serum levels should be obtained 72 hours after the final injection of Thyrogen.®

- ○ **Thyroid Cancer in Children:** The drug may be used in children >16 years of age in the same doses as given to adults.
- ○ **ADVERSE REACTIONS:**
  - ▪ **Minor:** The most common reaction is mild headache, which can occur in up to 10% of patients. A few patients develop fever, chills dizziness, nausea, and vomiting or muscle weakness, or a flu-like syndrome.
  - ▪ **Significant:** Edema or enlargement of tumor that can cause acute compression symptoms in the central nervous system, neck or elsewhere, resulting in respiratory distress, stridor or neurological symptoms. This has generally occurred in patients with known residual tumor.
- • **Liothyronine (T3)** (triiodothyronine): CYTOMEL® TRIOSTAT®
  - ○ **Hypothyroid adult under age 50 years without cardiac disease:** starting oral dose 25 mcg/day; increase by 12.5 mcg/day increments every 1–2 weeks to a maximum of 100 mcg. Usual maintenance dose is about 1 mcg/kg/day or 75 to 100 mcg/day.
  - ○ **TSH suppressive dose in adults under age 50 years without heart disease:**75 to 100 mcg/day for 7 to 14 days.
  - ○ **TSH suppressive dose in adults over age 50 years or anyone with heart disease:** 5 mcg/day increasing by 5 mcg every two weeks.
  - ○ **ADVERSE REACTIONS:** There are significant (1% to 10%) adverse cardiovascular reactions to this drug, including arrhythmias, tachycardia, myocardial infarctions, syncope, heart failure and sudden death.
- • **Levothyroxine (T4):** SYNTHROID,® LEVOXYL®, NOVOTHYROX®, UNITHROID® Generic Products are also available.
  - ○ **Hypothyroidism:** The usual oral dose is 1.7 mcg/kg/day in otherwise healthy adults under age 50 years and children in whom growth and puberty are complete. The dose should be titrated every 6 weeks until the target TSH is achieved. The average starting dose is ∼100 mcg.
  - ○ **Hypothyroid adults over age 50 years or anyone with cardiac disease:** Initial dose is 25 to 50 mcg/day, adjusted by 12.5 to 25 mcg increments at 4-6 week intervals.
  - ○ **TSH suppression with well differentiated thyroid cancer:** Highly individualized, but some patients require doses >2 mcg/dg/day to suppress TSH <0.1 mIU/L.
  - ○ **Pregnancy:** In women taking levothyroxine prior to pregnancy, the dose of levothyroxine increases about 30% immediately after conception (Alexander 2004).
  - ○ **Absorption:** Decreased by iron tablets or vitamins containing iron, aluminum- and magnesium-containing antacids, calcium carbonate, simethicone, sucralfate, raloxifene, cholestyramine, colestipol, Kayexalate® (Siraj 2003).
  - ○ **Factors altering dosage:** Should be taken on an empty stomach at least 30 minutes before food. Simultaneous food intake lowers absorption, estrogens require increased levothyroxine dosage.
  - ○ **Using different levothyroxine preparations:** Levothyroxine has a narrow therapeutic index. Products inappropriately deemed bioequivalent may put patients at

risk for iatrogenic hyperthyroidism or hypothyroidism. Thus, it is imperative that the patient remain on the same brand of thyroid hormone as initially prescribed because there may be important differences in TSH levels in patients receiving the same doses of different brands of levothyroxine.

- **Calcitriol (Vitamin D):** Rocaltrol® 0.25 mcg or 0.5 mcg tablets; Calcijex®; injection 1 mcg/1ml.
  - **Hypoparathyroidism in adults:** Oral dosage is individualized to maintain serum calcium levels of 9–10-mg/dL, which usually requires 0.5 to 2 mcg a day. Serum calcium levels must be monitored frequently until the patient has reached a stable dosage. Adequate daily calcium intake is necessary to maintain target serum calcium levels.
  - **Acute Hypocalcemia:** Patients may develop muscle cramps, circumoral or limb paresthesias, carpopedal spasm or laryngospasm, generalized or focal seizures, or hypotension. Chvostek's or Trousseau's signs are positive.
    - **Chvostek's sign** is elicited by tapping in the pretragal area and watching for an involuntary twitch of the lips. Up to 10% of patients who are normocalcemic will have a positive Chvostek's test.
    - **Trousseau's sign** is performed by occluding the brachial artery with a blood pressure cuff for 3 minutes. A positive test is carpopedal spasm.
  - Tetany is uncommon unless the serum ionized calcium concentration is less than 2.8 mg/dL.
  - Therapy is with intravenous calcium. Calcium should be diluted in dextrose and water or saline, because concentrated calcium solutions are irritating to veins. Calcium gluconate is preferred because calcium chloride may cause tissue necrosis.
    - **Calcium gluconate** is given intravenously 2–15 g/24 hours as a diluted solution.
    - **Major side effects:** Hypercalcemia with attendant symptoms of polyuria, polydipsia, fatigue, mood changes, altered consciousness and hypotension.
    - **Drug interactions:** Cholestyramine, colestipol may decrease absorption and the effects of Calcitrol; corticosteroids may decrease hypercalcemic effect of Calcitrol.

REFERENCES

Alexander, EK, E Marqusee, J Lawrence, P Jarolim, GA Fischer, and PR Larsen. 2004. Timing and magnitude of increases in levothyroxine requirements during pregnancy in women with hypothyroidism. N Engl J Med **351(3)**:241–249.

Compston, JE. 2000. Vitamin D. Molecular biology, physiology and clinical applications. Gut **46**:582C–582.

Eng, PH, GR Cardona, SL Fang, M Previti, S Alex, N Carrasco, WW Chin, and LE Braverman. 1999. Escape from the acute Wolff-Chaikoff effect is associated with a decrease in thyroid sodium/iodide symporter messenger ribonucleic acid and protein. Endocrinology **140**:3404–3410.

Engler, D, and AG Burger. 1984. The deiodination of the iodothyronines and of their derivatives in man. Endocr Rev **5**:151–184.

Felsenfeld, AJ. 1999. Bone, parathyroid hormone and the response to the rapid induction of hypocalcaemia. Eur J Clin Invest **29**:274–277.

Hollowell, JG, NW Staehling, WD Flanders, WH Hannon, EW Gunter, CA Spencer, and LE Braverman. 2002. Serum TSH, T(4), and thyroid antibodies in the United States population (1988 to 1994): National Health and Nutrition Examination Survey (NHANES III). J Clin Endocrinol Metab **87**:489–499.

Hollowell, JG, NW Staehling, WH Hannon, DW Flanders, EW Gunter, GF Maberly, LE Braverman, S Pino, DT Miller, PL Garbe, DM DeLozier, and RJ Jackson. 1998. Iodine nutrition in the United States. Trends and public health implications: Iodine excretion data from National Health and Nutrition Examination Surveys I and III (1971–1974 and 1988–1994). J Clin Endocrinol Metab **83:**3401–3408.

Machens, A,U Schneyer, HJ Holzhausen, and H Dralle. 2005. Prospects of remission in medullary thyroid carcinoma according to basal calcitonin level. J Clin Endocrinol Metab.

Santisteban, P. 2005. Development and anatomy of the hypothalamic–pituiatary–thyroid axis. In: Werner's & Ingbar's The Thyroid: A Fundamental and Clinical Text, 9th edn. Philadelphia: Lippincott Willams & Wilkins (Braverman LE, Utiger RD, eds) 8–25.

Shen, DH, RT Kloos, EL Mazzaferri, and SM Jhiang. 2001. Sodium iodide symporter in health and disease. Thyroid **11:**415–425.

Siraj, ES, MK Gupta, and SS Reddy. 2003. Raloxifene causing malabsorption of levothyroxine. Arch Intern Med **163(11):**1367–1370.

Smanik, PA, Q Liu, TL Furminger, K Ryu, S Xing,, EL Mazzaferri, and SM Jhiang. 1996. Cloning of the human sodium iodide symporter. Biochem Biophys Res Commun **226:**339–345.

Van Herle, AJ, and RP Uller. 1975. Elevated serum thyroglobulin. A marker of metastases in differentiated thyroid carcinomas. J Clin Invest **56:**272–277.

Van Herle, AJ, G Vassart, and JE Dumont. 1979. Control of thyroglobulin synthesis and secretion (first of two parts). N Engl J Med **301:**239–249.

1.3. PATHOLOGY AND CLASSIFICATION OF THYROID CARCINOMA

HEATHER M. BROWN, MD, ROBERT J. AMDUR, MD AND
ERNEST L. MAZZAFERRI, MD, MACP

The pathology of thyroid carcinomas plays a fundamental role in clinical management and patient outcome. This chapter presents a brief review of the essential features of pathology and classification of thyroid carcinomas. For an extensive review of surgical pathology, we refer the reader to the classic work by LiVolsi (1990), cited below.

CELL OF ORIGIN

Figure 1 presents a system for classifying thyroid cancer based on differences in the cell of origin of the tumor, the presence of cytologic features of neoplasia, and growth morphology. Medullary cancers arise from the parafollicular C-cells whereas all other thyroid carcinomas arise from follicular epithelium. This explains why medullary thyroid carcinoma is positive by immunohistochemical staining for calcitonin and why medullary carcinoma never concentrates radioiodine.

The nomenclature for thyroid cancer of follicular epithelial cell origin can be confusing because the term "follicular" is used in three different ways. All thyroid carcinomas other than medullary carcinoma are follicular tumors because they arise from epithelial cells of the thyroid follicle. The term follicular also describes the architectural growth pattern of a tumor, for example, the follicular variant of papillary carcinoma. Finally, follicular carcinoma is a distinct tumor.

THE THYROID CAPSULE VERSUS THE TUMOR CAPSULE

It is important to understand that there are two different capsules of interest when discussing the extent of invasion of a follicular thyroid cancer (Fig. 2). The thyroid

---

Classification of Thyroid Cancer Based on Histology

I. THE CELL OF ORIGIN IS THE FOLLICULAR EPITHELIAL CELL

    A. Differentiated Thyroid Cancer

        1. Papillary Cancer

           a) Classic morphology

           b) Encapsulated variant

           c) Follicular variant

           d) Aggressive variants

               1. Diffuse sclerosing variant

               2. Tall Cell variant

               3. Columnar Cell variant

        2. Follicular Cancer

           a) Classic morphology (called "Follicular Carcinoma")

             - minimally invasive versus widely invasive

           b) Hürthle Cell variant

             -minimally invasive versus widely invasive

    B. Poorly differentiated thyroid cancer (Insular Carcinoma)

    C. Undifferentiated thyroid cancer (Anaplastic Carcinoma)

II. THE CELL OF ORIGIN IS THE PARAFOLLICULAR C-CELL

Medullary carcinoma

Figure 1. Classification of thyroid cancer based on histology.

capsule is the thin layer of connective tissue that surrounds the normal thyroid gland. In most people the thyroid capsule is only a few cell layers thick and may be completely absent in some areas. Pathologists and clinicians who like to use the thyroid capsule as a point of reference describe tumors that extend outside the thyroid as tumors with "invasion beyond the thyroid capsule". We prefer to discuss tumors in terms of the presence

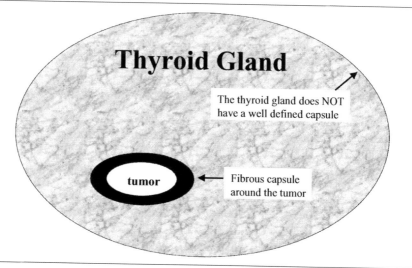

Figure 2. This diagram shows the difference between the tumor capsule and thyroid capsule.

or absence of "extrathyroidal extension". The question of extrathyroidal extension of tumor beyond the thyroid capsule is important for all types of thyroid cancer. However, the relationship of tumor to a second capsule—the tumor capsule—is relevant only when evaluating tumors that are defined by tumor capsule invasion (e.g., minimally invasive follicular and Hürthle cell carcinomas).

DIFFERENTIATED THYROID CANCER

The first major subdivision of follicular tumors is based on the degree of tumor differentiation. The term "differentiated thyroid cancer (DTC)" describes all well differentiated thyroid cancers of follicular cell origin. The two major subgroups of DTC are papillary carcinoma and follicular carcinoma. The architectural and cytologic features of the tumor distinguish papillary from follicular carcinoma.

Papillary Thyroid Carcinoma

The distinguishing feature of a papillary carcinoma is malignant cytologic (nuclear) changes. The typical nuclear changes include enlargement, hypochromasia, intranuclear cytoplasmic inclusions (nuclear pseudoinclusions), nuclear grooves and distinct nucleoli (Fig. 3). After formalin fixation, clearing of chromatin from the nuclei may cause the changes of "Orphan Annie eyes". Orphan Annie changes only develop after formalin fixation of the tissue. Psammoma bodies (laminated calcifications) may be present, but are not always specific for papillary thyroid carcinoma. However, we recommend that thyroid glands with non–tumor-associated psammoma bodies and no histologically identified carcinoma be entirely submitted to look for microscopic carcinoma. There

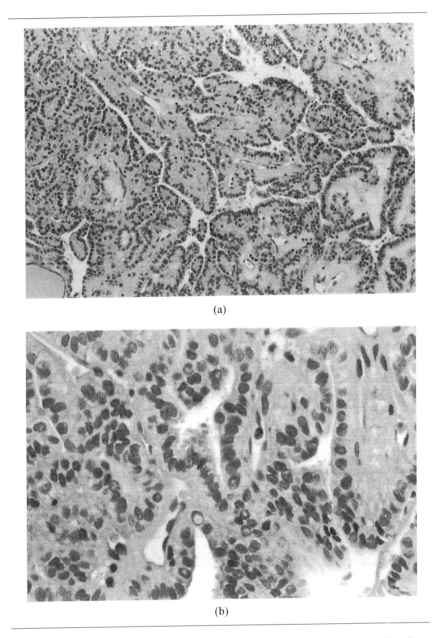

(a)

(b)

Figure 3. Papillary thyroid carcinoma, usual type: On medium power (200X) the classic form of papillary carcinoma is composed of papillae lined by cells with malignant cytologic features (A). Nuclear features on higher power (400X) that define papillary carcinoma are longitudinal nuclear grooves and pseudoinclusions (B).

are several different growth patterns of papillary cancer (classic, follicular, etc). In the classic type of papillary carcinoma, the tumor architecture consists of branching papillae with fibrovascular cores.

Encapsulated Variant of Papillary Thyroid Carcinoma

Most papillary thyroid cancers are nonencapsulated and infiltrate into the surrounding thyroid parenchyma. However, about 10% of cases of papillary thyroid cancers are surrounded by a well-defined fibrous capsule. These tumors otherwise have the typical architectural or nuclear changes of PTC. This variant is defined because it has a better prognosis than most other forms of PTC.

Follicular Variant of Papillary Thyroid Carcinoma

The follicular variant of papillary thyroid carcinoma lacks the papillary architecture seen in the usual type, and is defined only by the cytologic (nuclear) changes that are identical to those discussed in the section on the classic type. The architecture is that of follicle formation (Fig. 4), similar to those seen in other follicular lesions, such as follicular adenomas and follicular carcinomas. By definition, most of the tumor is composed of follicles, although most cases have some papillary structures present as well.

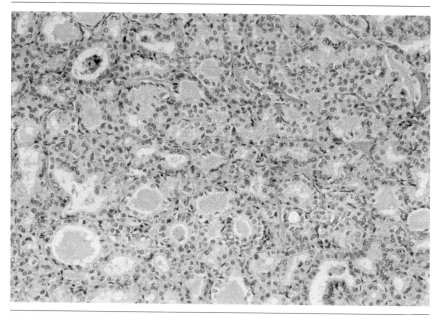

Figure 4. Papillary thyroid carcinoma, follicular variant (200X): This is a papillary carcinoma because the nuclear features are as described in Fig. 3. This is a follicular variant because the architectural pattern is that of follicle formation, not papillae.

Diffuse Sclerosing Variant of Papillary Carcinoma

This is a rare form of papillary carcinoma characterized by extensive sclerosis, lymphocytic infiltrate, and psammoma bodies. The tumor usually involves an entire lobe or the entire gland at presentation. Many reviews classify diffuse sclerosing papillary carcinoma as an "aggressive variant" because the percent of patients with extrathyroidal extension or metastasis appears to be greater with this variant than with the classic form of papillary carcinoma.

Tall Cell Variant of Papillary Thyroid Carcinoma

The tall cell variant maintains the papillary architecture and the cytologic (nuclear) features of the usual type of papillary carcinoma, but in addition, the cells have abundant cytoplasm, which makes the cells at least twice as tall as they are wide (Fig. 5). Focal tall cell features may be seen in otherwise conventional papillary thyroid carcinomas. By definition, a lesion should be composed of at least 70% tall cells to be designated as a tall cell variant. Unlike the classic type of papillary carcinoma, the tall cell variant usually has mitoses.

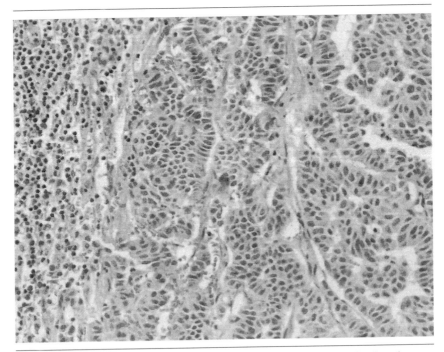

Figure 5. Papillary thyroid carcinoma, tall cell variant (400X): The nuclear changes define this to be a papillary carcinoma. The architectural pattern is that of the classic type with papillae. This is a tall cell variant because the malignant cells have excessive cytoplasm that results in an oval or rectangular shape.

Columnar Cell Variant of Papillary Carcinoma

Columnar cell is an extremely unusual variant and shows striking nuclear stratification, usually with papillary architecture. However, the usual nuclear features of papillary thyroid cancers may be absent. Some investigators prefer to classify tumors that exhibit columnar cell features as poorly differentiated carcinomas.

Follicular Carcinoma

Follicular carcinoma is the term for differentiated thyroid cancers that do not have the cytologic features of papillary carcinoma. As mentioned above, there is a form of papillary cancer called "follicular variant of papillary carcinoma" that is a distinct histologic and clinical entity from follicular carcinoma. The follicular form of differentiated thyroid cancer includes two main subtypes: Follicular and Hürthle cell.

Follicular carcinoma is a tumor that shows evidence of thyroid follicle formation and lacks the nuclear features of papillary thyroid carcinoma. In general, follicular carcinomas are classified as either minimally or widely invasive. In minimally invasive follicular carcinoma, the lesion is well circumscribed with a well defined fibrous tumor capsule. Grossly, follicular carcinoma is indistinguishable from a follicular adenoma, although the capsule of a follicular carcinoma is usually better defined and thicker than that surrounding a benign lesion. Microscopically the tumor is usually composed of microfollicles (small follicles with minimal colloid) or solid nests of tumor. The diagnosis of minimally invasive follicular carcinoma is made if one, or both, of the following features are present: 1) the tumor invades all of the way through the capsule around the tumor, or 2) the tumor invades into a blood vessel located in the tumor capsule or immediately outside of the tumor capsule (Fig. 6). Often the pathologist must examine multiple sections to find evidence of capsular or vascular invasion, as neither of these diagnostic features are visible on gross examination of this variant.

Widely invasive follicular carcinomas are obviously invasive tumors, grossly and microscopically. The thick capsule present in minimally invasive follicular carcinomas is often not discernible in the widely invasive type. Microscopically, widely invasive follicular carcinoma is composed of microfollicles or solid nests of tumor, usually with little colloid. Cytologic features, including mitotic figures and necrosis may be present.

The Hürthle Cell Tumors

Hürthle cells are follicular epithelial cells that are large with abundant granular eosinophilic cytoplasm, due to the accumulation of mitochondria in their cytoplasm (Fig. 7). Hürthle cells are not specific for any pathologic process and may be seen in non-neoplastic processes. A lesion is designated as a Hürthle cell neoplasm if it is composed of at least >75% Hürthle cells. Grossly and microscopically benign and malignant Hürthle cell neoplasms are diagnosed similarly to their follicular counterparts-meaning by the presence of invasion of vascular spaces or the tumor capsule. Hürthle cell lesions are traditionally included under follicular lesions but it is now clear that there is a Hürthle cell variant of both follicular and papillary carcinoma.

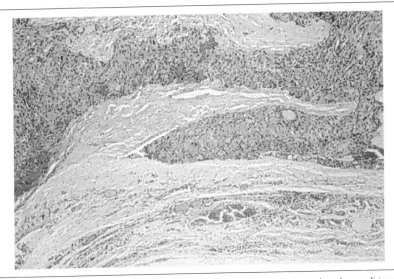

Figure 6. Follicular carcinoma, minimally invasive (100X): This tumor lacks the nuclear abnormalities that are characteristic of papillary carcinoma. Cytologically the tumor cells are indistinguishable from benign follicular cells. The finding that defines this as a follicular carcinoma is extension of tumor through the fibrous capsule that surrounds the tumor within the thyroid gland. See text for an explanation of minimally versus widely invasive follicular carcinoma.

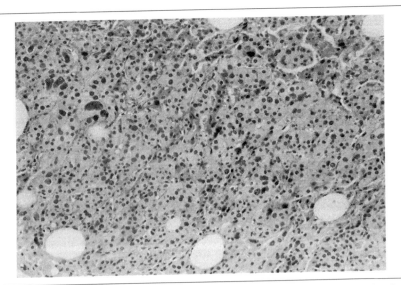

Figure 7. Hürthle cell carcinoma (200X): Hurthel cells have abundant cytoplasm that appears pink and grainy when stained with Hematoxylin and Eosin. In other locations in the body, cells with these features are called oncocytes. As in follicular thyroid tumors, malignancy in a Hürthle cell tumor is defined by invasion of tumor through the tumor capsule rather than nuclear abnormalities.

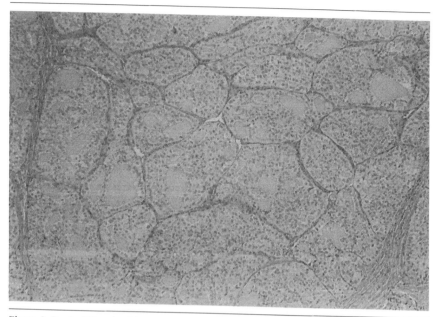

Figure 8. Poorly differentiated (Insular) carcinoma (100X): These tumors are thought to represent a poorly differentiated form of papillary carcinoma. Tumor cells have malignant nuclear characteristics and are organized in nests, or islands, separated by fibrous septae. Insula is the Latin word for island.

POORLY DIFFERENTIATED THYROID CANCER (INSULAR CARCINOMA)

These tumors are derived from follicular epithelial cells and are intermediate between differentiated and undifferentiated (anaplastic) thyroid carcinomas both histologically and in terms of biologic behavior. Most poorly differentiated thyroid carcinomas are widely invasive and may show extension beyond the thyroid gland.

Insular carcinoma refers to a distinct pattern of poorly differentiated thyroid carcinoma in which the tumor cells are arranged in discrete nests separated by fibrous stroma (nests or insulae, meaning islands) (Fig. 8). Microscopically, poorly differentiated and insular carcinomas are usually solid, and may show some evidence of follicle formation. Mitotic figures and necrosis are common. Evidence of a preexisting differentiated thyroid carcinoma may be found, suggesting that these represent "dedifferentiated" lesions.

UNDIFFERENTIATED (ANAPLASTIC) THYROID CARCINOMA

The undifferentiated or anaplastic thyroid carcinoma is a tumor that arises from the follicular epithelial cell but shows only minimal or no evidence of differentiation. At the time of diagnosis, these tumors are widely invasive, may replace most or all of the thyroid gland and infiltrate freely into perithyroidal soft tissues. Areas of necrosis and hemorrhage are seen grossly and microscopically. Microscopically, these tumors may show several different patterns, including spindle cell, squamoid, pleomorphic, or a mixture of these.

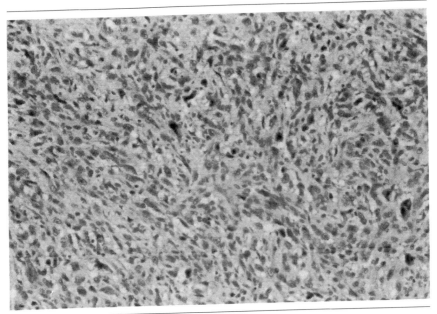

Figure 9. Anaplastic thyroid carcinoma (200X): These tumors are an undifferentiated form of either papillary or follicular carcinoma. The nuclear features of the tumor cells are those of high-grade malignancy (pleomorphism, hyperchromasia, and high mitotic rate). The architectural growth pattern is variable and includes spindle cell, squamoid, and giant cell patterns. Areas of necrosis are common.

The spindle pattern shows cigar shaped cells and may resemble a high-grade undifferentiated sarcoma. The squamoid pattern may make it difficult to rule out a squamous cell carcinoma in a small tissue sample. The pleomorphic (also called giant cell) pattern is composed of highly pleomorphic and bizarre cells. Regardless of the pattern, the cytology is malignant and a high mitotic count and necrosis are readily evident (Fig. 9). Because these tumors are undifferentiated it may be difficult to prove its origin from the follicular epithelial cell, as not all cases are routinely positive with markers seen in better differentiated thyroid carcinomas (e.g., immunohistochemical markers for cytokeratins or thyroglobulin). In these cases, the history (elderly patient, recent rapid enlargement of the thyroid, lack of evidence of another site of a primary tumor) and the appearance of a highly malignant neoplasm may be the only clues to the diagnosis. As with poorly differentiated thyroid carcinomas, anaplastic carcinoma may arise from dedifferentiation of a preexisting well-differentiated lesion.

MEDULLARY THYROID CARCINOMA

Medullary thyroid carcinoma is seen sporadically (~80% of cases) or in association with a familial syndrome. Familial cases of medullary thyroid carcinoma are more commonly

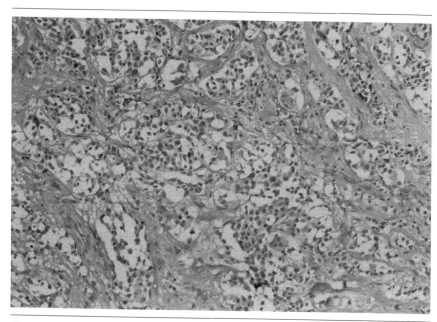

Figure 10. Medullary carcinoma (200X): The defining feature of medullary carcinoma is reactivity with immunohistochemical stains for Calcitonin or Chromogrannin. We do not show these stains because it is difficult to see them in a black and white figure. The growth pattern of medullary carcinoma is highly variable. In most cases, the architectural pattern is that of solid nests of tumor cells with a highly vascularized stroma.

multifocal and bilateral but otherwise relatively indistinguishable from their sporadic counterpart. Grossly, medullary thyroid carcinoma is usually non-encapsulated, but well-circumscribed. Because the normal C cells of the thyroid are located in the mid to upper thirds of the thyroid, this is where medullary thyroid carcinomas arise. Microscopically, these tumors can have several different patterns including patterns that mimic several other types of thyroid tumors. The most common pattern is of solid growth, or nests similar to the insulae seen in insular carcinoma.

Medullary thyroid carcinoma may appear more infiltrative into normal tissue at the microscopic level than is grossly appreciated. Individual tumor cells are spindled or plasmacytoid (eccentrically located nuclei resembling a plasma cell) (Fig. 10). One characteristic feature of medullary thyroid carcinoma is the presence of amyloid, seen in about 80% of cases. Amyloid appears as pink, amorphous material on routine H & E sections, and can be confirmed as amyloid with the use of the Congo Red stain which shows a characteristic apple-green color under polarized light. Immunohistochemical stains for calcitonin are specific for medullary thyroid carcinoma, but are positive in only ~80% of cases. Neuroendocrine markers such as chromogranin may also be useful.

Classification of Thyroid Cancer Based on Ability to Concentrate Radioiodine

I. USUALLY CONCENTRATE RADIOIODINE

   Differentiated Thyroid Carcinoma Other Than Hürthle, Tall, and Columnar Cell

   Variants

   1. Papillary carcinoma: Classic morphology

   2. Papillary carcinoma: Encapsulated and Follicular variant

   3. Papillary carcinoma: Diffuse sclerosing variant

   4. Follicular carcinoma other than Hürthle Cell

II. FREQUENTLY DO <u>NOT</u> CONCENTRATE RADIOIODINE

   A. Tall and Columnar Cell variants of Papillary Carcinoma

   B. Hürthle Cell Carcinoma

   C. Poorly differentiated (Insular) Carcinoma

III. NEVER CONCENTRATE RADIOIODINE

   A. Anaplastic Carcinoma

   B. Medullary Carcinoma

Figure 11. Classification of thyroid cancer based on ability to concentrate radioiodine.

CLASSIFICATION BASED ON ABILITY TO CONCENTRATE RADIOIODINE

Figure 11 presents a classification system that organizes the different histologic types of thyroid cancer based on their ability to concentrate radioiodine to a degree that is likely to result in tumor cure. A classification system of this kind is useful because it explains the treatment approach and relative prognosis of the different types of thyroid cancer. The common types of papillary and follicular carcinoma usually concentrate radioiodine. The follicular variant of papillary cancer has the same avidity for radioiodine as papillary cancer with classic morphology. Therefore, from the treatment standpoint, the distinction between the classic form of papillary cancer and the follicular variant of papillary cancer is not important.

The aggressive variants of papillary cancer, and the Hürthle cell variant of follicular carcinoma, concentrate radioiodine less well than the classic morphologies and there may be no measurable iodine uptake in metastases of these tumors. Anaplastic and medullary cancers never concentrate radioiodine to a degree that is useful for treatment purposes.

REFERENCE

LiVolsi, VA. 1990. Surgical Pathology of the Thyroid. WB Saunders Co.

1.4. THE AMERICAN JOINT COMMITTEE ON CANCER SYSTEM OF STAGING THYROID CANCER

ROBERT J. AMDUR, MD AND ERNEST L. MAZZAFERRI, MD, MACP

The purpose of a staging system is to stratify patients into groups that predict prognosis and determine treatment. There are multiple different stratification systems for thyroid cancer. This chapter will describe the staging system developed by the American Joint Committee on Cancer (AJCC) because it is updated frequently and incorporates the most useful features of other systems. The latest version of the AJCC staging system for thyroid cancer was published in 2002 in the sixth edition of the AJCC Cancer Staging Handbook. Tables 1 and 2 summarize these guidelines. Major points from this staging system are as follows:

- Extrathyroid extension makes the patient stage T3 or T4
- Metastatic nodes are either present (N1) or absent (N0). Node number or size does not change the stage.
- The overall AJCC grouping rules are different for Differentiated Thyroid Cancer (Papillary and Follicular), Medullary and Anaplastic Carcinoma.
- For Differentiated Thyroid Cancer, age (45 years) is a major determinant of the AJCC grouping. Age is presented as a dichotomous variable. All patients <45 years old are either stage I (no distant metastases) or stage II (distant metastases present), which means they should have an excellent prognosis.
- All Anaplastic Carcinomas are considered Stage IV.

Table 1. AJCC Staging System for Thyroid Cancer: TNM Definitions*.

Primary Tumor (T): All categories may be subdivided: (a) solitary, (b) multifocal

TX:	Primary tumor cannot be assessed
T0:	No evidence of primary tumor
T1:	Tumor 2 cm or less and limited to the thyroid
T2:	Tumor 2.1–4 cm and limited to the thyroid
T3:	Tumor >4 cm and limited to the thyroid, or
	Any tumor with minimal extrathyroid extension (e.g., sternothyroid muscle or perithyroid soft tissues)
T4a:	Tumor of any size with invasion of subcutaneous soft tissues, larynx, trachea, esophagus, or recurrent laryngeal nerve
T4b:	Tumor invades prevertebral fascia or encases carotid artery or mediastinal vessels

All anaplastic carcinomas are considered T4:

T4a:	Intrathyroid (surgically resectable)
T4b:	Extrathyroid extension (surgically unresectable)

Regional Nodes (N): central compartment, lateral cervical, and upper mediastinal

NX:	Regional nodes cannot be assessed
N0:	No regional node metastasis
N1a:	Metastasis limited to level VI (pretracheal, paratracheal, and prelaryngeal)
N1b:	Metastasis to unilateral, contralateral, or bilateral cervical or superior mediastinal lymph nodes

Distant Metastasis (M):

MX:	Distant metastasis cannot be assessed
M0:	No distant metastasis
M1:	Distant metastasis

* 6th edition of the American Joint Committee on Cancer, published in 2002.

Table 2. AJCC Staging System for Thyroid Cancer: Stage Groupings*.

Papillary and Follicular Carcinoma: Under 45 years:		
Stage I	Any T	Any N	M0
Stage II	Any T	Any N	M1

Papillary and Follicular Carcinoma: 45 years and older:		
Stage I	T1	N0	M0
Stage II	T2	N0	M0
Stage III	T3	N0	M0
	T1–3	N1a	M0
Stage IVA	T4a	N0–1a	M0
	T1–4a	N1b	M0
Stage IVB	T4b	Any N	M0
	Any T	Any N	M1

Medullary Carcinoma:		
Stage I	T1	N0	M0
Stage II	T2	N0	M0
Stage III	T3	N0	M0
	T1–3	N1a	M0
Stage IVA	T4a	N0–1a	M0
	T1–4a	N1b	M0
Stage IVB	T4b	Any N	M0
	Any T	Any N	M1

Anaplastic Carcinoma (All are considered stage IV):		
Stage IVA	T4a	Any N	M0
Stage IVB	T4b	Any N	M0
Stage IVC	Any T	Any N	M1

* 6th edition of the American Joint Committee on Cancer, published in 2002.

LIMITATIONS OF CURRENT STAGING SYSTEMS FOR DIFFERENTIATED THYROID CANCER

Ideally, a staging system will predict the chance of cure and guide treatment. In this regard the AJCC, and all other prominent staging systems, are severely limited when it comes to the management of papillary and follicular thyroid cancer. For this reason most clinicians are not familiar with the details of staging systems and many outcome studies do not report results by stage. There are three main reasons that current staging systems are of limited value in managing patients with differentiated thyroid cancer:

Current Staging systems do not accurately predict the risk of tumor recurrence: Most staging systems are based on multivariate analyses with the endpoint being survival. This approach does not reflect the fact that patients with differentiated thyroid cancer often live many years with recurrent disease. Tumor recurrence is an important event because it results in additional therapy and causes morbidity for the patient and their family. With an indolent disease like differentiated thyroid cancer, a staging system that more accurately predicts relapse-free survival would be desirable.

Current Staging systems rarely help to select therapy: The main questions in the treatment of differentiated thyroid cancer are the need for total thyroidectomy, the use of radioiodine following thyroidectomy, the use of radioiodine for recurrent disease, the dose of radioiodine in each of these settings, and the use of external beam radiotherapy.

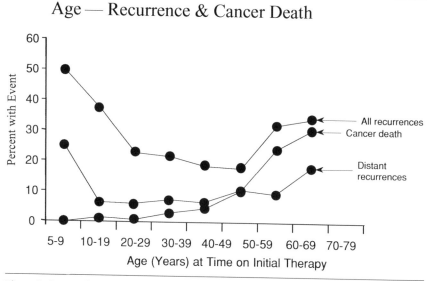

Figure 1. Age stratified by decade at the time of initial treatment as it affects the percentage of patients with tumor recurrence, distant recurrence and cancer deaths (From Mazzaferri EL and Kloos R.T. Current approaches to primary therapy for papillary and follicular thyroid cancer. J. Clin. Endocrinol. Metab 86(4), 1447–1463. 2001. Reproduced with permission of the Endocrine Society).

Making age the major factor in current staging systems is reasonable if the goal is to estimate 5–10 year overall survival but most clinicians do not use age to choose therapy for patients with differentiated thyroid cancer. As we will explain in subsequent chapters, the radioiodine is given to facilitate cancer surveillance and to prevent tumor recurrence. The primary goal of external beam radiotherapy is to prevent tumor recurrence in the neck. In a disease where there are major differences between overall and relapse-free survival rates, a staging system based on survival is of little value in guiding therapy.

Current Staging systems do not reflect the high recurrence rate in children: Current staging systems separate patients into only two groups based on age. This implies that that younger patients (age < 45years in the AJCC system) do well and older patients do poorly. The problem with this simplification is that the rate of tumor recurrence and cancer death in patients less than 10 years old is similar to that of patients over 60 years old (Fig. 1). Ignoring the poor prognosis of young children partially explains why approximately 10% of the patients dying of differentiated thyroid cancer present with AJCC stage I, or II, disease.

Most recent publications tend to reflect these facts in that initial therapy for patients with differential thyroid cancer is near-total thyroidectomy and I-131 remnant ablation, regardless of their age or tumor stage at the time of presentation.

REFERENCES

American Joint Committee on Cancer. 2002. AJCC Cancer Staging Manual, 6th edn. New York: Springer **22**:91–92.

Mazzaferri, EL, and RT Kloos. 2001. Current approaches to primary therapy for papillary and follicular thyroid cancer. J Clin Endocrinol Metab **86**(4):1447–1463.

PART 2. DIAGNOSIS AND IMAGING OF THYROID CANCER

2.1. THE DIAGNOSIS OF THYROID CANCER

ERNEST L. MAZZAFERRI, MD, MACP

Thyroid cancer usually presents as an asymptomatic thyroid nodule. The problem is that very few thyroid masses are malignant. Thyroid cancer is found in about 7 per 100,000 persons a year in the in the U.S., which is a prevalence of only 0.007% in the entire population. In contrast, palpable thyroid nodules are found in about 1% of persons during the first several decades of life and their frequency gradually rises, especially in women, to about 5% by age 50 years (Mazzaferri 1993). By palpation, most appear to be solitary nodules. The actual prevalence of thyroid nodules, however, is 10-fold that detected by palpation when the thyroid gland is examined by ultrasonography or by other imaging studies or at surgery or autopsy (Fig. 1). Most nodules discovered this way are multiple and benign. The problem is seriously worsened by the fact that there is a relatively high prevalence (about 3%) of indolent papillary microcarcinomas ($\leq$1 cm) in the population, which are identified in surgical and autopsy thyroid specimens. Under usual circumstances these small papillary cancers never become clinically evident but when serendipitously identified by imaging studies and biopsy their presence may lead to unnecessary surgery.

Thus, identifying a cancer among the many benign nodules is like finding a needle in a haystack (Mazzaferri 1993). Still, a methodical diagnostic approach ordinarily will sort out those that require therapy from tumors that are best left alone. This chapter will describe the diagnostic approach used to identify malignant thyroid nodules. Certain questions provide a guide to identifying and managing malignant tumors:

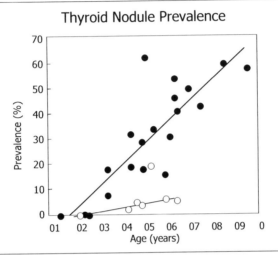

Figure 1. Prevalence of palpable thyroid nodules detected at autopsy or by ultrasonography (o) or by palpation (•) in persons without radiation exposure or known thyroid disease. Data are updated from (Mazzaferri 1993) and now also includes recent studies (Ezzat 1994; Kang 2004).

HOW WAS THE THYROID MASS DISCOVERED?

A thyroid mass is commonly found by an imaging study performed for another condition, termed an incidentaloma. Whether it is palpable is related to its size and location. Most 2-cm nodules are palpable but 60% of 1 cm nodules are not felt, even by experienced examiners (Takahashi 1997). Large thyroid nodules deep in the neck close to the lateral aspects of the trachea are not easily felt while isthmus nodules or those in the anterior thyroid smaller than 1 cm are usually palpable.

WHAT IS THE IMPLICATION OF FINDING AN INCIDENTALOMA?

Incidentalomas are found in 19% to 67% of prospective randomized studies of CT, MRI or ultrasound (Tan 1997). The risk of cancer in this setting ranges from <1% to 13% (Tan 1997; Nam–Goong 2004). In contrast, only 2% of FDG PET scans have thyroid incidentalomas, but 25% to 50% of them are malignant (Cohen 2001; Kang 2003). Thyroid masses discovered by CT, MRI or ultrasonography are often quite small, making them difficult to biopsy and often yielding insufficient material for diagnosis (Hatipoglu 2000).

Incidentalomas seen on imaging studies are common but they are not necessarily benign or low grade tumors. A study of 36 patients with incidentalomas that were well differentiated thyroid cancers found extrathyroidal extension in 44%, regional lymph node metastasis in 50% and multifocal tumors in 39% (Nam–Goong 2004).

WHAT IS THE DIFFERENTIAL DIAGNOSIS OF A THYROID NODULE?

The main disorders that produce thyroid nodules are shown in Figure 2, but many other things can cause them, such as tumors metastasizing from other sites or congenital cystic

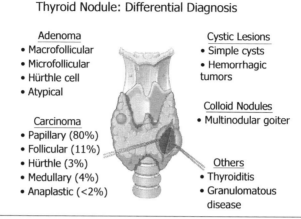

Thyroid Nodule: Differential Diagnosis

Adenoma
- Macrofollicular
- Microfollicular
- Hürthle cell
- Atypical

Carcinoma
- Papillary (80%)
- Follicular (11%)
- Hürthle (3%)
- Medullary (4%)
- Anaplastic (<2%)

Cystic Lesions
- Simple cysts
- Hemorrhagic tumors

Colloid Nodules
- Multinodular goiter

Others
- Thyroiditis
- Granulomatous disease

Figure 2. The main disorders that should be considered in the differential diagnosis of thyroid nodules are shown in this figure.

lesions. The most common cause of a thyroid nodule is a benign colloid multinodular goiter that by palpation often presents as a solitary thyroid nodule in a gland that does not appear to be enlarged.

WHAT ARE THE MAIN HISTORICAL AND PHYSICAL EXAMINATION FINDINGS OF THYROID CANCER?

The history and physical examination are the cornerstones of the clinical evaluation of a thyroid nodule. A study by Hamming et al. (1990) evaluated the accuracy of the clinical diagnosis in 199 patients with nodular thyroid disease and retrospectively divided them into high, moderate and low-risk of having thyroid cancer as verified by surgery (Table 1). Most of the patients with highly suspicious clinical findings had thyroid cancer, and if any two of the high risk features were present the likelihood of cancer approached 100%. Not included in this study was a family history of thyroid cancer, stridor, and symptoms to suggest invasion of other regional structures such as dysphagia or neurologic complaints. The main point of this study is that all patients with highly suspicious thyroid nodules need surgery regardless of the fine needle aspiration (FNA) result, which in this case is done mainly to obtain important information that will guide the surgeon's choice of procedures.

Still, only a minority of patients with malignant nodules has suggestive clinical findings, and conversely, some patients with benign thyroid disorders have symptoms that suggest malignancy. For example, vocal cord paralysis can occur with benign cystic thyroid nodules (Massoll 2002), whereas the risk of thyroid cancer in asymptomatic thyroid incidentalomas (asymptomatic nodules found by imaging) is as high as that in

Table 1. Suspicious Signs and Symptoms of Thyroid Cancer in 199 Patients with a Thyroid Nodule.

	Probability of cancer		
Percent of patients	High 20%	Moderate 35%	Low 45%
Symptoms or Signs	Rapid growth* Hard nodule* Fixation to tissue* Vocal cord paralysis* Cervical lymph nodes* Stridor† Esophageal obstruction† Other symptoms of invasion (neurologic, vascular)†	Age < 20 or > 60 years* Head & neck irradiation* Male* Dubious nodule fixation* Nodule > 4cm & cystic*	No suspicious* signs or symptoms
Percent Malignant*	71%	14%	11%

* The criteria marked with an asterisk and the percent with malignancy are from (Hamming 1990). The signs and symptoms marked with † were not included in the Hamming study.

larger nodules (Papini 2002). This may explain why an increasing number of endocrinologists use ultrasonography as part of the diagnostic evaluation and why its use is recommended by most experts (Hegedus 2004). The fact that ultrasonography detects nodules—a third of which are more than 20 mm in diameter—in up to half the patients with a normal neck examination highlights the low specificity and sensitivity of clinical examination.

WHAT ARE THE KEY TESTS USED TO IDENTIFY AND STAGE A MALIGNANT MASS?

Neck ultrasonography with Doppler studies and ultrasound-guided FNA are becoming the standard approach to the diagnosis of thyroid nodules. Routine calcitonin testing has been suggested in the initial diagnostic workup of a thyroid mass (Elisei 2004) but this has not become routine practice in the USA, although it has major implications in the initial surgical management of medullary thyroid carcinoma. Baseline serum thyroglobulin measurements may be helpful when an FNA diagnosis of papillary thyroid carcinoma has been established (Baloch 2003). A CT (without contrast!) may be informative when the mass is very large and extends into the mediastinum or is potentially invading neck structures, but is otherwise usually unnecessary.

A 1999 survey (Bennedbaek 2000) of clinical members of the American Thyroid Association found all respondents routinely used FNA but 87% guided it by palpation. Yet when clinical factors suggested malignancy (e.g., rapid nodule growth and a large nodule of 5 cm) about half the clinicians disregarded FNA biopsy results to choose surgery. Compared with European endocrinologist, those in North American used scintigraphy and ultrasonography less and ordered fewer calcitonin measurements in the evaluation of a nodule (Bennedbaek 2000).

WHAT SIZE NODULE SHOULD BE BIOPSIED?

For many years the problem of incidentalomas was solved by simply not biopsying nodules smaller than 1 cm, but the answer is not this simple. For example, Ito et al. (2003) performed a prospective study of 732 patients in whom papillary microcarcinomas were found by ultrasonography and verified by FNA. Of this group, 78% opted for immediate surgery. The other 162 patients underwent follow-up, during which most (70%) of the tumors did not change or decreased in size. A few (10%) of the tumors enlarged by more that 10 mm and 1% of the patients developed enlarged lateral neck compartment lymph nodes. Among the 626 patients (86%) who eventually underwent surgery, histologically confirmed lymph node metastases were found in half of the patients who underwent lymph node dissections and many (43%) had multifocal tumors. The 5 and 8 year recurrence rates in the treated group were, respectively, 2.7% and 5%, but none died of thyroid cancer. Thus, the majority of papillary microcarcinomas do not become clinically apparent and patients can choose observation as long as their tumors are not progressing, but ongoing follow-up is necessary because a substantial number of such patients have tumors that are multifocal and involve regional lymph nodes.

These observations underscore several points. First, palpation of nodules has a low sensitivity. Second, the high sensitivity of imaging studies, especially ultrasonography, creates important diagnostic problems. Third, simply using nodule size as the only criterion for biopsy will miss some potentially serious thyroid cancers. Fourth, biopsying every small thyroid nodule found by ultrasonography is not necessary because most of them will never threaten the patient's life. Fifth, there are criteria in addition to nodule size that must be factored into the decision to perform an FNA, not the least of which is a careful discussion with the patient about the potential outcomes of doing procedure.

WHAT IS THE ROLE OF ULTRASONOGRAPHY?

Ultrasonography should not be used for screening. However, when a nodule has been discovered either by palpation or an imaging study, ultrasonography can estimate size nodule size and can differentiate simple cysts, which have a low risk of being malignant, from mixed cystic solid nodules and solid nodules, which have about a 5% risk of being malignant. Ultrasonography also plays a major role in guiding FNA. Indeed, the most accurate means of identifying malignant thyroid nodules is to perform an ultrasound-guided FNA on suspicious thyroid nodules.

HOW SHOULD A NODULE BE SELECTED FOR FNA?

Ultrasonography plays a major role in selecting nodules for FNA. For example, in the study by Marqusee et al. (2000), ultrasonography altered the course of clinical management in two thirds of the patients who had been referred for evaluation of a palpable thyroid abnormality, mainly by identifying nodules smaller than 1 cm, which in 20% of the patients were not considered to require further evaluation and by discovering additional nodules that required FNA in 24% of the patients.

Table 2. Ultrasonographic or Other Patient Characteristics Used to Select Thyroid Nodules for FNA.

Ultrasound or other characteristic	Tumor size to biopsy	Comments
Size > 1m in at least one dimension	All	All nodules including those in MNG
Spherical Shape	> 1 cm	Ratio of the longest to shortest dimension
Hypoechoic	> 1 cm	Particularly mixed echogenicity Seen also in benign nodules
Microcalcifications	> 1 cm	Seen also in benign nodules
Irregular nodule margins in nodule	> 8 cm	Key finding*
Blurred (indistinct) nodule margins	> 8 cm	Key finding
Increased Doppler Flow in nodule	> 8 cm	Absent Doppler does not rule out cancer
Evidence of invasion of surrounding tissues by a nodule	> 8 cm	Key finding*
Suspicious lymph node with nodule	> 8 cm	Key finding*
Suspicious history[†]	> 8 cm	Key finding*

* These findings are particularly important, regardless of nodule size, but performing FNA in nodules smaller than about 8 mm increases the risk of inadequate cytology specimens. It is best to follow nodules with ultrasonography that show these characteristics but are too small to biopsy.
[†] Familial papillary thyroid carcinoma, head and neck irradiation. Note if history is highly suspicious, patients should have FNA, but will need surgery regardless of cytology findings.

Ultrasonographic characteristics of a nodule that are associated with an increased risk of cancer include hypoechogenicity, microcalcifications, irregular nodule margins, blurred nodule margins, increased nodular blood flow visualized by Doppler, and evidence of tumor invasion or regional lymph node metastases (Table 2). Solid nodules with hypervascular Doppler flow have a high likelihood of malignancy that was nearly 42% in the series by Frates et al. (2003), but the color characteristics of a thyroid nodule cannot be used to exclude malignancy because 14% of solid non–hypervascular nodules were found to be malignant. Another study by Alexander et al. (2004) found that spherical shape of the nodule estimated by calculating a ratio of the longest to shortest dimensions was independently correlated with risk of malignancy. Still, sonographic findings cannot reliably distinguish between benign and malignant lesions.

Nodules found in the setting of a multinodular goiter have the same incidence of thyroid cancer (about 5%) as do isolated thyroid cancers. For example, the large prospective study by Belfiore et al. (1992) found that the incidence of thyroid cancer was 4.7% in 4,485 patients with single thyroid nodules and 4.1% in 1,152 patients with multinodular goiter.

Thus the criteria for biopsying a thyroid nodule is the same whether found in a patient with a single nodule or a multinodular gland: every nodule that is larger than 1 cm or that is ultrasonographically suspicious of cancer should be biopsied.

HOW SHOULD CYSTIC THYROID NODULES BE MANAGED?

Cystic thyroid nodules are common, comprising as many as 40% of thyroid nodules (Massoll 2002). Their differential diagnosis is relatively broad, and includes lesions that often do not fit a stereotypical presentation such as intrathyroidal thyroglossal duct cysts, branchial cleft cysts near the midline, and cystic lesions that are malignant. Benign cystic thyroid nodules not infrequently present with symptoms and signs that mimic an aggressive thyroid cancer, including pressure symptoms and rapid growth, whereas a cystic papillary thyroid carcinoma may provide no clues to its malignant nature, featuring a soft consistency to palpation and little or no apparent growth over several years.

The physical and biochemical features of the aspirated fluid of a cystic nodule provide little diagnostic information; both benign and malignant lesions may yield grossly bloody aspirates or translucent yellow fluid. Cystic thyroid nodules not only have a higher than usual likelihood of yielding a cytology specimen that is inadequate for diagnosis, but also have higher than usual rates of false negative cytology specimens. Using a careful clinical assessment, ultrasonography, Doppler studies and ultrasound-guided FNA, the malignant or benign nature of most cystic thyroid nodules can be identified.

WHAT ARE THE POTENTIAL BENEFITS OF ULTRASOUND-GUIDED FNA?

Fine-needle aspiration of a thyroid nodule is best done under ultrasound guidance for several reasons. First, the operator knows exactly where the tip of the needle is located, which avoids inadvertently placing the needle through the malignant nodule and biopsying normal tissue. Second, this is the only way to accurately biopsy cystic thyroid nodules and to lower the rate of inadequate specimens. Third, it is the only way to biopsy impalpable thyroid nodules found by imaging studies. Fourth, it facilitates the biopsy of lymph nodes near important structures such as the carotid artery. Fifth, it provides Doppler information that gives an estimate of the anticipated bleeding that will occur when a solid nodule is biopsied. Thyroid ultrasonography is especially useful to guide FNA in nodules that are small or partly cystic nodules that initially yield insufficient material for diagnosis.

The diagnostic algorithm for the evaluation and treatment of thyroid nodules is shown in Fig. 3. Diagnostically useful results are obtained in about 90% of cases, typically with three to four needle passes.

WHAT ARE THE DIAGNOSTIC CATEGORIES OF CYTOLOGY OBTAINED BY FNA?

While there are several ways to group FNA cytology results, the easiest way is to divide them into four categories. (Mazzaferri 1993; Hegedus 2004).

Insufficient for diagnosis (about 5% to 10%) The probability of obtaining a sufficient sample increases if aspiration is guided by ultrasonography, especially in nodules that are partly cystic. Repeat biopsy reduces by half the rate of insufficient samples to a final rate of 10% or less. If the cytology continues to be insufficient after several attempts to biopsy the nodule under ultrasound guidance, the patient should undergo surgery, usually lobectomy on the side of the lesion with completion thyroidectomy for the 5% found to have thyroid cancer.

Benign cytology (about 65% to 75%) The cytology in benign specimens shows normal follicular cells, abundant colloid, and when the tumor has undergone cystic degeneration, macrophages or benign appearing Hürthle cells.

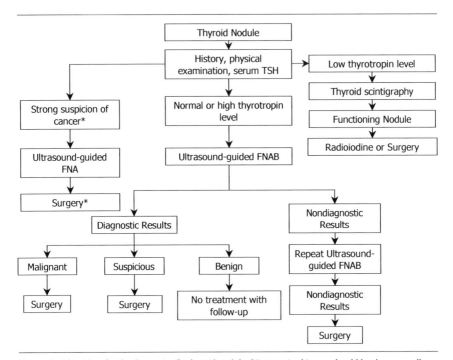

Figure 3. Algorithm for the diagnosis of a thyroid nodule. *Surgery in this case should be done regardless of the FNA findings.

Positive for cancer (about 5%) The accuracy rates are highest for papillary thyroid cancer because the cytology specimens show typical cytologic features that the cytopathologist can identify in nearly all the cases. FNA accuracy is also highly accurate for anaplastic and medullary thyroid cancer and other poorly differentiated tumors. All patients with an FNA diagnosis of thyroid cancer should undergo total thyroidectomy.

Indeterminate for diagnosis (about 15–20%) This is sometimes termed a "Suspicious" specimen but is probably most commonly reported as being "compatible with a follicular neoplasm" or as a "follicular tumor." The cytology specimen shows sheets of normal appearing follicular or Hürthle cells without colloid. About 20% of these specimens are from follicular or Hürthle cell carcinomas. If the patient's TSH is suppressed, radionuclide scanning should be performed. All other patients with indeterminate cytology specimens should undergo lobectomy on the side of the lesion, with completion thyroidectomy immediately thereafter for the 20% who on the final histopathologic sections are found to have follicular or Hürthle cell thyroid carcinoma.

WHAT IS THE DIAGNOSTIC ACCURACY OF FNA?

The diagnostic accuracy of fine-needle aspiration depends upon the skill and experience of the person doing the FNA and the cytopathologist reading the specimen. It also depends upon how indeterminate (suspicious) lesions are handled. Viewing them as "positive" increases the sensitivity of FNA, but decreases specificity. The rate of unsatisfactory cytology specimens was only 0.7% among 1,153 ultrasound-guided thyroid FNA specimens performed by Yang et al. (2001) who are highly skilled in this technique. Among the satisfactory specimens in this study, about 6% were cancer or suspicious for cancer, 10% were follicular neoplasms, and 82% were benign lesions. After 2 to 6 years follow-up of the 1,127 cases with satisfactory FNA specimens, the false-negative rate was 0% and a false-positive rate was 1.5%. Of the 169 surgical follow-ups, the sensitivity was 100%, and the specificity was 67%, the positive predictive value was 87%, and the negative predictive value was 100%. The global accuracy in this study was 90%. This study shows how accurate this technique is in the hands of highly skilled people.

WHAT ARE THE MAJOR WEAKNESSES OF FINE-NEEDLE ASPIRATION?

The main limitations of FNA are the difficulty in distinguishing benign follicular tumors from follicular carcinoma and follicular variant papillary thyroid carcinomas. The other limitations are that some biopsies yield insufficient material for diagnosis and the accuracy of the procedure depends heavily upon the skill and experience of the operator and cytopathologist.

In our clinic, where we do ultrasound-guided FNA and have a cytopathologist assisting and preliminarily assessing the cytology specimen for accuracy, we get results comparable to those reported by Yang et al. (2001) after doing an average of 2 to 3 needle sticks per nodule.

REFERENCES

Alexander, EK, E Marqusee, J Orcutt, CB Benson, MC Frates, PM Doubilet, ES Cibas, and A Atri. 2004. Thyroid nodule shape and prediction of malignancy. Thyroid **14**:953–958.

Baloch, Z, P Carayon, B Conte-Devolx, LM Demers, U Feldt-Rasmussen, JF Henry, VA LiVosli, P Niccoli-Sire, R John, J Ruf, PP Smyth, CA Spencer, and JR Stockigt. 2003. Laboratory medicine practice guidelines. Laboratory support for the diagnosis and monitoring of thyroid disease. Thyroid **13**:3–126.

Belfiore, A, GL La Rosa, GA LaPorta, D Giuffrida, G Milazzo, L Lupo, C Regalbuto, and R Vigneri. 1992. Cancer risk in patients with cold thyroid nodules: relevance of iodine intake, sex, age and multinodularity. Am J Med **93**:363–369.

Bennedbaek, FN, and L Hegedus. 2000. Management of the solitary thyroid nodule: results of a North American survey. J Clin Endocrinol Metab **85**:2493–2498.

Cohen, MS, N Arslan, F Dehdashti, GM Doherty, TC Lairmore, LM Brunt, and JF Moley. 2001. Risk of malignancy in thyroid incidentalomas identified by fluorodeoxyglucose-positron emission tomography. Surgery **130**:941–946.

Elisei, R,V Bottici, F Luchetti, G Di Coscio, C Romei, L Grasso, P Miccoli, P Iacconi, F Basolo, A Pinchera, and F Pacini. 2004. Impact of routine measurement of serum calcitonin on the diagnosis and outcome of medullary thyroid cancer: experience in 10,864 patients with nodular thyroid disorders. J Clin Endocrinol Metab **89**:163–168.

Ezzat, S, DA Sarti, DR Cain, and GD Braunstein. 1994. Thyroid incidentalomas: prevalence by palpation and ultrasonography. Arch Int Med **154**:1838–1840.

Frates, MC, CB Benson, PM Doubilet, ES Cibas, and E Marqusee. 2003. Can color Doppler sonography aid in the prediction of malignancy of thyroid nodules? J Ultrasound Med **22**:127–131.

Hamming, JF, BM Goslings, GJ vanSteenis, H Claasen, J Hermans, and JH Velde. 1990. The value of fine-needle aspiration biopsy in patients with nodular thyroid disease divided into groups of suspicion of malignant neoplasms on clinical grounds. Arch Int Med **150**:113–116.

Hatipoglu, BA, T Gierlowski, E Shore-Freedman, W Recant, and AB Schneider. 2000. Fine-needle aspiration of thyroid nodules in radiation-exposed patients. Thyroid **10**:63–69.

Hegedus, L. 2004. Clinical practice. The thyroid nodule. N Engl J Med **351**:1764–1771.

Ito, Y, T Uruno, K Nakano, Y Takamura, A Miya, K Kobayashi, T Yokozawa, F Matsuzuka, S Kuma, K Kuma, and A Miyauchi. 2003. An observation trial without surgical treatment in patients with papillary microcarcinoma of the thyroid. Thyroid **13**:381–387.

Kang, KW, SK Kim, HS Kang, ES Lee, JS Sim, IG Lee, SY Jeong, and SW Kim. 2003. Prevalence and risk of cancer of focal thyroid incidentaloma identified by 18F-fluorodeoxyglucose positron emission tomography for metastasis evaluation and cancer screening in healthy subjects. J Clin Endocrinol Metab **88**:4100–4104.

Kang, HW, JH No, JH Chung, YK Min, MS Lee, MK Lee, JH Yang, and KW Kim. 2004. Prevalence, clinical and ultrasonographic characteristics of thyroid incidentalomas. Thyroid **14**:29–33.

Marqusee, E, CB Benson, MC Frates, PM Doubilet, PR Larsen, ES Cibas, and SJ Mandel. 2000. Usefulness of ultrasonography in the management of nodular thyroid disease. Ann Int Med **133**:696–700.

Massoll, N, MS Nizam, and EL Mazzaferri. 2002. Cystic thyroid nodules: diagnostic and therapeutic dilemmas. Endocrinologist **12**:185–198.

Mazzaferri, EL. 1993. Management of a solitary thyroid nodule. N Engl J Med **328**:553–559.

Nam-Goong, IS, HY Kim, G Gong, HK Lee, SJ Hong, WB Kim, and YK Shong. 2004. Ultrasonography-guided fine-needle aspiration of thyroid incidentaloma: correlation with pathological findings. Clin Endocrinol (Oxford) **60**:21–28.

Papini, E, R Guglielmi, A Bianchini, A Crescenzi, S Taccogna, F Nardi, C Panunzi, R Rinaldi, V Toscano, and CM Pacella. 2002. Risk of malignancy in nonpalpable thyroid nodules: predictive value of ultrasound and color-Doppler features. J Clin Endocrinol Metab **87**:1941–1946.

Takahashi, T, KR Trott, K Fujimori, SL Simon, H Ohtomo, N Nakashima, K Takaya, N Kimurea, S Satomi, and MJ Schoemaker. 1997. An investigation into the prevalence of thyroid disease on Kwajalein Atoll, Marshall Islands. Health Phys **73**:199–213.

Tan, GH, and H Gharib. 1997. Thyroid incidentalomas: management approaches to nonpalpable nodules discovered incidentally on thyroid imaging. Ann Int Med **126**:226–231.

Yang, GC, D Liebeskind, and AV Messina. 2001. Ultrasound-guided fine-needle aspiration of the thyroid assessed by Ultrafast Papanicolaou stain: data from 1135 biopsies with a two- to six-year follow-up. Thyroid **11**:581–589.

2.2. DEFINITIONS: THYROID UPTAKE MEASUREMENT, THYROID SCAN, AND WHOLE BODY SCAN

ROBERT J. AMDUR, MD AND ERNEST L. MAZZAFERRI, MD, MACP

The purpose of this chapter is to explain the terms that describe the four studies that use radioactive iodine (I-131 and I-123) to evaluate thyroid cancer. These studies are: Measurement of thyroid uptake (Radioactive Iodine Uptake [RAIU]), Thyroid scan, Diagnostic Whole Body Scan (DxWBS), and Post-treatment Whole Body Scan (RxWBS). The major points from this chapter are summarized in Table 1. The roles of DxWBS and RxWBS in the management of patients with thyroid cancer are the subjects of seperate chapters.

THYROID UPTAKE MEASUREMENT (RAIU)

The result of this study is a number, not an image. Its main purpose is to quantitate how avidly thyroid tissue is concentrating iodine but it is also used to estimate the amount of residual thyroid tissue following thyroidectomy. The study consists of measuring the amount of radioiodine that remains in the thyroid bed after 2–24 hours. Here are the basic components of the procedure as it is used to evaluate a patient who has undergone a thyroidectomy for thyroid cancer:

- Prepare the patient by restricting dietary iodine for 2 weeks and elevating serum TSH to >30 U/mL with levothyroxine deprivation or rhTSH
- The patient swallows tablets containing I-123 or I-131 (we use I-123, 200–300 μCi)
- Measure radioactive iodine activity in the low neck 2–24 hours after radioiodine ingestion

Table 1. Definitions: Thyroid Uptake Measurement, Thyroid Scan, and Whole Body Scan.

Thyroid Uptake = Radioactive Iodine Uptake (RAIU):
- A number not an image
- RAIU = % radioiodine remaining in the low neck 2,6, or 24 hours after administration (2 hours in our program)
- Normal value after near total thyroidectomy: 0.5–5%
- Usual Isotope: I-123 (200–400 μCi)
- We measure RAIU only when delivering I-131 as an outpatient as this value is required by federal regulations to release a patient from the hospital

Thyroid Scan:
- An image of the pattern of radioiodine concentration in the thyroid or low neck
- Often done in conjunction with measurement of RAIU
- Usual isotope: I-123 (400–600 μCi)
- Historically, a thyroid scan is done as part of the workup for a thyroid nodule
- In our program we do not use a thyroid scan to evaluate thyroid nodules or to manage patients following the diagnosis of thyroid cancer

Radioiodine Whole Body Scan:
- An image of the pattern of radioiodine concentration throughout the entire body
- The image is acquired 4–7 days after administration (7 days in our program)
- Usual isotope: I-131

Abbreviations: DxWBS and RxWBS:
DxWBS: An image of the distribution of radioiodine when radioiodine is administered purely for diagnostic purposes. Radioiodine dose is usually 2–5 mCi I-131
RxWBS: An image of the distribution of radioiodine when the main reason for administering radioiodine is to destroy residual thyroid tissue or cancer. Radioiodine dose is usually 50–200 mCi I-131

- Thyroid uptake or RAIU = Activity in the thyroid area/activity administered
- Thyroid uptake is usually 0.5–5% following near-total or total thyroidectomy as compared to 5–20% for an intact thyroid gland that is functioning normally.

The Society of Nuclear Medicine has published guidelines for the use of scintigraphy in the diagnosis of residual functioning thyroid tissue or cancer (Becker 1996). For the purposes of this chapter it is not necessary to understand the technical details involved with measuring radioactive iodine activity in the thyroid area (e.g., camera specifications, normalization measurements, etc.). Basically, a device that measures radioactive emissions is placed over the low neck for about 2 minutes (Fig. 1). The number of counts detected is proportional to the amount of radioactive iodine in the low neck.

Many departments record thyroid uptake values at 6 and 24 hours after administering radioactive Iodine. The only reason that we measure RAIU is that this value is required by federal regulations to deliver I-131 therapy as an outpatient. The regulations permit a 2 hour RAIU value for the calculation related to patient release. We measure RAIU at 2 hours because it is inconvenient for the patient to return at later intervals. The requirements for outpatient I-131 therapy are the subject of a separate chapter.

THYROID SCAN

Thyroid scans have a role in the evaluation of a thyroid nodule but have no role in the management of a patient with thyroid cancer. This is the only place in this book

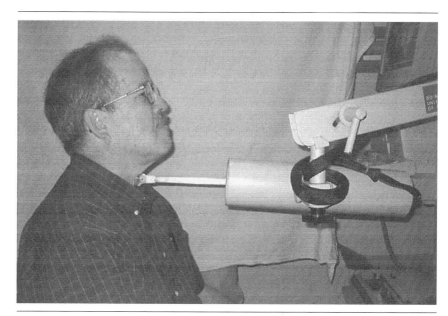

Figure 1. Illustration of the basic setup used to measure thyroid uptake (Radioactive Iodine Uptake, RAIU).

where we will mention a thyroid scan. The reason for discussing it here is to help readers remember that the terms Thyroid Uptake, Thyroid Scan, and Whole Body Scan describe three different kinds of studies that are done for different purposes.

The purpose of a thyroid scan is to produce an image that demonstrates the pattern of concentration of a radioactive probe in the thyroid gland. The most commonly used probes for thyroid scanning are I-123, I-131 and Tc-99. A thyroid scan is done with the same basic procedure that is used to measure thyroid uptake with the exception that radioactive emissions are measured with a device that can generate an image (Fig. 2). In a patient with an intact thyroid, a thyroid scan produces an image that shows the basic shape of the thyroid gland and the pattern of distribution of radioactive probe within the gland (Fig. 3). We do not evaluate thyroid nodules in euthyroid patients with a thyroid scan. Some prefer I-123 for this study (400–600 mCi). We do this study occasionally in patients with low TSH levels to identify a hyperfunctional (hot) nodule.

WHOLE BODY SCAN

When discussing thyroid cancer management the term Whole Body Scan is usually used to describe a study that records the distribution of I-131 (or I-123) throughout the entire body (Fig. 4). A scan that uses a probe other than I-131 is usually identified by the imaging probe. For example, a scan of the entire body with Tc-99 is called a

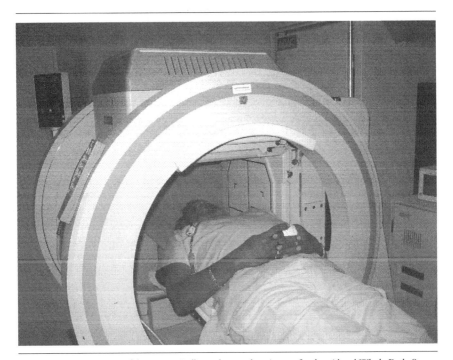

Figure 2. Gamma camera of the type typically used to produce images for thyroid and Whole Body Scans.

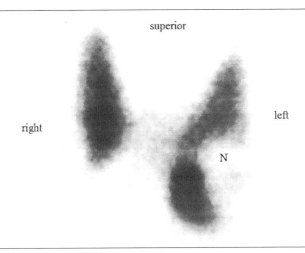

Figure 3. Radioiodine thyroid scan in a patient with an intact thyroid gland. There is a cold nodule (N) in the left lower pole.

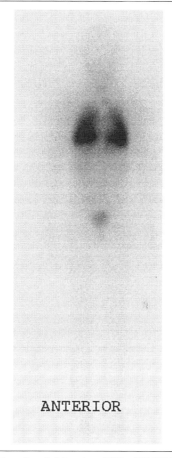

ANTERIOR

Figure 4. Whole body Scan 7 days after administration of 100 mCi I-131 in a patient who has previously undergone total thyroidectomy and remnant ablation. This scan demonstrates diffuse metastases in both lung fields.

Technetium Scan, and a scan with 18-Flouro Deoxy Glucose is called an FDG PET scan.

The equipment that is used to perform an I-131 whole body scan is similar to that used for a thyroid scan with the exception that the radioactive emissions are recorded over larger areas of the body than just the thyroid bed (by using larger cameras and/or moving the patient past imaging portals at a set rate). Patients are prepared for a whole body scan with a low-iodine diet and elevation in TSH. Images are recorded 4–7 days after radioiodine administration. This kind of delay is required to allow the radioiodine to wash out of normal tissues. The dose and isotope of radioiodine are different when a total body scan is being done purely for diagnostic purposes as opposed to a scan done following a therapeutic dose of I-131. Diagnostic and post-treatment radioiodine scans are the subjects of the next two chapters.

DIAGNOSTIC WHOLE BODY SCAN (DxWBS) VERSUS POSTTREATMENT WHOLE BODY SCAN (RxWBS)

The final point about terminology is that it is common to refer to a radioiodine Whole Body Scan as a DxWBS when radioiodine is administered purely for diagnostic purposes and as an RxWBS when the main reason for administering radioiodine is to destroy residual thyroid tissue or cancer.

REFERENCE

Becker, D, ND Charkes, H Sworkin, et al. 1996. Procedure guideline for extended scintigraphy for differentiated thyroid cancer: 1.0. J Nucl Med **37**:1269–1271.

2.3. THYROID STUNNING

ROBERT J. AMDUR, MD AND ERNEST L. MAZZAFERRI, MD, MACP

First described by Rawson et al. in 1951, thyroid stunning has become a subject of considerable controversy. Diagnostic whole body scan (DxWBS) images are usually obtained with the oral administration of 2 to 5 mCi of I-131. However, in 1994, Park and his associates at the University of Indiana showed that amounts of I-131 larger than 2 mCi have a sufficiently harmful effect on thyroid tissues to interfere with subsequent uptake of therapeutic amounts of I-131 on the posttreatment whole body scan (RxWBS)(Fig. 1). This effect occurred in both thyroid remnants and in tumor foci, and was observed with activities as small as 3 mCi, becoming progressively greater with larger amounts of I-131 but was not produced by I-123. The term "stunning" was used to describe this observation because the thinking was that the relatively low activities of I-131 used for DxWBS images (2–10 mCi I-131) temporarily decreased a cell's ability to concentrate iodine, but did not kill the cell (Fig. 2). The possibility of thyroid stunning is of concern because if it occurs to any significant degree it has the potential to decrease the efficacy of I-131 therapy for cancer.

The existence and potential importance of thyroid stunning have been debated for the past decade and continues to spark controversy in the literature. Our opinion is that thyroid stunning is a real phenomenon to the point that DxWBS images performed with 3 mCi or more I-131 have the capacity to compromise the effectiveness of subsequent I-131 therapy. The major studies on thyroid stunning are summarized in the articles listed in the reference section of this chapter. We will focus on the following issues: The mechanism of decreased iodine concentration as a result of a diagnostic I-131 scan (stunning versus cell killing), the frequency of thyroid stunning based on the activity

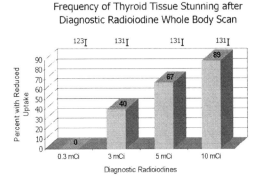

Figure 1. Degree of thyroid stunning with I-123 and progressively larger doses of I-131. Drawn from the data of Park et al. Influence of diagnostic radioiodines on the uptake of ablative dose of iodine-131. Thyroid 1994; 4:49–54.

of I-131, and the use of I-123 to avoid thyroid stunning. In the final section we will summarize our view of the role of diagnostic whole-body iodine scans (DxWBS) in the management of patients with thyroid cancer.

CELL KILLING VERSUS CELL STUNNING

Some authorities argue that diagnostic scanning does not compromise I-131 therapy because the decreased uptake that has been attributed to temporary stunning is actually due to radiation damage that will ultimately result in cell death. If this "kill rather than stun" theory is true then thyroid stunning is likely to enhance I-131 cancer therapy because a DxWBS study would in fact be the first step in ablating cells that concentrate I-131.

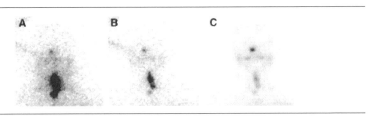

Figure 2. Sequential I-131 scans from a patient treated on the protocol described by Lassmann et al. (2004) (Fig. 3 reproduced with permission from J Nucl Med 2004; 45:619–625). (A) After 2 mCi with the patient hypothyroid, (B) After 2 mCi with the patient euthyroid and prepared with two rhTSH injections, and (C) After 100 mCi ablation prepared with additional injections of rhTSH. There was 6 weeks between scans A and B, and 12 days between scan B and C. In scan C the grey scale was adjusted to the diagnostic activity. The decrease in intensity of uptake of I-131 with each subsequent scan demonstrates the phenomenon of thyroid stunning.

We believe this theory is flawed insofar as it relates to the use of diagnostic I-131 scans in clinical practice. There are now data from animal models and *in-vitro* experimental systems demonstrateing that stunning—meaning a temporary reduction in iodine transport capacity in viable thyroid cells—is a real phenomenon that occurs as a result of radiation exposure in a dose-dependent fashion. Diagnostic amounts of I-131 appear to stun but not kill a large percentage of the cells that concentrate iodine.

The study that most clearly evaluates the kill versus stun issue is that of Postgard et al. (2002) This study used a transwell bicameral culture chamber to evaluate iodine transport across a monolayer of porcine thyroid cells following stimulation with TSH and different amounts of I-131. A dose of approximately 3 Gy resulted in a 50% decrease in iodine transport across the monolayer. This is an alarming finding considering that the mean dose to the thyroid remnant from a 2–3 mCi diagnostic scan with I-131 is approximately 14 Gy. The observed decrease in iodine transport following I-131 exposure was not associated with cell death and there was no change in transport kinetics in a control group treated with I-127, which is not radioactive.

FREQUENCY OF THYROID STUNNING BASED ON DOSE OF I-131

Studies on the relationship between stunning and I-131 DxWBS administered in amounts less than 10 mCi are conflicting. The recent study by Lassmann et al. (2004) makes several important observations regarding the serious effects that small amounts of I-131 may have on thyroid tissues. In this multicenter trial, DxWBS studies were done with 2 mCi I-131 during which a variety of biokinetic parameters where meticulously evaluated. A single 2 mCi I-131 scan resulted in an approximately 40% decrease in 24 hour uptake and half-time values that translated into a ~25% decrease in overall iodine residence time in the thyroid remnant. Values of this magnitude are likely to compromise the effectiveness of I-131 therapy to an important degree. Still, this is indirect evidence that subsequent I-131 therapy in these patients would have been unsuccessful.

In a recent retrospective study, Morris et al. (2001, 2003) compared ablation rates in patients who received 3 to 5 mCi I-131 DxWBSs (n = 37) with the ablation rates in patients who received no I-131 studies before the initial I-131 treatment (n = 63). Both groups underwent postoperative therapy with 100 to 200 mCi of I-131. The criterion for successful ablation was a visually negative 3 to 5 mCi I-131 DxWBS performed between 4 and 42 monthspt after the first I-131 treatment (mean, ~12 months). According to these criteria, ablation rates were nearly 65% for patients who had undergone DxWBS and 67% for those who did not undergo DxWBS, a difference that was not statistically significant. Patients who had not undergone DxWBS but had metastatic lesions (n = 23) achieved a higher success rate (78%) than patients (n = 9) who had undergone a DxWBS (67% rate), but the difference was not statistically significant. Still, this was a retrospective study in which serum thyroglobulin data were not used to support the diagnosis of successful I-131 ablation. Moreover, the shortcomings of DxWBS have been widely recognized in the past several years.

In terms of scan quality, there is little question that decreasing the amount of I-131 below 10 mCi compromises the sensitivity of cancer detection. Many studies demonstrate a major decrease in scan sensitivity as the amount of I-131 is lowered from 10 to

5 mCi or from 5 to 2 mCi. For this reason, our interpretation of the literature is that diagnostic scanning with I-131 involves a major tradeoff between scan sensitivity and the potential efficacy of I-131 therapy. A diagnostic scan that is acceptably sensitive in terms of cancer detection is likely to cause an unacceptable degree of thyroid stunning.

USING I-123 INSTEAD OF I-131 TO AVOID THYROID STUNNING

I-123 is a gamma emitter that deposits little radiation in the surrounding tissues. The main argument for using I-123 instead of I-131 in patients with thyroid cancer is less risk of thyroid stunning. Multiple studies confirm that thyroid stunning is virtually nonexistent with I-123 over the range of activities that are used in diagnostic imaging. There are several problems with using I-123 to look for thyroid cancer metastases: early studies suggested that I-123 was inferior to I-131 scanning, I-123 is much more expensive than I-131, and I-123 half-life is so short that it cannot be used effectively for total body scanning without administering large doses. Still, I-123 has better imaging characteristics than I-131 and in recent studies has been shown to be equivalent or superior to low-dose I-131. For example, in the large study by Shankar et al. (2002), the diagnostic yield of planar 1.5 mCi I-123 DxWBS scintigraphy done at 24 hr (this is superior to 5 hr images for lesion detection and image quality) when compared with images obtained after I-131 therapy detected all the metastatic foci seen on RxWBS (i.e., there was no stunning and I-123 was highly accurate). The study by Mandel et al. (2001) found I-123 imaging of thyroid remnants to be superior to that of I-131. Also, the study by Anderson et al. (2003) found that I-123 DxWBS can be done after preparation with recombinant human TSH. But, the 1.5 to 3.0 mCi of I-123 that is necessary to produce optimal results in terms of cancer detection is both unavailable and prohibitively expensive in many areas of the country. As its availability increases and the cost decreases, this agent might replace I-131 for imaging of patients with suspected recurrent or metastatic thyroid cancer when a DxWBS is necessary.

OMITTING DIAGNOSTIC I-131 WHOLE BODY SCANS

Despite the differences of opinion regarding the pathophysiology of stunning and its ultimate effects on therapy, we believe that it is prudent to accept that stunning is a real phenomenon that has the potential to seriously impair the efficacy of I-131 therapy. The potential clinical value of an I-131 DxWBS rarely outweighs the risk of compromising the effectiveness of I-131 cancer therapy by causing thyroid stunning. The alternative view of this is that some patients may not require I-131 ablation or should receive larger than usual amounts of I-131 therapy based on the results of the DxWBS. Morris et al. (2001, 2003) found that of 7 studies that based the need for I-131 treatment on the basis of a DxWBS, only 8 of 880 patients were eliminated from I-131 therapy for remnant ablation because of negative postsurgical DxWBS.

We measure thyroid uptake (RAIU) of 200–400 uCi I-123 without performing imaging studies and rarely do a radioiodine scan purely for diagnostic purposes. When we do perform a DxWBS, we use 5 mCi of I-131.

REFERENCES

Anderson, GS, S Fish, K Nakhoda, H Zhuang, A Alavi, and SJ Mandel. 2003. Comparison of I-123 and I-131 for whole-body imaging after stimulation by recombinant human thyrotropin: a preliminary report. Nucl Med **28(2):**93–96.

Lassmann, M, M Luster, H Hanscheid, and C Reiners. 2004. Impact of I-131 diagnostic activities on the biokinetics of thyroid remnants. J Nucl Med **45:**619–625.

Mandel, SJ, LK Shankar, F Benard, A Yamamoto, and A Alavi. 2001. Superiority of iodine-123 compared with iodine-131 scanning for thyroid remnants in patients with differentiated thyroid cancer. Clin Nucl Med **26(1):**6–9.

Morris, LF, AD Waxman, and GD Braunstein. 2001. The nonimpact of thyroid stunning: remnant ablation rates in I-131-scanned and nonscanned individuals. J Clin Endocrinol Metab **86(8):**3507–3511.

Morris, LF, AD Waxman, and GD Braustein. 2003. Thyroid stunning. Thyroid **13(4):**333–340.

Postgard, P, J Himmelman, U Lindencrona, N Bhogal, D Wiberg, G Berg, S Jansson, E Nystrom, E Forsssell-Aronsson, and M Nilsson. 2002. Stunning of iodine transport by I-131 irradiation in cultured thyroid epithelial cells. J Nucl Med **43:**828–834.

Shankar, LK, AJ Yamamoto, MDA Alavi, and SJ Mandel. 2002. Comparison of (123)I scintigraphy at 5 and 24 hours in patients with differentiated thyroid cancer. J Nucl Med **43(1):**72–76.

2.4. THE ROLE OF A DIAGNOSTIC RADIOIODINE WHOLE BODY SCAN (DxWBS)

ROBERT J. AMDUR, MD AND ERNEST L. MAZZAFERRI, MD, MACP

The term diagnostic whole body scan (DxWBS) is used when radioiodine (I-131 or I-123) is administered for the sole purpose of detecting normal remnant thyroid tissue or residual cancer. The term post-treatment whole body scan (RxWBS) is used when the scan is done following I-131 therapy. A DxWBS is usually done with 2–5 mCi I-131. The purpose of this chapter is to explain the role of a DxWBS in the management of patients with thyroid cancer. Table 1 summarizes the main points.

THYROID STUNNING AND THE USE OF I-123

DxWBS images are usually obtained 48 hours after the oral administration of 2 to 5 mCi of I-131. However, 2 mCi of I-131 may fail to show thyroid bed or tumor uptake on the DxWBS, whereas larger amounts interfere with subsequent uptake of therapeutic amounts of I-131. This effect, referred to as "thyroid stunning," occurs with activities as small as 3 mCi and becomes progressively greater with larger amounts of I-131, but is not produced by I-123 (Park 1994). Thus, one rationale for not performing a DxWBS prior to I-131 therapy is to avoid thyroid stunning that may decrease the chance of successful ablation of the thyroid remnant or cancer. Concern about thyroid stunning is the main argument for using I-123 instead of I-131 for diagnostic studies prior to I-131 therapy (Mandel 2001). I-123 has better imaging characteristics than I-131 and has been shown to be equivalent or superior to low-dose I-131 in recent studies; however, it is expensive and not widely available for this purpose. As the availability of I-123 increases and the cost decreases, this agent may replace I-131 in imaging for recurrent

Table 1. The Role of a Diagnostic Radioiodine Whole Body Scan.

Definition of a diagnostic radioiodine whole body scan (DxWBS):
DxWBS: An image of the distribution of radioiodine when radioiodine is administered purely for diagnostic purposes
Usual isotope and radioiodine dose for a DxWBS:
Most departments use 2–5 mCi I-131
The use of higher amounts of I-131 or of I-123 is discussed in the chapter on thyroid stunning
Historic role of a DxWBS:
To determine the need for I-131 therapy and to determine I-131 activity.
At 6–12 month intervals following therapy to check for residual cancer
Changes that have decreased the value of a DxWBS:
Ultrasonography is used to detect and quantitate thyroid tissue or tumor in the neck
Serum thyroglobulin level, together with ultrasonography, is the most sensitive way to detect residual tumor
The indications for a DxWBS in our program:
Determination of iodine avidity of gross disease that is unlikely to concentrate radioiodine (e.g., recurrent following prior treatment with I-131).
To obtain approval for insurance coverage for payment for a PET scan (uncommon)

or metastatic thyroid cancer when a DxWBS is required (Anderson 2003). The results of a DxWBS, however, contribute so little to patient management that the question of thyroid stunning is often moot.

THE LIMITED VALUE OF A DxWBS

Historically, a DxWBS was routinely done at 6-12 month intervals following I-131 therapy to check for residual cancer. The purpose of the DxWBS was to determine the need for I-131 therapy or the amount of I-131 for therapy. In our opinion, improved access to high-quality ultrasonography and the sensitivity of serum thyroglobulin assays for detecting recurrent tumor, has decreased the value of a DxWBS to the point that the role of this study in the management of patients with thyroid cancer is now extremely limited. Many studies support this point of view (Haugen 2002; Mazzaferri 2002; Mazzaferri 2003; Taylor 2004; Torlontano 2003; Torre 2004; Pacini 2002; Schlumberger 2004). The policies that we use in our program reflect the view that ultrasonography and thyroglobulin measurement usually make it unnecessary to perform a DxWBS:

DxWBS Prior to Thyroid Remnant Ablation

We rarely perform a DxWBS prior to remnant ablation. In our opinion the results of a DxWBS should not determine the need for I-131 therapy following thyroidectomy for differentiated thyroid cancer. We usually recommend I-131 therapy in all patients who have undergone near-total or total thyroidectomy regardless of stage of disease, RAIU value, DxWBS results or basal thyroglobulin level.

The chance that a DxWBS will change the amount of I-131 that we administer after thyroidectomy is too low to justify the risk of thyroid stunning, added cost and patient inconvenience associated with this study. We rely on the surgeon's operative report and our office ultrasound study to determine if there is a large thyroid remnant or gross residual tumor in the neck. We also use ultrasound to measure tumor volume when residual thyroid tissue exists. We use a chest x-ray (followed by noncontrast Computerized Tomography if indicated) to determine if there are visible metastases in the mediastinum or lungs. When a DxWBS is done in a way that is unlikely to stun residual tissue (< 3 mCi I-131 or I-123), the chance of detecting lung or bone metastases is extremely low in a patient with a negative chest x-ray and no symptoms of a distant metastasis.

DxWBS After Remnant Ablation

We rarely perform a DxWBS for thyroid cancer surveillance or to determine the need for, or amount of, I-131 required for therapy in a patient with an elevated thyroglobulin level following thyroidectomy and I-131 remnant ablation. Thyroglobulin measurements and neck ultrasonography together provide a more sensitive indicator of disease activity than does a DxWBS, which is not indicated in the majority of patients either before initial I-131 therapy or during follow-up. As described in subsequent chapters, our standard follow-up of patients who are at low risk of recurrence and are clinically free of tumor is usually limited to neck ultrasonography and measurements of baseline serum thyroglobulin values during thyroid hormone suppression of TSH. If under these circumstances the Tg is < 1 ng/mL, then an rhTSH-stimulated or thyroid hormone withdrawal-stimulated serum thyroglobulin measurement is made at 6–12 months following remnant ablation. If we are concerned about distant metastases we evaluate the patient with other imaging studies, usually noncontrast chest CT scans and/or FDG PET scan, or a technetium bone scan, or an MR scan of the neck or brain.

INDICATIONS FOR A DxWBS

There are two relatively infrequent reasons to perform DxWBS in patients at low risk of having residual disease, which is the majority of patients following initial therapy.

Brain or Spinal Cord Metastases

Although a DxWBS may sometimes help determine the potential value of additional radioiodine therapy in a patient with gross, unresectable disease that has recurred following treatment with I-131, the RxWBS is far more likely to give a clear answer to this question. We rarely perform a DxWBS unless we have reason to believe that the patient has brain or spinal cord metastases that might be adversely affected by a therapeutic dose of I-131.

Insurance Coverage for a FDG PET Scan

Medicare, and many commercial insurance plans will not approve payment for an FDG-PET scan to evaluate the extent of thyroid cancer unless a recent radioiodine whole body scan is negative for tumor and the serum thyroglobulin level is elevated. The usual scenario in which we encounter this problem is in a patient with a rising serum thyroglobulin level following one or more I-131 treatments that show no evidence of uptake on the RxWBS. In this setting, we want to determine if the patient has measurable disease that does not take up radioiodine. The most sensitive study in this setting is an FDG PET scan performed with TSH elevation (usually with rhTSH injections). In such patients we may have to obtain a DxWBS to demonstrate that it is negative for tumor uptake before the patient's insurance plan will approve payment for a PET scan. DxWBS is not necessary if a recent RxWBS was negative.

REFERENCES

Anderson, GS, S Fish, K Nakhoda, H Zhuang, A Alavi, and SJ Mandel. 2003. Comparison of I-123 and I-131 for whole-body imaging after stimulation by recombinant human thyrotropin: a preliminary report. Clin Nucl Med **28**:93–96.

Haugen, BR, EC Ridgway, BA McLaughlin, and MT McDermott. 2002. Clinical comparison of whole-body radioiodine scan and serum thyroglobulin after stimulation with recombinant human thyrotropin. Thyroid **12(1)**:37–43.

Mandel, SJ, LK Shankar, F Benard, A Yamamoto, and A Alavi. 2001. Superiority of iodine-123 compared with iodine-131 scanning for thyroid remnants in patients with differentiated thyroid cancer. Clin Nucl Med **26**:6–9.

Mazzaferri, EL, and RT Kloos. 2002. Is diagnostic iodine-131 scanning with recombinant human TSH (rhTSH) useful in the follow-up of differentiated thyroid cancer after thyroid ablation? J Clin Endocrinol Metab **87**:1490–1498.

Mazzaferri, EL, RJ Robbins, CA Spencer, LE Braverman, F Pacini, L Wartofsky, et al. 2003. A consensus report of the role of serum thyroglobulin as a monitoring method for low-risk patients with papillary thyroid carcinoma. J Clin Endocrinol Metab **88(4)**:1433–1441.

Pacini, F, M Capezzone, R Elisei, C Ceccarelli, D Taddei, and A Pinchera. 2002. Diagnostic 131-iodine whole-body scan may be avoided in thyroid cancer patients who have undetectable stimulated serum tg levels after initial treatment. J Clin Endocrinol Metab **87(4)**:1499–1501.

Park, HM, OW Perkins, JW Edmondson, RB Schnute, and A Manatunga. 1994. Influence of diagnostic radioiodines on the uptake of ablative dose of iodine-131. Thyroid **4**:49–54.

Schlumberger, M, G Berg, O Cohen, L Duntas, F Jamar, B Jarzab, E Limbert, P Lind, F Pacini, C Reiners, F S Franco, A Toft, and WM Wiersinga. 2004. Follow-up of low-risk patients with differentiated thyroid carcinoma: a European perspective. Eur J Endocrinol **150(2)**:105–112.

Taylor, H, S Hyer, L Vini, B Pratt, G Cook, and C Harmer. 2004. Diagnostic I whole body scanning after thyroidectomy and ablation for differentiated thyroid cancer. Eur J Endocrinol **150(5)**:649–653.

Torlontano, M, U Crocetti, L D'Aloiso, N Bonfitto, A Di Giorgio, S Modoni, G Valle, V Frusciante, M Bisceglia, S Filetti, M Schlumberger, and V Trischitta. 2003. Serum thyroglobulin and I-131 whole body scan after recombinant human TSH stimulation in the follow-up of low-risk patients with differentiated thyroid cancer. Eur J Endocrinol **148(1)**:19–24.

Torre, EM, MT Carballo, RM Erdozain, LF Llenas, MJ Iriarte, and JJ Layana. 2004. Prognostic value of thyroglobulin serum levels and (131)I whole-body scan after initial treatment of low-risk differentiated thyroid cancer. Thyroid **14(4)**:301–306.

2.5. THE VALUE OF A POST-TREATMENT WHOLE BODY SCAN

ROBERT J. AMDUR, MD AND ERNEST L. MAZZAFERRI, MD, MACP

The term post-treatment whole body scan (RxWBS) is used to define the whole body scan performed when the sole purpose of I-131 administration is to destroy a normal thyroid remnant or residual cancer. Unlike a diagnostic whole body scan (DxWBS), which is done 72 hours after administration of I-123 or I-131, an RxWBS is performed 4–7 days after I-131 therapy so that the isotope is cleared from normal tissues. The purpose of this chapter is to explain the rationale for performing an RxWBS when therapeutic I-131 is administered. Table 1 summarizes the main points from this chapter.

THE POTENTIAL ADVERSE ASPECTS OF A RxWBS

A RxWBS is an extremely low risk procedure but there is a chance that a false positive finding will lead to additional testing or treatment. The conditions that may result in a false positive interpretation of a radioiodine whole body scan are summarized by Shapiro et al. (2002) and Carlisle et al. (2003) and summarized in Table 2. In our experience, false positive interpretations of an RxWBS can be minimized and generally cause little morbidity. Still, there is always a risk of administering I-131 therapy unnecessarily because of a false positive RxWBS study, which is probably the main negative aspect of performing the study. This can be avoided if the scan is interpreted in light of the clinical findings, especially the serum thyroglobulin levels. The other issues are the added expense and inconvenience associated with acquiring and interpreting RxWBS images.

Table 1. The value of a post-treatment whole body scan (RxWBS).

A RxWBS:
RxWBS: An image of the distribution of I-131 throughout the body when the main reason for administering radioiodine is to destroy residual thyroid tissue or cancer.
Radioiodine activity for an RxWBS is usually 50–200 mCi I-131.
Images are performed 4–7 days following I-131 administration.

A RxWBS is a procedure that involves very little discomfort or risk:
The only "discomfort" associated with an RxWBS is the cost of the procedure and the inconvenience of coming for a 30 minute scan.
The only risk of RxWBS is the risk that a false positive interpretation will lead to additional workup or treatment.

The potential value of a RxWBS:
Evaluation of the quality of therapy in a patient with a thyroid remnant.
In a patient who is being treated for subclinical disease, diffuse hepatic uptake indicates that residual thyroid or tumor cells are metabolizing radioiodine.
A RxWBS is more sensitive than a DxWBS.
Results of a RxWBS may indicate the need for additional studies. For example, when a RxWBS demonstrates a brain, spine or long bone metastasis.
A RxWBS identifies patients who will probably need another radioiodine treatment in the near future.

Our policy:
We perform a RxWBS in all patients 7 days after radioiodine therapy.

THE POTENTIAL VALUE OF A RxWBS

We perform RxWBS 7 days after I-131 administration in all patients who receive a therapeutic dose of I-131 ($\geq$30 mCi). A RxWBS shows the degree of I-131 uptake, determines the extent of disease, identifies situations that require additional workup, and predicts prognosis.

An RxWBS Evaluates the Quality of I-131 Therapy for Remnant Ablation

Even the most thorough surgical resection usually leaves a small amount of residual thyroid tissue next to the larynx or trachea after near-total thyroidectomy. For this reason, almost all RxWBS studies done after the initial thyroid surgery demonstrate uptake in the thyroid bed. When we do not see clear evidence of thyroid bed uptake on a RxWBS following thyroidectomy, it suggests that the patient was not optimally prepared for I-131 therapy. The most common reasons for a poor quality RxWBS studies are noncompliance with the low-iodine diet, a recent history of having a radiology study with intravenous iodinated contrast, or inadequate TSH elevation prior to therapy.

Diffuse Hepatic Uptake in a Patient with a Negative RxWBS

Diffuse homogenous hepatic uptake of I-131 on a whole body scan without visible uptake by the thyroid or tumor suggests hidden metastases. Diffuse hepatic uptake of I-131 indicates that the liver is metabolizing I-131-labelled fragments of thyroglobulin secreted by the tumor. In the study by Chung et al. (1997), diffuse hepatic uptake on DxWBS was seen in 12% of the patients, but following RxWBS, it increased according to the amount of administered I-131, ranging from 39% of the patients treated with

Table 2. False Positive I-131 Uptake on Whole Body Radioiodine Scans.

Site	Clinical cause	Mimics
Head	Meningioma Scalp inflammation Dacryocystitis Venous lakes skull Hair contamination Tears	Brain metastases
Nose	Nasal secretions Sinusitis Mucocele	Facial bone metastases
Facial area	Salivary glands Warthin's tumor Saliva Tears Urine contamination	Facial bone metastases
Oropharyngeal area	Periodontal disease Oral inflammation Lingual thyroid	Facial bone metastases
Neck	Tracheostomy Thyroglossal duct	Neck metastases
Mediastinum	Thymus	Mediastinal metastases
Lungs	Adenocarcinoma, Squamous cell carcinoma Bronchiectasis Pleural effusions, Struma cordis, Pleuropericardial cyst, Fungal infections Any infection	Lung metastases
Chest Wall	Breast uptake (lactating), Breast cyst, Urine contamination, Skin infections	Lung, bone metastases
Esophageal area	Barrett's esophagus, Zenker's diverticulum, Hiatal hernia, Esophageal inflammation/scarring.	Lung, bone metastases
Liver	Physiologic diffuse hepatic uptake, Gallbladder disease	Hepatic metastases
Stomach	Physiologic uptake, Gastritis	Bone metastases, intraabdominal metastases
Abdomen	Abdominal nonthyroidal tumors Cholecystitis	Bone metastases, intraabdominal metastases
Colon	Meckel's diverticulum Colonic bypass Abdominal wall mesh	Bone metastases, intraabdominal metastases
Urinary tact	Renal cysts Polycystic kidneys Ectopic kidney	Bone metastases, intraabdominal metastases
Ovary	Ovarian cystadenoma, struma ovarii, ovarian cysts	Bone metastases, intraabdominal metastases
Testicular area	Epididymitis, Skin contamination	Testicular metastases
Contamination	Pelvis Low back Anywhere within reach of the hands	Bone metastases
Perspiration Skin	Axilla Sebaceous cysts	Distant metastases

30 mCi of I-131 to 71% given 150 mCi. This is important information when the main indication for radioiodine therapy is an elevated serum thyroglobulin level.

A RxWBS is More Sensitive than a DxWBS

RxWBS done after a I-131 therapy often demonstrates tumor that was not visualized on a diagnostic study (DxWBS). In most cases a RxWBS will demonstrate all functional foci of tumor > 1 cc and often pick up diffuse lung metastases with sub centimeter nodules. The RxWBS identifies twice the number of malignant lymph nodes and four-fold the number of lung metastases than does the DxWBS. The false negative rate of DxWBS after thyroid hormone withdrawal or rhTSH stimulation is 80% in low-risk patients with baseline serum thyroglobulin levels <1 ng/mL during TSH suppression (Mazzaferri 2003).

Result of a RxWBS May Indicate the Need for Additional Studies

Brain, spine, and long bone metastases require additional evaluation and monitoring to determine if treatment other than radioiodine therapy is needed. A metastasis to one of these areas may be discovered on a RxWBS.

Results of the RxWBS Helps to Predict Prognosis

The RxWBS frequently helps to predict the likelihood that additional therapy will be needed in the future. For example, finding nodal or distant metastases on the RxWBS after remnant ablation indicates that the patient will likely need additional therapy over the next 12 to 24 months.

REFERENCES

Carlisle, MR, C Lu, and IR McDougall. 2003. The interpretation of I-131 scans in the evaluation of thyroid cancer, with an emphasis on false positive findings. Nucl Med Commun **24(6):**715–735.

Chung, JK, YJ Lee, JM Jeong, DS Lee, MC Lee, BY Cho, et al. 1997. Clinical significance of hepatic visualization on iodine-131 whole-body scan in patients with thyroid carcinoma. J Nucl Med **38:**1191–1195.

Mazzaferri, EL, and RT Kloos. 2001. Current approaches to primary therapy for papillary and follicular thyroid cancer. J Clin Endocrinol Metab **86(4):**1447–1463.

Mazzaferri, EL, RJ Robbins, CA Spencer, LE Braverman, F Pacini, L Wartofsky, BR Haugen, SI Sherman, DS Cooper, GD Braunstein, S Lee, TF Davies, BM Arafah, PW Ladenson, and A Pinchera. 2003. A consensus report of the role of serum thyroglobulin as a monitoring method for low-risk patients with papillary thyroid carcinoma. J Clin Endocrinol Metab **88(4):**1433–1441.

Shapiro, B, V Rufini, A Jarwan, O Geatti, KJ Kearfott, LM Fig, ID Kirkwood, and MD Gross. 2000. Artifacts, anatomical and physiological variants, and unrelated diseases that might cause false-positive whole-body 131-I scans in patients with thyroid cancer. Semin Nucl Med **30(2):**115–32.

2.6. EXAMPLES OF RADIOIODINE WHOLE BODY SCANS

ROBERT J. AMDUR, MD AND ERNEST L. MAZZAFERRI, MD, MACP

The purpose of this chapter is to help clinicians learn how to interpret radioiodine whole body scans. The figures in this chapter demonstrate a wide range of normal and abnormal findings (Figs. 1–19). The review article listed in the reference section presents a detailed description of artifacts and normal variants that may cause a false-positive interpretation of a whole body iodine scan (Shapiro 2000). Table 1 lists the basic questions that help direct scan review. Two questions require further explanation:

HAS THE PATIENT RECEIVED I-131 THERAPY ≥6 MONTHS PRIOR TO THIS SCAN?

When interpreting a radioiodine scan it is important to know if you expect to see residual thyroid tissue. Following a near total thyroidectomy, ≥30 mCi of I-131 usually destroys all the residual normal thyroid tissue. Therefore, in a patient who has previously received I-131 therapy, an area of radioiodine concentration in the thyroid bed is tumor until proven otherwise. Conversely, a scan done immediately before or after the first I-131 treatment (ablation of the thyroid remnant) is expected to show radioiodine uptake in the thyroid bed to the point that it is usually not possible to differentiate tumor from residual normal tissue in this area.

IS THERE DIFFUSE, HOMOGENEOUS UPTAKE IN THE LIVER?

Diffuse, homogeneous radioiodine uptake in the liver occurs when thyroid tissue or differentiated thyroid cancer is present (Chung 1997). This is described in detail in the

Table 1. Questions that direct the review of a radioiodine whole body scan.

Has the patient received I-131 therapy ≥6 months prior to this scan?
YES: Areas of nonphysiologic uptake of radioiodine in a patient with a history of remnant ablation are tumor until proven otherwise.
NO: Uptake in the thyroid bed is an expected finding in a patient who has not been previously treated with I-131.

Is there radioiodine uptake in the neck outside the thyroid bed?
YES: radioiodine uptake in the neck outside the thyroid bed indicates metastasis to cervical nodes or soft tissue of the neck.

Is there radioiodine uptake in the mediastinum?
YES: radioiodine uptake in the central chest that is clearly separate from the thyroid bed indicates metastasis to mediastinal nodes or a residual thymus gland.

Is there radioiodine uptake in the lungs?
YES: diffuse radioiodine uptake in the lungs indicates lung metastases. A solitary area of uptake likely represents a nonneoplastic process.

Is there radioiodine uptake in bone?
YES: multiple areas of radioiodine uptake in bone indicate bone metastases. A solitary area of uptake in bone requires further evaluation.

Is there radioiodine uptake in the brain?
YES: uptake in the region of the saggital sinus often represents a normal variant. Focal uptake in the brain suggests metastasis.

Is there diffuse, homogeneous concentration of radioiodine in the liver?
YES: Diffuse, homogeneous hepatic uptake is an expected finding anytime there is normal thyroid tissue or functioning thyroid cancer anywhere in the patient's body.
NO: The absence of diffuse hepatic uptake of radioiodine means that the patient has no residual thyroid tissue or thyroid cancer, or that the patient was not prepared properly for the scan or that residual cancer do not concentrate radioiodine.

---

chapter on diagnostic whole body scans. There are three possible explanations for an absence of hepatic uptake of radioiodine on a total body scan:

- There is no residual thyroid tissue or thyroid cancer
- The residual thyroid cancer does not trap radioiodine
- The patient was not prepared properly for the scan

EXAMPLES OF I-131 WHOLE BODY SCANS

The figures in this chapter are post-treatment whole body scans (RxWBS) performed seven days after 100–200 mCi I-131 in patients who have previously undergone near-total thyroidectomy. Unless specified otherwise, all images are anterior views with the image cropped above the knees. In most of the scans there is concentration of radioiodine in the nasal cavity, oral cavity, liver, bowel, and bladder. Radioiodine concentration in the nasal area is caused by radioiodine secretion by the serous glands lining the nasal cavity. Radioiodine concentration in the bowel is a physiologic but undesirable finding. Areas of mild, diffuse uptake in the left upper quadrant or lower quadrants of the abdomen are common findings even in patients who have multiple bowel movements each day. Larger areas of intense concentration of radioiodine in the bowel are a reflection of poor bowel clearance during the week following I-131 therapy. Patients should be instructed to take cathartics if they are constipated to avoid unnecessary bowel irradiation.

Radioiodine is excreted from the serous glands lining the nasal cavity. Saliva produced during eating is mainly from the parotid glands. The submandibular glands, the sublingual glands, and the minor salivary glands lining the mouth produce most of the saliva between meals. Radioiodine whole body scans usually demonstrate radioiodine concentration in the region of the nasal cavity and mouth. Radioiodine uptake in the nasal cavity and submandibular glands often appears as intense, well-defined areas of radioiodine uptake.

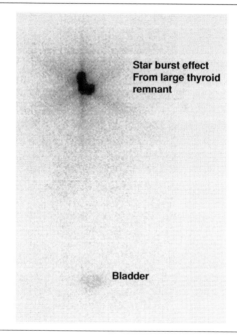

Figure 1. Posttreatment scan (RxWBS) showing a large thyroid remnant giving a star burst effect that is sufficient enough to obscure metastases in the neck.

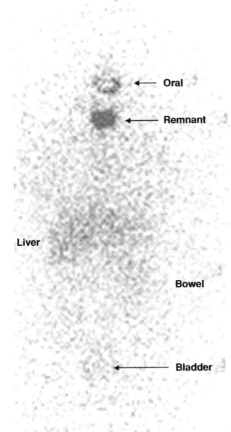

Figure 2. This is an RxWBS after 100 mCi of I-131 given to a 32 year-old woman with Graves' disease and a small papillary thyroid carcinoma confined to the thyroid gland. I-131 was administered after preparation with rhTSH, lithium and a two-week low-iodine diet. This image demonstrates the typical findings when a low-risk patient is given I-131 to ablate the thyroid remnant. The RxWBS shows no uptake outside the thyroid bed. Her serum Tg level one year later is undetectable <0.9 ng/mL but she had high anti-Tg antibody (TgAb) levels of >90 IU/L. Her serum TgAb levels have been falling and a Tg measured by RIA is 1 ng/mL. Neck ultrasonography is negative and she appears to be free of disease. Radioiodine uptake is seen in the oral cavity, thyroid bed, diffusely in the liver, and is barely visible in the bowel and bladder. The pattern of uptake in the thyroid bed is homogeneous and symmetrical. As will be seen in subsequent examples, the pattern of radioiodine concentration in residual thyroid tissue is extremely variable. Absence of uptake in the bowel is typical in euthyroid patients prepared by rhTSH for remnant ablation.

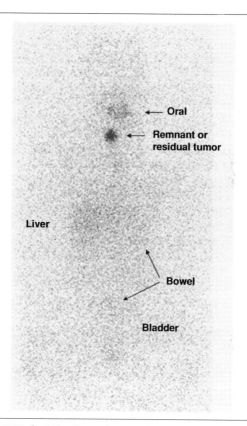

Figure 3. This is a RxWBS after 205 mCi was administered to a 36 year-old woman with a 1.2 cm thyroid papillary carcinoma in the left thyroid lobe. The tumor was invading the thyroid capsule and was not completely resected because of its involvement with the left recurrent laryngeal nerve. A small amount of tumor tissue was left at the cricotracheal junction at the insertion of the recurrent laryngeal nerve. Postoperatively this patient was prepared with rhTSH and a low-iodine diet. There is physiologic uptake in the oral cavity, thyroid remnant and liver. There are faint areas of uptake in the bowel and bladder. There is faint radioiodine uptake in the mediastinal area but we did not think this was definitive enough to call a metastasis. There is a focal area of intense uptake in the right side of the thyroid bed. This is labeled remnant or residual tumor because it is not possible to distinguish tumor from normal thyroid tissue when there is uptake in the thyroid bed in a patient who has not previously received I-131 therapy. It is likely that this was normal thyroid remnant. The patients serum Tg level is undetectable (<0.9 ng/mL) with negative TgAb and fails to rise with rhTSH stimulation, and her neck ultrasonography is negative. We believe she is free of disease. Radioiodine uptake in the thyroid remnant is often asymmetrical.

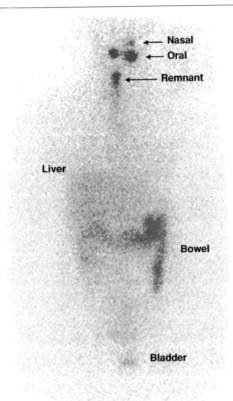

Figure 4. This is a RxWBS done with thyroid hormone withdrawal 48 hours after the administration of 100 mCi of I-131 to a 38 year-old woman with a 3.5 cm papillary thyroid carcinoma. The considerable radioiodine in the bowel indicates poor bowel evacuation in a hypothyroid patient. The patient was instructed to take cathartics but failed to do so. There is also physiologic radioiodine concentration in the nasal and oropharyngeal cavities and uptake in the thyroid bed and liver and residual I-131 in the bladder. Asymmetric uptake in the nose, mouth, or thyroid bed is not unusual and does not identify residual tumor.

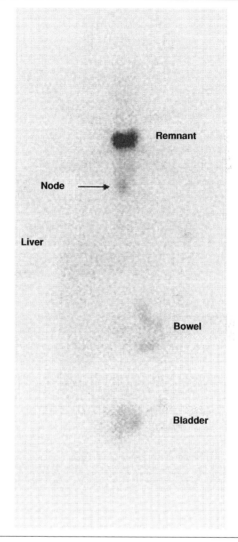

Figure 5. This is a RxWBS of a 68 year-old woman with no prior history of I-131 therapy. Her papillary thyroid carcinoma was resected with hemithyroidectomy and right radical neck dissection about 40 years before she had a recurrence of tumor in the right lateral neck compartments at levels III, IV and VI, which contained multiple 2 to 3 cm lymph node metastases. The surgeon resected several malignant upper mediastinal lymph nodes through a cervical incision. The patient was prepared with a low-iodine diet, lithium and rhTSH. There is physiologic radioiodine uptake in the thyroid bed, liver, bowel and bladder. The lack of radioiodine uptake in the nasal cavity and oral cavity is unusual but not indicative of pathology. The focus of I-131 in the mediastinum is in the area in which a mediastinal lymph node metastasis was resected. Her serum Tg level was 14.8 ng/mL with a TSH of <0.1 mIU/L before I-131 therapy, and 12 months later was 0.9 ng/mL during thyroid hormone suppression of TSH and failed to rise with rhTSH stimulation. Her neck ultrasonography is negative and we think that she is free of disease.

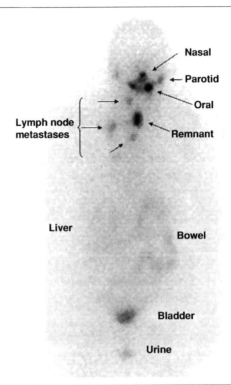

Figure 6. This is a RxWBS after 200 mCi of I-131 in an 81 year-old woman with no prior history of I-131 therapy. She had a multifocal, bilateral papillary thyroid carcinoma with a small area (5%) of tall cell carcinoma in the tumor. The largest tumor was 2.5 cm in the right lobe that was metastatic to five level V lymph nodes on the right. She was prepared with low-iodine diet and rhTSH stimulation. Prior to treatment her serum Tg (Tg) level was 49 ng/mL with a TSH of 2.8 mIU/L. There is physiologic concentration of I-131 in the nasal cavity, oral cavity, thyroid remnant, liver, bowel, and bladder. The area of uptake inferior to the bladder is urine on the perineum. There is physiologic radioiodine uptake in the parotid glands. Nodal metastases are identified in the right neck (arrows). There is I-131 uptake in the mediastinum that is clearly separate from the thyroid bed. One year after treatment her serum Tg is gradually falling and was 18 ng/mL during thyroid hormone suppression of TSH.

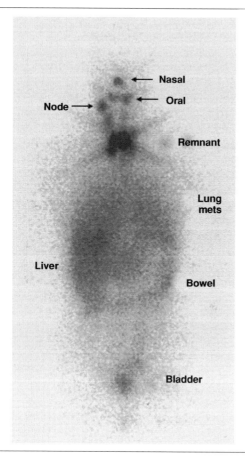

Figure 7. This is a RxWBS of an 18 year-old woman with no prior history of I-131 therapy. The patient had a negative 5 mCi diagnostic whole body scan done in another hospital and had a negative chest x-ray and neck CT without contrast. There is physiologic uptake of radioiodine in the nasal cavity, oral cavity, and a star burst effect of uptake in the thyroid bed indicative of a large thyroid remnant, and uptake in the liver, bowel, and bladder. A cervical lymph node metastasis is identified in the right upper neck and diffuse lung metastases are seen bilaterally. This patient has been treated with a total of nearly 500 mCi of I-131 and has no uptake in the lungs on RxWBS and has a serum Tg of 1 ng/mL on thyroid hormone suppression of TSH that rises to 2.3 ng/mL with rhTSH stimulation.

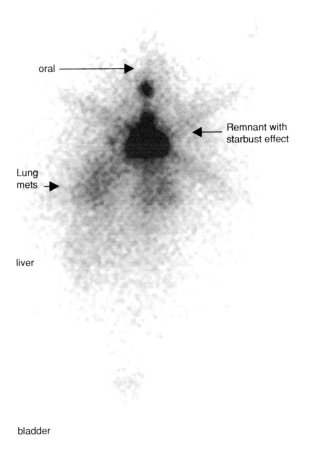

oral

Remnant with
starbust effect

Lung
mets

liver

bladder

Figure 8. This is a RxWBS after 100 mCi I-131 given to an 11 year-old girl with no prior history of I-131 therapy, who had a papillary thyroid carcinoma involving the entire right thyroid lobe and the lower pole of the left lobe, the isthmus and pyramidal lobe. The tumor extended into perithyroid soft tissues and extended into the inked soft tissue margins. The right level III cervical neck lymph node chain contained multiple matted lymph nodes with metastatic papillary thyroid carcinoma and extranodal extension. Her serum Tg was 1,710 ng/mL when this RxWBS was performed. There is physiologic uptake of radioiodine in the nasal cavity and oral cavity. A large tumor deposit in the neck or superior mediastinum on the left is so intense that the star burst effect almost obliterates the bilateral diffuse lung uptake indicative of pulmonary metastases.

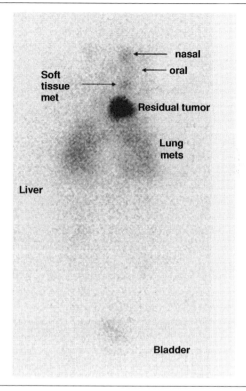

Figure 9. This is an RxWBS after 150 mCi I-131given to the same patient shown in Figure 8. This scan was done after lithium pretreatment and thyroid hormone withdrawal. It shows uptake in residual tumor in the left upper mediastinum and in both lungs. The patient's Tg following the second treatment was 4,408 ng/mL with a TSH of 250 mIU/L.

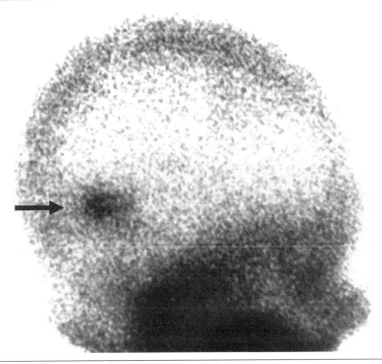

Figure 10. Oblique view of the head on a RxWBS in an asymptomatic patient with no neurological symptoms. There is a focal area of uptake in the cerebellum (arrow) It is important to evaluate a suspected brain metastasis with MR as there are normal variants that can cause focal uptake in the skull region (see figure 9). This patient underwent surgical resection of her tumor.

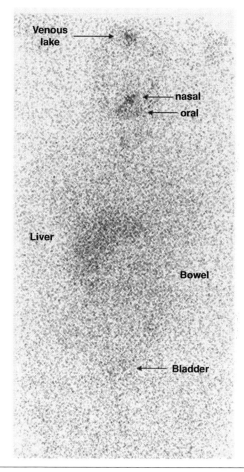

Figure 11. This is a RxWBS in a 22 year-old woman with a 1.5 cm papillary thyroid carcinoma confined to the right thyroid lobe. The tumor was originally treated with total thyroidectomy and 100 mCi I-131 for remnant ablation after which the RxWBS showed uptake only in the thyroid bed. Six months later her serum Tg was <0.9 ng/mL with negative TgAb and neck ultrasonography. However, over the next year her serum Tg gradually began to rise and peaked at 37 ng/mL with a serum TSH of 25.9 mIU/L. Based on the rising Tg concentrations and a negative neck ultrasound examination, the patient underwent a second treatment with 157 mCi I-131 after being pretreated with lithium and rhTSH. The RxWBS, which is shown, has uptake in the nasal cavity, oral cavity, liver, bowel and bladder, although the bowel and bladder uptake is difficult to see on this image. The diffuse hepatic uptake of I-131 indicates that there is functional thyroid tissue or tumor somewhere in the patient's body. There is faint uptake in the thyroid bed. Also, there is a focal area of I-131 that appears to be in the superior aspect of the skull or brain, which is seen in the midline. MR and FDG-PET scans were negative for metastasis. This finding is a normal variant that represents a venous lake in the sagittal sinus. The patient's serum Tg level has gradually declined to 3.5 ng/mL with a TSH of 2.04 mIU/L within the last year after I-131 treatment.

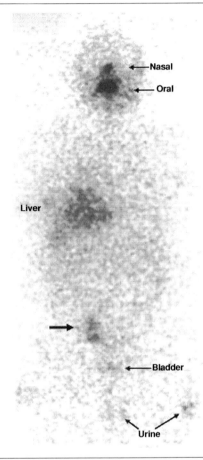

Figure 12. This is a RxWBS of a 64 year-old man who underwent total thyroidectomy six years previously for a 1.7 cm papillary thyroid carcinoma that was focally extending into the adjacent connective tissue, but was not otherwise noted to be metastatic. He was given 150 mCi of I-131 for remnant ablation at another hospital but a posttreatment scan was not done. Because of rising serum Tg levels, a CT was done at the same hospital with radiographic contrast that showed 1 cm discrete nodules in the peripheral lung fields. Administration of I-131 therapy shortly thereafter resulted in no visible uptake in the lungs and he was referred to our clinic for further evaluation. His serum Tg was 59.4 ng/mL on 200 mcg of levothyroxine daily. The RxWBS shown here was done after urine iodine levels had fallen to less than 100 mcg/g Cr and after thyroid hormone withdrawal and lithium pretreatment. There is physiologic concentration of radioiodine in the nasal cavity, oral cavity, liver, and bladder. Diffuse radioiodine concentration in the liver, no matter how faint, indicates that there is residual thyroid tissue or functional cancer cells somewhere in the body. There are two small areas of radioiodine concentration inferior to the bladder from urine on the patient or the table. There is no uptake in the neck or lung. The area of radioiodine concentration in the right pelvis was initially interpreted as a pelvis metastasis; however, subsequent imaging (99mTechnetium bone scan, CT scan) was negative for tumor. The finding of a solitary area of uptake in the abdomen or pelvis usually represents retained feces rather than metastasis. This represents a case of lung metastases that are now visible on chest x-ray which do not take up I-131, a fact that was not certain until he underwent a stringent low-iodine diet and lithium pretreatment. He has been enrolled in a clinical trial of a promising new drug (17-AAG).

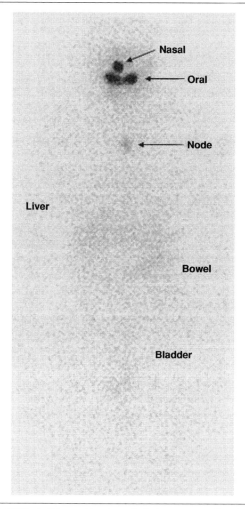

Figure 13. This is a RxWBS of a 76 year-old patient who had a 5.5 cm papillary thyroid carcinoma with metastatic level VI lymph nodes that were resected through a cervical incision. She was initially treated with 200 mCi I-131 and after which the RxWBS showed uptake in the upper mediastinum. Because of a rising serum Tg level one year later, she was treated with 148 mCi I-131. The RxWBS done with the second treatment is shown. There is physiologic radioiodine concentration in the nasal cavity, oral cavity, and barely visible in the liver, bowel, and bladder. There is a focal area of uptake in the mid chest that identifies tumor in the mediastinum. It is not entirely clear if this is a tumor in a lymph node or free in the soft tissues. This represents a case of a lady with a large primary tumor that was metastatic to the mediastinum. She will receive additional I-131 therapy.

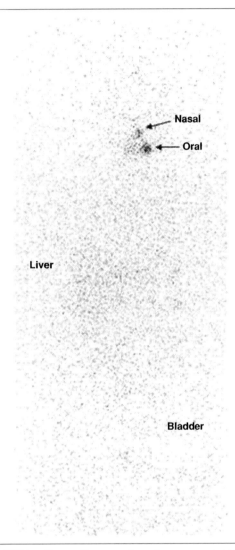

Figure 14. This is a RxWBS in a 31 year–old woman who underwent a near-total thyroidectomy and right modified neck dissection for bilateral multifocal papillary thyroid carcinoma, with the largest tumor being 1 cm in the right lobe, and with tumor metastatic to seven left levels II, to IV and VI lymph nodes. She was treated with 155 mCi of I-131 but the RxWBS showed only hepatic uptake, consistent with a small amount of thyroid tissue having been treated. Her serum Tg has been undetectable (<0.9 ng/mL) on three tests since her therapy and does not rise with rhTSH stimulation.

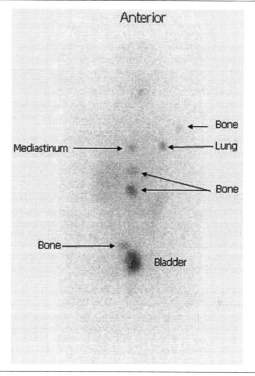

Figure 15. This is a RxWBS of a 22 year-old woman who at age 18 underwent right thyroid lobectomy for a 3.5 cm follicular variant papillary thyroid carcinoma. Two years later she developed a 2 cm palpable frontal bone metastasis from this tumor that was surgically resected and shortly thereafter a 9 mm brain frontal lobe metastatic lesion was discovered and treated with stereotactic radiosurgery. Since then she has felt well but her serum Tg has been steadily rising. The present RxWBS was performed after she was given 170 mCi I-131 after thyroid hormone withdrawal and lithium pretreatment. The scan shows uptake of I-131 in numerous metastatic lesions as labeled on the picture.

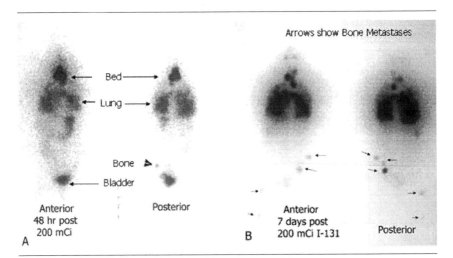

Figure 16. This is a series of studies on a 47 year-old lady who presented with a long standing multinodular goiter that seemed to be enlarging, which turned out to be a large bilateral multicentric follicular variant papillary thyroid carcinoma that was invading surrounding tissues in the neck and was metastatic to lung and bone. She was referred to our medical center and underwent total thyroidectomy and was treated with a total of about 1100 mCi I-131 over a 10 year span, during which she was functional and pain free until near the end or her life. The scans show multiple bone and lung metastases.

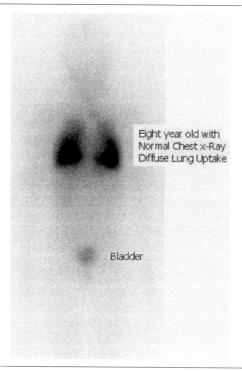

Figure 17. This is a RxWBS of an 8 year-old boy who presented with a history of visible cervical lymph nodes since age 2 years. He recently underwent open biopsy of a cervical lymph node and was found to have follicular variant papillary thyroid carcinoma for which he underwent total thyroidectomy for a tumor that was occupying the entire left thyroid lobe but was not invading the thyroid capsule. Shortly thereafter he was referred to our center and underwent further surgery because persistent lymph node metastases were found on neck ultrasonography, for which he underwent left modified neck dissection. Twelve of 36 level II, III, IV and V lymph nodes were positive for tumor and all of them showed extracapsular extension of tumor into the soft tissues. Two months after surgery his serum Tg was >25,000 ng/mL and he was treated with 100 mCi I-131. The RxWBS shows diffuse lung uptake by metastases but no visible tumor in the neck.

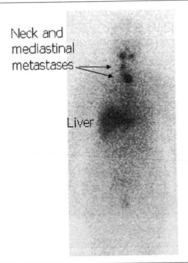

Figure 18. This is a RxWBS of a 36 year-old woman with residual tumor in her neck and mediastinum. Note the intense hepatic uptake of iodinated thyroid hormone and thyroid hormone degradation products, which is typically seen when large treatment doses of I-131 are administered to patients with residual tumor.

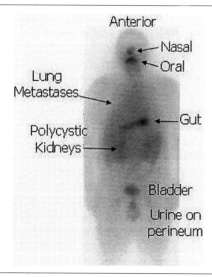

Figure 19. This is a RxWBS of a 38 year-old man with papillary thyroid carcinoma and renal fail due to polycystic kidney disease. The scan shows uptake in both lungs from diffuse pulmonary metastases, and large polycystic kidneys.

REFERENCES

Chung, JK, YJ Lee, JM Jeong, DS Lee, MC Lee, BY Cho, et al. 1997. Clinical significance of hepatic visualization on iodine-131 whole-body scan in patients with thyroid carcinoma. J Nucl Med **38**:1191–1195.

Shapiro, B, V Rufini, A Jarwan, O Geatti, KJ Kearfott, LM Fig, ID Kirkwood, and MD Gross. 2000. Artifacts, anatomical and physiological variants, and unrelated diseases that might cause false-positive whole-body 131-I scans in patients with thyroid cancer.
Semin Nucl Med **30(2)**:115–32.

2.7. COMPUTERIZED TOMOGRAPHY (CT) AND MAGNETIC RESONANCE (MR) IMAGING OF THYROID CANCER

ILLONA M. SCHMALLFUSS, MD, ROBERT J. AMDUR, MD, DOUGLAS B. VILLARET, MD AND ERNEST L. MAZZAFERRI, MD, MACP

The role of Computerized Tomography (CT) and Magnetic Resonance (MR) imaging in the evaluation of a patient with thyroid cancer is small compared to other head and neck, or thoracic malignancies. We use MR imaging to plan the surgical procedure in a patient with symptoms of extrathyroidal tumor extension (usually voice change or dysphagia) and we use a non-contrast CT of the chest in selected cases to evaluate the presence or extent of mediastinal and lung metastases. Table 1 and the bullet points in the remainder of this chapter summarize the major concepts:

- **In the majority of cases we do not perform a CT or MR scan prior to thyroidectomy:** In the absence of symptoms of tumor invasion of adjacent structures, preoperative CT or MR imaging does not add useful information.
- **Prior to thyroidectomy, it is not necessary to obtain a CT or MR scan to look for adenopathy:** Unlike other head and neck malignancies, it is not necessary to stage the neck prior to surgery with CT or MR scans. The extent of node dissection is determined by cervical ultrasonography and palpation of the nodes prior to and during the thyroidectomy procedure.
- **An MR scan is the preferred imaging test to evaluate the extent of tumor relative to adjacent structures in the neck:** MR is better than CT for evaluating the relationship of tumor to the larynx, esophagus, trachea, spine, and major vessels. This is true both at the time of initial thyroidectomy and at the time of local-regional recurrence. Another advantage of MR imaging is that it does not

Table 1. Guidelines for CT and MR Imaging in Patients with Thyroid Cancer.

Prior to thyroidectomy:
Most patients do not need CT or MR imaging
It is not necessary to obtain a CT or MR scan of the neck to look for adenopathy
MR is better than CT for evaluating extrathyroidal tumor extension
An MR scan of the neck is done only when there are symptoms of extrathyroidal tumor extension
  (e.g., hoarseness, dysphagia, stridor, cough)
There is no indication for a CT scan of the neck in a patient who can undergo an MR scan
Do not perform a CT scan with intravenous contrast if radioiodine therapy may be needed within the next
  6 months
In general, the only role for CT imaging is the evaluation for lung metastases

At the time of tumor recurrence in the neck after thyroidectomy:
An MR scan of the neck is often useful even in the absence of symptoms of extrathyroidal extension to help
  define the relationship of tumor to important normal structures
A non-contrast CT of the chest is often done to look for lung metastases

To evaluate signs or symptoms of a brain metastasis:
MR is much better than CT at detecting brain metastases

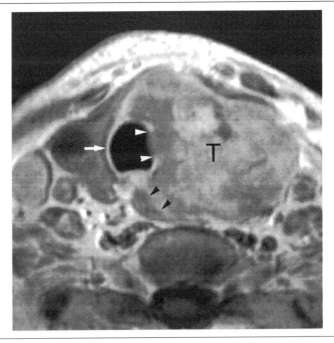

Figure 1. Gadolinium enhanced, axial T1 weighted image through the level of the thyroid gland shows a large mass (T) involving the left thyroid lobe that severely compresses the upper esophagus (black arrowheads). There is tumor infiltration of the tracheal cartilage on the left noticeable as subtle bulge (between white arrowheads) along the left lateral tracheal wall and replacement of the normal high signal intensity (white arrow) of the tracheal cartilage by hypointense signal (between white arrowheads).

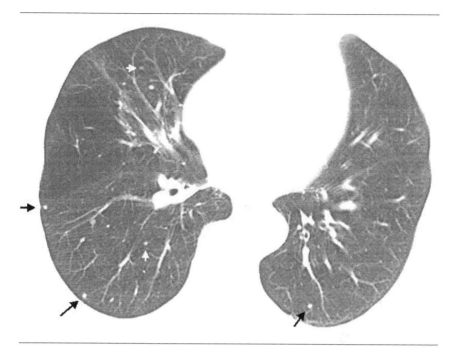

Figure 2. Axial CT images at the level of the carina show subcentimeter parenchymal lung lesions consistent with metastatic disease in a patient with known thyroid cancer. Several lesions are marked with an arrow.

use iodinated contrast, which is a factor in patients who may subsequently need I-131 therapy. MR is less sensitive than neck ultrasonography in identifying cervical metastases.

- **The indication for MR scan of the low neck and upper mediastinum is clinical signs or symptoms of tumor extension to these areas:** Extension of tumor to the larynx, esophagus, trachea, prevertebral fascia, or great vessels may change the length or nature of the procedure that is needed to remove a primary thyroid cancer. For this reason we image the neck with MR prior to surgery in any patient with vocal cord dysfunction, dysphagia, suspicious cough, Horner's syndrome, vascular congestion, or other findings that suggest extension of tumor to adjacent structures (Fig. 1). MR scan is used in patients with suspected recurrence to determine the relationship of tumor to the major normal tissue structures.
- **Do not administer intravenous contrast containing iodine if radioiodine therapy may be needed within the next 6 months:** The intravenous contrast agents that are used with a CT scan contain a high concentration of iodine. Residual iodine compromises the effectiveness of I-131 therapy. It usually takes a minimum

of three months for a patient to metabolize all of the iodine that has been received with a CT scan that includes intravenous contrast. This is discussed in more detail in a separate chapter.

- **The main role for CT is the evaluation of the lung or the skeletal system for metastases:** In patients with differentiated thyroid cancer it is important to avoid iodinated contrast if I-131 therapy is potentially required. A non-contrast chest study is adequate to detect lung metastases in most cases and should be obtained in any situation where it is important to detect metastases that may not concentrate radioiodine or in situations where it is important to determine the location and volume of metastases in the neck prior to surgery or radioiodine therapy (Fig. 2). CT-FDG PET fusion studies may be useful for identifying the extent and volume of metastases in bone and soft tissues.

- **Prior to thyroidectomy, there is usually no need to image the chest with CT if the chest radiograph is negative for metastases:** The presence of lung metastases will not change the plan for the resection of disease at the primary site unless lung metastases compromise pulmonary function or compress the major bronchi or blood vessels in the chest. For this reason CT of the chest prior to thyroidectomy is not required unless the chest radiograph suggests large volume metastases, particularly in the mediastinum.

- **MR is much better than CT in evaluating brain metastases:** A patient with signs or symptoms of a brain metastasis should have a brain MR scan done with both T1 and T2 weighted echo sequences.

2.8. POSITRON EMISSION TOMOGRAPHY (PET) OF THYROID CANCER

ROBERT J. AMDUR, MD AND ERNEST L. MAZZAFERRI, MD, MACP

Positron Emission Tomography (PET) has been evaluated with several different isotopes in patients with thyroid cancer but the discussion in this chapter will be limited to the role of PET with 18-Flourodeoxyglucose (FDG PET). Table 1 summarizes the main points from this chapter and the reference list cites major studies related to this subject.

FDG PET FOR DIFFERENTIATED THYROID CANCER THAT DOES NOT CONCENTRATE RADIOIODINE

Although FDG PET is highly accurate in a wide range of situations, many studies focused on the detection of differentiated thyroid cancer metastases that do not concentrate radioiodine (Fig. 1). FDG PET accurately detects tumors with high thyroglobulin (Tg) levels (Chung 1999; DeGroot 2004; Gotthardt 2004; Helal 2001; Pacak 2004).

The large European multicenter study by Grünwald et al. (2001) found the sensitivity of FDG PET for identifying differentiated thyroid carcinoma was 75% for the entire study population and 85% in a subset with a negative diagnostic whole body I-131 scans. The study by Wang et al. (2000, 2001) also found that FDG PET was able to localize residual thyroid cancer lesions in patients who have negative diagnostic I-131 whole body scans and elevated Tg levels, but was not sensitive enough to detect minimal residual disease in cervical nodes. Although FDG PET has the highest sensitivity in this group of patients and is the preferred imaging agent, its availability and cost are still major issues.

Table 1. FDG PET in Patients with Thyroid Cancer.

FDG PET is the nuclear medicine study of choice with cancers that may not concentrate radioiodine:
We use FDG PET instead of Thallium or Technetium scans for radioiodine negative disease

The accuracy of FDG PET increases with TSH stimulation:
We elevate TSH prior to FDG PET in patients with cancers that may respond to TSH stimulation using rhTSH or T4 deprivation as described for radioiodine studies or therapy

Issues related to the use of FDG PET in place of a diagnostic radioiodine scan:
Advantages of FDG PET over a diagnostic radioiodine scan are: ability to detect metastases that do not concentrate iodine, no need for a low-iodine diet, and reasonable accuracy if TSH elevation is undesirable.
It is currently standard practice in most centers to perform a diagnostic radioiodine scan prior to considering FDG PET in patients with a cancer than may concentrate radioiodine
All currently published guidelines recommend a diagnostic radioiodine scan in patients with differentiated cancers prior to considering FDG PET
Medicare, and many commercial insurance carries, currently will not approve payment for FDG PET in a patient with differentiated thyroid cancer unless a recent radioiodine scan is negative for tumor

The role of FDG PET in our program:
We use FDG PET to rule out distant metastases prior to recommending external beam radiotherapy in situations where the histologic subtype of the cancer, or a history of resistance to radioiodine, suggests that metastases may not concentrate radioiodine
In patients with papillary or follicular carcinoma we perform FDG PET with TSH stimulation, usually with rhTSH injections on the two days preceding the scan
FDG PET is used in patients with medullary thyroid cancer who have high plasma calcitonin levels

---

THE ACCURACY OF FDG PET INCREASES WITH TSH STIMULATION

The accuracy of FDG PET imaging in patients with differentiated thyroid carcinoma increases with TSH stimulation. The prospective randomized study by Chin et al. (2004) compared FDG PET scans both during thyroid hormone suppression and after recombinant human TSH (rhTSH) stimulation found that the rhTSH stimulation studies identified additional lesions not seen on TSH suppression. They concluded that rhTSH improves the detectability of occult thyroid metastases with FDG PET compared with scans performed on TSH suppression. For this reason we use the same protocols to elevate serum TSH levels that we use for radioiodine studies or therapy, and prefer rhTSH because of patient comfort. We give a 0.9 mg rhTSH IM injection on each of the two days prior to the FDG PET scan to spare the patient the problems of hypothyroidism.

THE ACCURACY OF FDG PET IN MEDULLARY THYROID CARCINOMA (MTC)

MTC belongs in the group of neuroendocrine tumors with early lymphatic and hepatic dissemination. Liver metastases are particularly difficult to identify and probably account for the majority of undetectable metastases and are usually responsible for the frequent mismatch between the apparent relatively small tumor burden and the elevated plasma calcitonin level.

Although FDG PET can identify metastases in MTC patients with high plasma calcitonin levels (Fig. 2), studies find that computed tomography (CT) is similar to or even better than FDG PET scanning in the diagnosis of metastatic MTC. In the study by

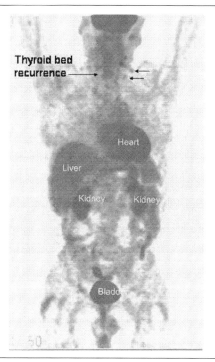

Figure 1. Coronal FDG PET images demonstrating recurrent cancer in the thyroid bed (R) and metastatic lesions in both side of the neck (arrows). All lesions were negative by I-131 scintigraphy.

Gotthardt et al. (2004), if the results were classified as "sure," 57% of the MTC tumor sites were clearly demonstrated by FDG PET, 65% by CT and 48% by SSR (somatostatin receptor scintigraphy). A combination of CT and FDG PET seems to be the most appropriate non-invasive diagnostic approach in patients with MTC.

FDG PET AS COMPARED WITH OTHER RADIONUCLIDE IMAGING STUDIES

Many other radiopharmaceutical imaging studies have the ability to detect suspected thyroid cancer recurrence or metastases but we have not discussed them in detail because considerable data suggests that FDG PET is better for imaging patients with radioiodine negative whole body scans than the other options, including 18-flourodeoxyglucose scintigraphy with a triple head camera. Radiopharmaceuticals that have some utility for this purpose are as follows: 99m-Tecnitium (Tc) MIBI, 99m-Tc perchlorate, 99mTc furifosmin and 99mTc tetrofosmin, 201-Thalium and somatostatin receptor scintigraphy. The review by Haugen et al. (2001) concluded that radiopharmaceuticals other than I-131 and FDG PET have a limited role in the follow-up diagnostic algorithms used in the surveillance of patients for recurrent or metastatic thyroid cancer. We rarely

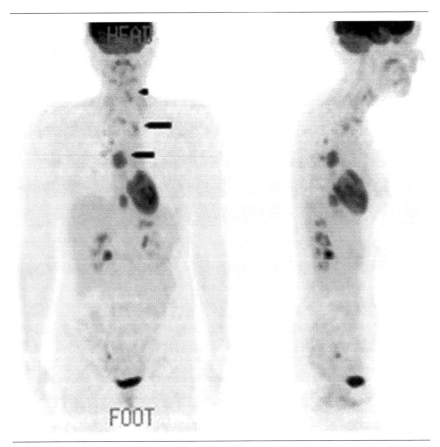

Figure 2. These are coronal and lateral FDG PET images in a 36 year-old woman with medullary thyroid carcinoma showing multiple foci of abnormal FDG accumulation throughout both lungs, representing multiple pulmonary metastases. There is a very prominent area of uptake in the left paratracheal region, in the right azygous region, and less prominently in the right paratracheal region. There also is activity in the midline of the neck, and an intense focus in the lower chest near the gastroesophageal junction that probably represents a nodal metastasis. The area of intense uptake in the pelvis likely represents gut activity.

use radiopharmaceutical studies in patients with differentiated thyroid carcinoma other than I-131 scans and FDG PET.

FDG PET INSTEAD OF A DIAGNOSTIC RADIOIODINE SCAN

At present (January 2005) published guidelines on the management of patients with differentiated thyroid cancer recommend a radioiodine scan prior to considering FDG PET scans. Medicare and many other insurance carriers will not approve payment for an FDG PET scan unless a recent radioiodine scan is negative for residual cancer and the serum thyroglobulin level is above 10 ng/mL. While there are reasons to believe that this may not be the optimal place in the evaluation to do an FDG PET scan, we rarely use FDG PET other than as described in this chapter.

FDG PET POSITIVITY AND SUBSEQUENT PROGNOSIS

There are good studies showing that the results of an FDG PET scan provide important prognostic information and guide subsequent therapeutic decisions. In the study by Wang et al. (2000, 2001), FDG PET scanning was incorporated into the routine follow-up of a cohort of thyroid cancer patients undergoing annual evaluations. The single strongest predictor of survival was the volume of FDG-avid tumor. The 3-yr probability of survival was 96% among patients with FDG volumes of 125 mL or less compared with 18% in patients with FDG volume greater than 125 mL. No cancer deaths occurred in the PET-negative group, including 10 patients with distant metastases.

INDICATIONS FOR A FDG PET SCAN IN OUR PROGRAM

The main role for this study in our program is to locate disease in a patient with an elevated serum thyroglobulin level and a negative RxWBS and neck ultrasonography. This provides prognostic information and also helps guide the decision to proceed with further therapy.

FDG PET POSITIVITY AND SUBSEQUENT THERAPY

Persistent tumor identified as a hot spot on a FDG PET scan is typically resistant to I-131 therapy. For this reason, it is usually not wise to administer I-131 therapy to someone who has intense uptake of FDG. For example, the study by Wang et al. (2000, 2001) found no significant changes in maximum standard FDG uptake values or serum thyroglobulin levels after I-131 therapy in the FDG PET-positive group, whereas in a control group of FDG PET-negative patients, the serum thyroglobulin decreased to 38% of baseline after I-131 therapy. They concluded that high-dose I-131 therapy appears to have little or no effect on the viability of metastatic FDG-avid differentiated thyroid cancer lesions.

On the other hand, surgical therapy or External Beam Radiotherapy (EBRT) to the neck and upper mediastinum may be beneficial to some patients with positive FDG PET studies. In the large study by Chung et al. (1999), FDG PET detected cervical lymph node metastasis in 88% of the patients with high serum Tg levels and a negative I-131 whole body scan, and found lung metastasis in 27%, mediastinal metastasis in 33% and bone metastasis in 9% of the patients. It was possible to dissect the cervical lymph nodes identified by FDG PET. Likewise, in the study by Wang et al. (2000, 2001) the FDG PET result changed the clinical management in 51% of the patients. When the tumor is amenable to surgery, this is our first choice of therapy.

In most situations the tumor is not resectable and EBERT may be the best therapy. In patients with locoregional tumor that is not surgically resectable, FDG PET plays a major role in identifying patients without distant metastases in whom EBRT may be helpful. The patients in whom this decision is applicable are described in detail in the chapters in this book that focus on the indications for EBRT in different subtypes of thyroid cancer. We usually recommend EBRT when it is not possible to eliminate residual cancer with additional surgery or radioiodine therapy in a patient over age 45 and when there is no evidence of metastasis beyond the neck and upper mediastinum. PET is usually the only study that is needed in this setting because it has a high negative predictive value for metastases >1 cm anywhere in the body.

REFERENCES

Chin, BB, P Patel, C Cohade, M Ewertz, R Wahl, and P Ladenson. 2004. Recombinant human thyrotropin stimulation of fluoro-D-glucose positron emission tomography uptake in well-differentiated thyroid carcinoma. J Clin Endocrinol Metab **89(1)**:91–95.

Chung, JK, Y So, JS Lee, CW Choi, SM Lim, DS Lee, SW Hong, YK Youn, MC Lee, and BY Cho. 1999. Value of FDG PET in papillary thyroid carcinoma with negative ^{131}I whole-body scan. J Nucl Med **40**:986–992.

de Groot, JW, TP Links, PL Jager, T Kahraman, and JT Plukker. 2004. Impact of ^{18}F-fluoro-2-deoxy-D-glucose positron emission tomography (FDG-PET) in patients with biochemical evidence of recurrent or residual medullary thyroid cancer. Ann Surg Oncol **11(8)**:786–794.

Gotthardt, M, A Battmann, H Hoffken, T Schurrat, H Pollum, D Beuter, S Gratz, M Behe, A Bauhofer, KJ Klose, and TM Behr. 2004. ^{18}F-FDG PET, somatostatin receptor scintigraphy, and CT in metastatic medullary thyroid carcinoma: a clinical study and an analysis of the literature. Nucl Med Commun **25(5)**:439–443.

Grünwald, F, T Kaelicke, U Feine, R Lietzenmayer, K Scheidhauer, M Dietlein, et al. 1999. Fluorine-18 fluorodeoxyglucose positron emission tomography in thyroid cancer: results of a multicentre study. Eur J Nucl Med **26(12)**:1547–1552.

Haugen, BR, and EC Lin. 2001. Isotope imaging for metastatic thyroid cancer. Endocrinol Metab Clin North Am **30(2)**:469–492.

Helal, BO, P Merlet, ME Toubert, B Franc, C Schvartz, H Gauthier-Koelesnikov, A Prigent, and A Syrota. 2001. Clinical impact of (18)F-FDG PET in thyroid carcinoma patients with elevated thyroglobulin levels and negative (131)I scanning results after therapy. J Nucl Med **42(10)**:1464–1469.

Pacak, K, G Eisenhofer, and DS Goldstein. 2004. Functional imaging of endocrine tumors: role of positron emission tomography. Endocr Rev **25(4)**:568–580.

Wang, W, SM Larson, M Fazzari, SK Tickoo, K Kolbert, G Sgouros, H Yeung, H Macapinlac, J Rosai, and RJ Robbins. 2000. Prognostic value of ^{18}F-fluorodeoxyglucose positron emission tomographic scanning in patients with thyroid cancer. J Clin Endocrinol Metab **85(3)**:1107–1113.

Wang, W, SM Larson, RM Tuttle, H Kalaigian, K Kolbert, M Sonenberg, and RJ Robbins. 2001. Resistance of [^{18}F]-fluorodeoxyglucose-avid metastatic thyroid cancer lesions to treatment with high-dose radioactive iodine. **11(12)**:1169–1175.

2.9. NECK ULTRASONOGRAPHY IN PATIENTS WITH THYROID CANCER

ERNEST L. MAZZAFERRI, MD, MACP

Ultrasonography is a key part of the initial diagnostic evaluation of a patient with a thyroid nodule and in the follow-up of patients who have undergone initial surgery and remnant ablation for thyroid cancer. In this chapter I will summarize the ultrasonographic findings that identify malignancy in a thyroid nodule and in cervical lymph nodes.

THE ROLE OF CERVICAL ULTRASONOGRAPHY

There is good evidence that this test, performed by competent ultrasonographers, is highly sensitive in the detection of cervical metastases in patients with differentiated thyroid cancer. A study by Papini et al. (2002) shows that rhTSH-stimulated serum thyroglobulin combined with neck ultrasonography has the highest sensitivity in monitoring patients with differentiated thyroid carcinoma. However, this was marginally better than rhTSH-stimulated serum thyroglobulin combined with a diagnostic whole body scan. Still, on a cost-basis alone, ultrasonography is the test of choice, given its performance in detecting neck lymph node metastases. Other studies show that cervical metastases are sometimes detected by neck ultrasonography even when TSH-stimulated serum thyroglobulin levels remain undetectable (Frasoldati et al.; Torlontano et al.; Antonelli et al.) however, all three of these studies used recovery thyroglobulin assays about which there remains some controversy. In one study by Kouvaraki, preoperative ultrasonography detected lymph node or soft-tissue metastases in neck compartments believed to be uninvolved by physical examination in 39% of patients and altered the operative procedure in these patients, facilitating complete resection of tumor. Neck ultrasonography has clearly enriched the evaluation of cervical masses for malignancy,

Transverse View

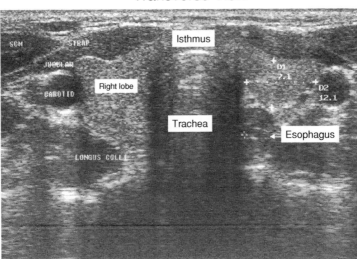

Figure 1. Transverse view, normal neck ultrasound.

which has become increasingly more important as newer and more sensitive means of detecting residual thyroid cancer have been developed. This is particularly important since the most common place for recurrence is in the neck (Mazzaferri 2003).

THE NORMAL THYROID GLAND

The thyroid gland is a highly vascular organ. There is a right and left thyroid lobe, with the right being normally slightly larger than the left. About half the time a pyramidal lobe is found extending up from the isthmus slightly to the left of the midline, which is a remnant of the distal end of the thyroglossal duct. It may be confused with a Delphian lymph node, which is found in the same area overlying the thyroid cartilage. By ultrasonography, the right and left thyroid lobes normally measure about 5 cm long and 3 cm in their greatest width and 2 cm in greatest thickness (Figs. 1, 2, and 3). The isthmus measures about 1.2 to 1.5 cm in breadth and depth. Laterally, the thyroid lies just medial to the common carotid arteries and wraps around 75% of the circumference of the trachea. The most posterior aspects of the left lateral lobe may touch the esophagus, which at the level of the thyroid gland lies just to the left of the trachea (Figs. 4 and 5) and may be confused with a thyroid nodule by the novice ultrasonographer. The anterior surface of the thyroid is just deep to the strap muscles of the neck. Figs. 6–28 are images of patients with thyroid findings.

Right Lateral View

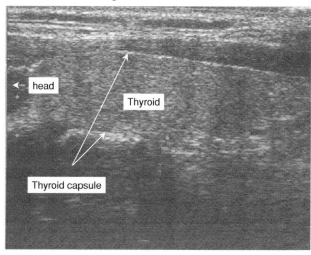

Figure 2. Longitudinal view, normal neck ultrasound.

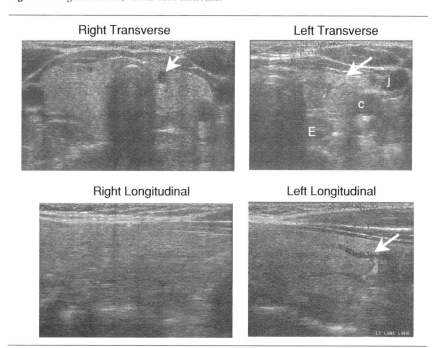

Figure 3. Normal ultrasound showing superior thyroid artery (arrow) and small cyst (dash).

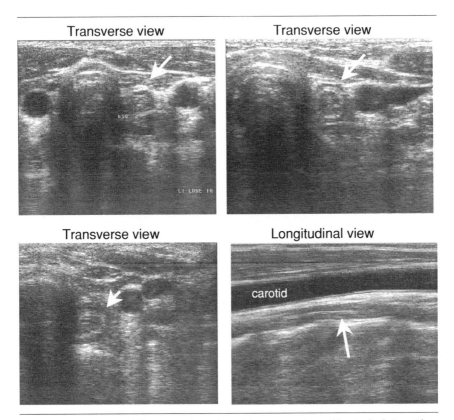

Figure 4. Normal ultrasound showing esophagus (arrows) in transverse view and longitudinal views. The bright spot in the lower pictures is taken with fluid in the esophagus during swallowing.

CONVENTIONS ABOUT DISPLAYING ULTRASONOGRAPHY RESULTS

When performing neck ultrasonography, the convention is to display the thyroid in the transverse ultrasonographic view with the left lobe on the right side of the picture (Fig. 1). In the lateral view the convention is to have the patient's head to the left of the picture (Fig. 2). Doppler color flow, which helps to identify the blood flow pattern in the thyroid and in thyroid nodules, is an indispensable feature of neck ultrasonography that helps to identify hyperfunctional nodules and can help identify malignant tumors, which often shows brisk Doppler flow. Also, Doppler helps identify arteries seen end on that may look like a malignant tumor.

ULTRASOUND FEATURES SUGGESTING MALIGNANCY IN A THYROID NODULE

The ultrasound features that suggest a thyroid nodule or lymph node is malignant are shown in a series of figures in this chapter. The ultrasonographic features of a nodule that are associated with an increased risk of cancer include hypoechogenicity,

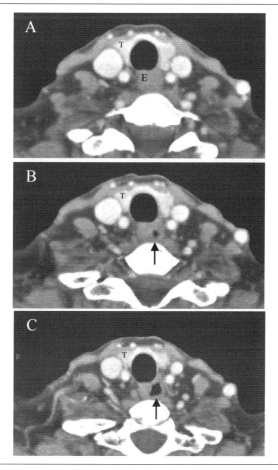

Figure 5. Axial contrast-enhanced CT scan at 5 mm intervals through the neck at the level of the thyroid gland (T) in a patient with normal anatomy. Note how the esophagus moves to left of midline as the images go from superior (A) to inferior (C). The arrows in images B and C indicate air in the esophagus.

microcalcifications, irregular or blurred nodule margins, increased nodular blood flow visualized by Doppler, and evidence of tumor invasion or regional lymph node metastases (see Chapter 2, Table 1).

ULTRASOUND FEATURES SUGGESTING MALIGNANCY IN A CERVICAL LYMPH NODE

Ultrasonography has become an important diagnostic modality in the follow-up of patients with thyroid cancer and is particularly important in identifying malignant cervical lymph nodes. More recently, color flow Doppler has been described as an

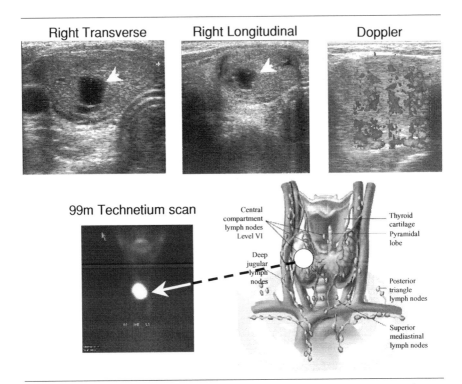

Figure 6. This is a hyperfunctional (hot) nodule in an asymptomatic 14 year old girl with a TSH of 0.001 mIU/L. The ultrasound shows a large (3.5 cm) nodule in the right lobe with a small hypoechoic area of degeneration (arrowheads). The nodule shows intense Doppler flow and uptake of technetium 99m scan only in the nodule.

additional tool for differentiating benign from malignant thyroid tumors (Ahuja 2001; Papini 2002; Frates 2003). Over the last few years, a new generation of high-resolution ultrasound platforms with the 'power-mode' feature has become available, enabling the imaging of blood flow in small vessels.

In an important study, Gorges et al. looked for ways of optimizing the ultrasono-graphic differences between benign and malignant cervical tumors in the follow-up of patients with thyroid cancer. In this study, the Solbiati index (SI), which is the ratio of largest to smallest diameter of a lymph node, and the nodule configuration, echogenicity, intranodular structures, and margins of cervical tumors were assessed by B-Mode ultrasonography performed at a frequency of 8 MHz with a small-part trans-ducer. Perinodular and intranodular blood flow was evaluated by color flow power-mode Doppler. The investigators found that a complex echo pattern or irregular hyperechoic small intranodular structures **(criterion A)** and irregular diffuse intranodular blood flow **(criterion B)** are the best indicators of malignancy, whereas an SI greater than 2

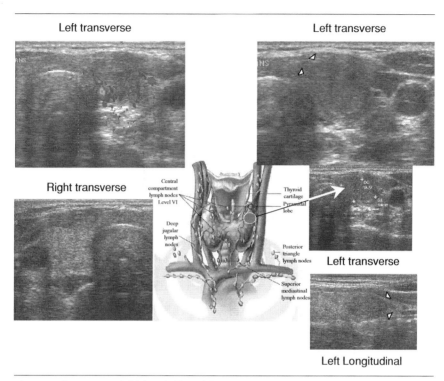

Figure 7. This is a 2.5 cm left lobe palpable nodule in a 42 year-old woman. The nodule is slightly hypoechoic and shows mixed echogenicity in the longitudinal view, has irregular and blurred (arrowheads) margins and shows moderate Doppler flow. The right thyroid lobe is normal. US-guided FNA revealed a papillary thyroid carcinoma. The patient underwent total thyroidectomy and I-131 ablation and was free of disease at one year after treatment. This is a classic US view of thyroid carcinoma.

(*i.e., the nodule is long, not round) is highly indicative of benign findings. The patterns of color flow Doppler in benign and malignant lymph nodes are seen in Figs. 6 and 7. Gorges et al. found that power-mode Doppler sonography improves imaging of perinodular and intranodular blood flow when compared with conventional color flow Doppler. Based upon their findings, they propose the following decision rules:

1) If the nodule shows irregular hyperechoic small intranodular structures (criterion A) with irregular diffuse intranodular blood flow (criterion B), the configuration of the node is not so important and malignancy is present as long as the SI is ≤ 4.
2) If only criterion B is present, then the SI should be ≤3 in malignant nodes.
3) If neither criterion is present then the SI should be about 1.

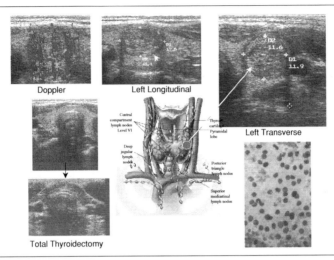

Figure 8. This is a 28 year-old woman referred to out clinic for follow-up of a left lobed thyroid nodule previously diagnosed as having Hashimoto's thyroiditis on the basis of a FNA that showed Hürthle cells and reactive lymphocytes. Our ultrasound examination showed this to be more compatible with an isolated thyroid nodule that has a thick halo sign (the dark area surrounding the nodule), intense Doppler flow and an otherwise normal thyroid gland. Rebiopsy of the nodule showed sheets of Hürthle cells without colloid consistent with a Hürthle cell tumor for which she underwent left lobectomy. The final histopathologic sections showed this to be a low grade Hürthle cell carcinoma with malignant cells invading the entire tumor capsule. There is a suggestion of tumor capsule disruption in the longitudinal view (arrow).

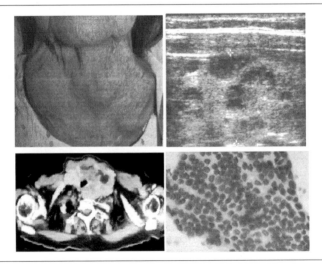

Figure 9. Long standing multinodular goiter in a 76 year-old woman who had an enlarging thyroid gland over the past three years. The ultrasound shows this to be goiter with multiple a mixed solid cystic nodules with hypoechoic and isoechoic areas. Many of the nodules had poorly demarcated margins as does the one shown. The CT scan shows displacement of the trachea and areas of hemorrhage into the nodule. The US-guided FNA cytology shows papillary thyroid carcinoma.

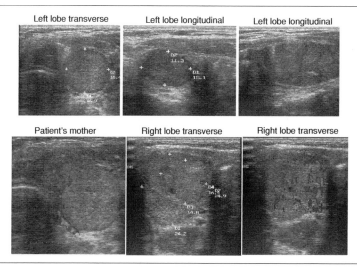

Figure 10. A 28 year-old woman with Cowden's disease. The US shows multiple isoechoic thyroid nodules with well defined margins and intense Doppler flow. The FNA was consistent with a benign nodule, but the patient was advised to undergo total thyroidectomy because the nodules were growing. At surgery these were adenomatoid nodules. The patient's mother's US is shown in the left lower corner. She has the same disease and has had thyroidectomy on two occasions (the last being a total thyroidectomy) and two I-131 treatments for benign adenomatoid nodules, but continues to have thyroid nodules.

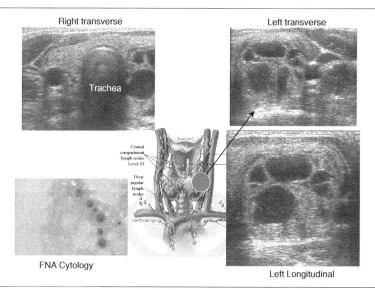

Figure 11. This is a 39 year-old woman with a long standing multinodular goiter. The goiter was enlarging, and despite several attempts to obtain cytology by FNA under US-guidance, the cytology simply showed proteinaceous fluid and macrophages and histiocytes and was insufficient for diagnosis. She underwent total thyroidectomy for what turned out to be a benign multinodular colloid goiter.

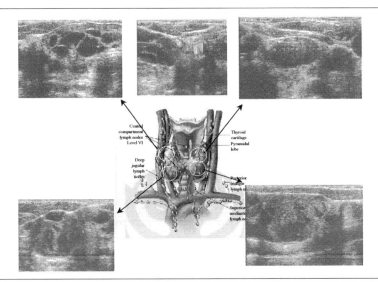

Figure 12. This is a 36 year-old woman with a small asymptomatic goiter of uncertain duration found on routine physical examination. The gland has the appearance of a benign multinodular goiter, but has some areas of increased Doppler flow over solid tissue. Also there are bilateral large cystic nodules (lower figures). The FNA showed papillary thyroid carcinoma. A CT scan showed several large (2–3 cm) cystic mediastinal lymph nodes. She underwent total thyroidectomy with removal of all the cervical and mediastinal lymph nodes (with limited sternotomy) and underwent I-131 therapy. Two years after treatment she is free of disease.

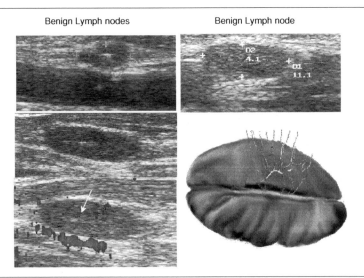

Figure 13. Benign cervical lymph nodes showing a hilar stripe and a small area of Doppler flow in the lymph node hilum. The hilar stripe is from a small area of fat and lymph node channels and blood vessels entering the lymph node in the same area of the lymph node, which is shown in the cartoon. The lymph nodes are slightly hypoechoic, are longer than they are wide and have an Solbiati (SI) index of about 2 (see text).

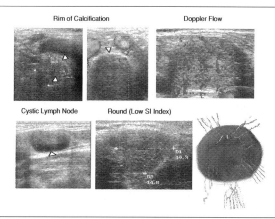

Figure 14. Malignant lymph nodes from different patients showing 1) round appearance (SI index ~1), chaotic intranodal Doppler flow, and irregular blurred margins. The cartoon shows how blood vessels enter lymph nodes with tumor causing a haphazard Doppler appearance. The left lower lymph node shows cystic degeneration, which is classic of papillary thyroid carcinoma. The two lymph nodes with a rim of calcification, which are also characteristic of papillary carcinoma, are from a 68 year-old woman with recurrent papillary thyroid carcinoma 40 years after she underwent hemithyroidectomy, radical right neck dissection and EBRT without I-131 therapy or having further follow-up. The FNA cytology was insufficient for diagnosis because of the dense calcifications but she was advised to have surgery anyway because this pattern of calcification is classic for this tumor. At surgery she was found to have multiple lymph node metastases in the right lateral neck compartments and in the upper mediastinum, some of which were completely invading the lymph node capsule.

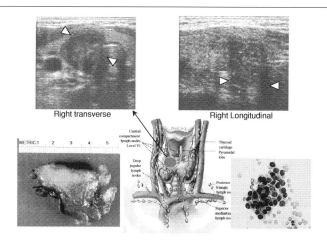

Figure 15. Papillary thyroid carcinoma in a 32 year-old woman. The right transverse view shows a hypoechoic nodule with internal microcalcifications, an irregular margin and tumor abutting the trachea. The longitudinal view showed tumor that appeared to be growing through the posterior capsule of the thyroid. FNA was positive for papillary thyroid carcinoma (cytology shown has inclusion bodies, nuclear groves and classic morphology of papillary carcinoma). At surgery the tumor was microscopically invading the trachea and was grossly invading the posterior capsule of the thyroid. The gross specimen shown shows why tumor margins with this neoplasm are often blurred and irregular.

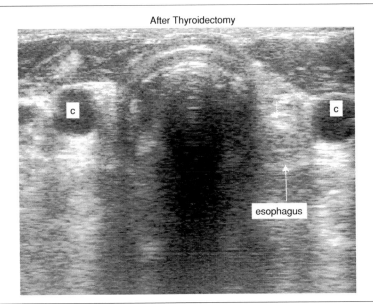

Figure 16. This is an ultrasound on the same patient shown in Fig. 14, done 6 months after total thyroidectomy and I-131 therapy. This is a typical US appearance after total thyroidectomy: the carotid artery marked (c) on the right is lying next to the trachea and the one on the left is lying close to the esophagus.

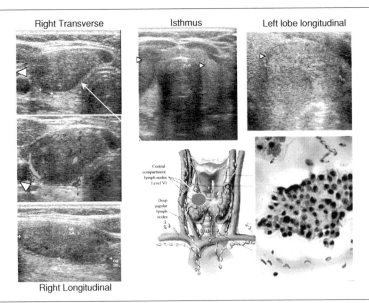

Figure 17. This is a benign multinodular goiter. The nodules are well demarcated, have clear margins, are isoechoic and have Doppler flow around the periphery of the nodule but not within it, and the US-guided FNA cytology shows colloid and normal follicular cells.

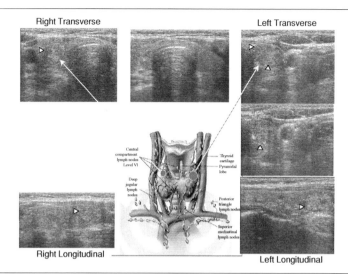

Figure 18. This is a benign multinodular goiter with several nodules larger than 1 cm. The nodules have internal microcalcifications (arrowhead) and appear to be encapsulated. The Doppler shows a small amount of intranodular flow. The US-guided FNA was consistent with a benign colloid multinodular goiter.

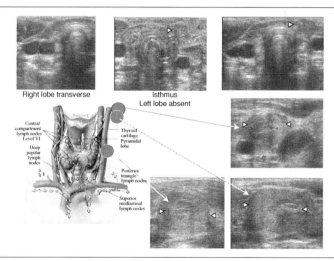

Figure 19. This is a US from a child with papillary thyroid carcinoma that was referred to out clinica after he was treated with total thyroidectomy several months before this US was obtained. The upper transverse views are consistent with his having undergone a total thyroidectomy however, however, there were palpable lymph nodes in left compartment levels II and III, and the 1–2 cm lymph nodes are compatible with metastatic disease, showing an SI index of ∼1, mixed echogenicity, Doppler flow, and irregular blurred margins. The child refused lymph node biopsy and he was sent to surgery on the strength of the history and this ultrasound examination. He had malignant lymph nodes removed form levels II III and IV and VI, some of which showed tumor cells invading the lymph node capsule. He also has bilateral diffuse lung uptake on the posttreatment whole body scan.

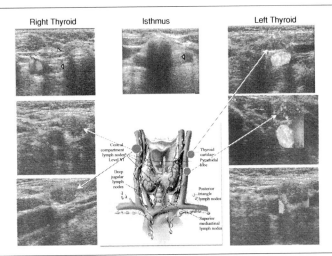

Figure 20. This is a US from a 55 year-old woman with a history of papillary thyroid carcinoma and a palpable lump on the left neck at level III. The top row shows transverse views and the figures below them are the longitudinal views. There are tumors the right at level II and on the left at levels II, III, IV and V, which were confirmed by US-guided FNA and bilateral modified neck dissections.

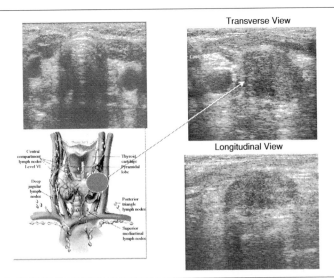

Figure 21. This is a 60 year-old woman referred for evaluation of a high serum thyroglobulin level (40 ng/mL with a suppressed TSH) and a negative whole-body scan. The patient had been treated with lobectomy and EBRT about 45 years previously and until recently had not undergone follow-up. There is a ~3 cm mass lateral to the left carotid at level III. At surgery this tumor was in the soft tissues that was not a lymph node metastasis, but was completely resected. It is hypoechoic, has mixed echogenicity, an irregular shape and blurred margins, and is close to the carotid and surrounding muscles, the latter being microscopically invaded by tumor.

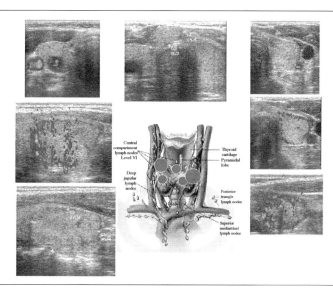

Figure 22. This is a 55 year-old lady with a multinodular goiter. The Transverse views in the top row show a thickened isthmus , a 14.4 × 8.2 mm nodule at the junction of the isthmus and left lobe, and large nodules in both the right and left lobes. The well demarcated nodules showed clear margins, perinodular Doppler flow and were all biopsied under ultrasound guidance and were compatible with a benign multinodular colloid goiter.

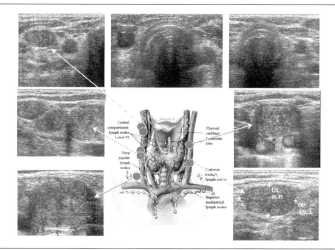

Figure 23. This is a 50 year-old woman with papillary thyroid carcinoma was referred to our clinic because of an elevated serum Tg of 17 ng/mL on thyroid hormone suppression of TSH and a negative diagnostic whole body scan. There are three level III lymph nodes on the left longitudinal views and one level II lymph node on the left transverse view. The lymph nodes are of mixed echogenicity with an SI of ∼1.5, clear margins and positive intranodal Doppler flow. US–guided FNA was positive for papillary thyroid carcinoma and she underwent left modified radical neck dissection that showed tumor confined to the lymph nodes.

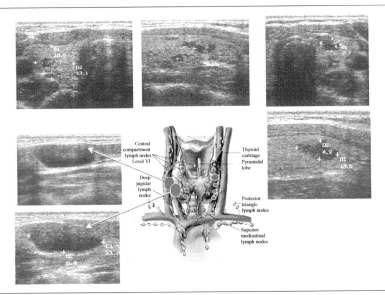

Figure 24. This is an 18 year-old woman with papillary thyroid carcinoma. The patient presented with a palpable lymph node on the right, which is the cystic lymph node seen at the bottom left of the figure. In addition another cystic lymph node was found as well as multifocal bilateral 3–4 mm hypoechoic areas. Ultrasonography-guided FNA on the palpable cystic lymph node was positive for papillary thyroid carcinoma. A cystic lymph node in a young person, even in children, has a high likelihood of being a papillary thyroid carcinoma.

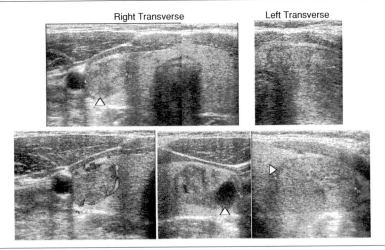

Figure 25. This is a 62 year-old woman with a large multinodular goiter of long standing. Her TSH was 0.5 mIU/L and the thyroidal radioiodine scan showed heterogeneous uptake of I-123. The nodules are isoechoic and show areas of cystic degeneration (arrows) and perinodular Doppler flow. FNA was done in all nodules >1 cm, all of which were compatible with a benign colloid multinodular goiter.

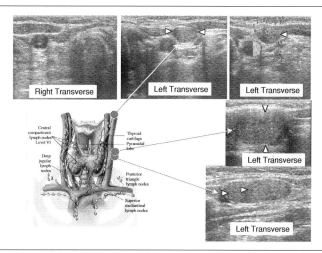

Figure 26. This is a 49 year-old woman with tall cell papillary thyroid carcinoma who underwent near-total thyroidectomy 8 years before she was referred to our clinic because of an elevated serum Tg (14 ng/mL) during thyroid hormone suppression of TSH and a negative diagnostic whole body scan. Tumor is present in level II lymph nodes on the right, which is seen on the transverse US view (arrows) and in the right longitudinal views (markers). There also is tumor on the left, posterior to the carotid artery (arrow), which is also seen in the longitudinal view (arrow). Brisk Doppler flow is seen in the lateral view of the tumor. She underwent bilateral modified neck dissections. The residual tumor was tall cell variant papillary thyroid carcinoma which was extending through the tumor capsule.

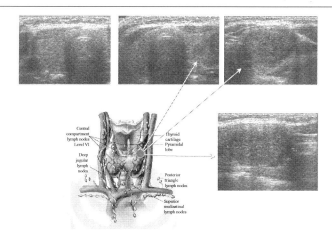

Figure 27. This is a 41 year-old woman who was referred to our clinic because of a palpable left lobe nodule, which is easily seen on the left transverse view. There is a thick dark ring around the tumor, a halo sign. The US-guided FNA showed sheets of Hürthle cells and no colloid. The cytologic diagnosis was a Hürthle cell tumor and because of this she underwent left hemithyroidectomy. The final histopathologic sections showed the tumor to be a Hürthle cell adenoma. However, a 5 mm papillary thyroid carcinoma was found in the isthmus that was invading through the thyroid capsule into the surrounding fibrofatty tissues. She accordingly underwent completion thyroidectomy and I-131 ablation and is now free of disease.

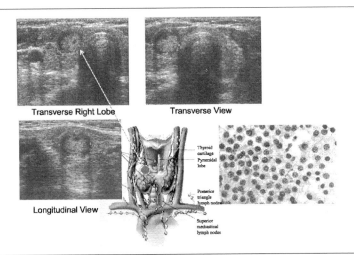

Figure 28. This is a 54 year-old woman who was referred to us because of a thyroid nodule found on a CT scan done for another reason. The nodule, which was not palpable, is seen in the right thyroid lobe. It has a thick halo and intranodular Doppler flow. The cytology was consistent with a follicular neoplasm and is shown at the bottom right of the figure. After undergoing right hemithyroidectomy, the pathology showed this to be a low-grade follicular carcinoma, for which she underwent completion thyroidectomy and I-131 ablation.

A

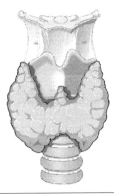

Thyroid Ultrasound
University of Florida
Thyroid Clinic

Patient:
UF Patient No:
Date of Ultrasound
Physician: Ernest L. Mazzaferri, MD

Palpation Findings

Figure 29. Forms to document (A) palpable and (B) ultrasonographic findings.

B

Thyroid Ultrasound
University of Florida
Thyroid Clinic

Patient:
UF Patient No:
Date of Ultrasound
Physician: Ernest L. Mazzaferri, MD

Transverse View

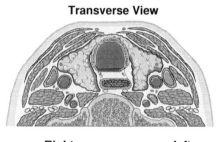

Right   left

Sagittal View

Right

Left

Impression:

Signature _____

❑ Hyperechoic
❑ Isoechoic
❑ Hypoechoic

❑ Solid
❑ Mixed
❑ Cyst

Margins
❑ Well defined
❑ Irregular
❑ Blurred

Calcification
❑ Yes
❑ Uncertain
❑ No

Color Doppler Flow
❑ Absence
❑ Peripheral
❑ Intranodular

Figure 29. Continued.

Using these decision rules, the sensitivity was 90% and the specificity is 82% for identifying malignant nodules. This study shows the clinical value of high-resolution ultrasonography and power-mode Doppler studies.

We find it helpful to use a hand written ultrasound report that includes drawing and notes concerning our findings. Figure 29 shows the forms that we use.

REFERENCES

Ahuja, AT, M Ying, HY Yuen, and C Metreweli. 2001. Power Doppler sonography of metastatic nodes from papillary carcinoma of the thyroid. Clin Radiol 56:284–288.

Frates, MC, CB Benson, PM Doubilet, ES Cibas, and E Marqusee. 2003. Can color Doppler sonography aid in the prediction of malignancy of thyroid nodules? J Ultrasound Med 22:127–131.

Gorges, R, EG Eising, D Fotescu, K Renzing-Kohler, A Frilling, KW Schmid, A Bockisch, and O Dirsch. 2003. Diagnostic value of high-resolution B-mode and power-mode sonography in the follow-up of thyroid cancer. Eur J Ultrasound 16:191–206.

Mazzaferri, EL, RJ Robbins, CA Spencer, LE Braverman, F Pacini, L Wartofsky, BR Haugen, SI Sherman, DS Cooper, GD Braunstein, S Lee, TF Davies, BM Arafah, PW Ladenson, and A Pinchera. 2003. A consensus report of the role of serum thyroglobulin as a monitoring method for low-risk patients with papillary thyroid carcinoma. J Clin Endocrinol Metab 88:1433–1441.

Papini, E, R Guglielmi, A Bianchini, A Crescenzi, S Taccogna, F Nardi, C Panunzi, R Rinaldi, V Toscano, and CM Pacella. 2002. Risk of malignancy in nonpalpable thyroid nodules: predictive value of ultrasound and color-Doppler features. J Clin Endocrinol Metab 87:1941–1946.

PART 3. INCIDENCE AND PROGNOSIS OF DIFFERENTIATED THYROID CANCER

3.1. INCIDENCE, PREVALENCE, RECURRENCE, AND MORTALITY OF DIFFERENTIATED THYROID CANCER

ROBERT J. AMDUR, MD AND ERNEST L. MAZZAFERRI, MD, MACP

The purpose of this chapter is to summarize data on the incidence, prevalence, mortality and recurrence rate of differentiated thyroid cancer (DTC) in a way that gives an overall picture of the impact of this disease on American society. Almost all the data presented in this chapter comes from the Surveillance, Epidemiology, and End Results (SEER) Program or the National Cancer Data Base (2004). The results that we present from the SEER database include all types of thyroid cancer, unless otherwise stated. Data that we summarize in this chapter applies mainly to differentiated thyroid cancer (Papillary, Follicular, and Hürthle Cell carcinoma) because these histologies account for approximately 94% of all thyroid cancer cases. Major points from this chapter are summarized in Tables 1 and 2.

INCIDENCE (NEW CASES DIAGNOSED OVER A SPECIFIC TIME PERIOD)

In the year 2003 there were approximately 20,000 new cases of DTC in the United States. This translates to an incidence of approximately 7 new cases per 100, 000 people in the general population per year (approximately 0.07% of the population developed DTC in 2003). In 2003, thyroid cancer accounted for approximately 1.6% of new cancer cases.

DTC is about three times more common in women than in men and may occur at any age (Fig. 1). Peak incidence of all thyroid cancers occurs at age 40–44 years in women and age 65–69 years in men, observations largely attributable to DTC. The

Table 1. Incidence, Prevalence, Recurrence, and Mortality of Differentiated Thyroid Cancer.

Incidence (new cases diagnosed over a specific time period):
In 2003: 20,000 new cases = 7 new cases per 100,000 people per year
Incidence is 3 times higher in women than men
Peak incidence occurs at age 40–44 years in women and age 65–69 years in men
Between 1992 and 2001 annual incidence increased by 57% in women and 33% in men

Prevalence (people living with the diagnosis at a given point in time):
On January 1, 2001 there were approximately 300,000 people in the United States who were living with a
   diagnosis of differentiated thyroid cancer

Rate of cancer recurrence following initial treatment:
Within 30 years of initial diagnosis approximately 30% of patients have experienced at least one episode of
   recurrent cancer based on a positive imaging study or biopsy. The recurrence rate would be much higher
   if the calculation included patients in whom an elevated serum thyroglobulin level was the only evidence
   of cancer

Time to detection of recurrent cancer following initial treatment:
Just over half (53%) of all recurrences present within five years of diagnosis, about three quarters (77%)
   present within 10 years, and 16% of recurrences present >15 years following initial diagnosis
The above numbers refer to recurrences that are documented with a positive scan or biopsy. Time to
   recurrence is likely to be much shorter if the calculations included recurrent disease based only on
   elevated serum thyroglobulin

Death from differentiated thyroid cancer:
Approximately 4000 people died of papillary or follicular thyroid cancer during the ten-year period ending
   in 1995
Papillary carcinoma causes the great majority (53%) of deaths from thyroid cancer
The 10-year risk of dying from papillary carcinoma is 7% and 15% from follicular carcinoma

peak incidence of anaplastic thyroid carcinoma occurs at about age 60 years, and that for medullary thyroid carcinoma varies according to whether it is sporadic or familial. The incidence of thyroid cancer rose continuously during the decade between 1992 and 2001 (Fig. 2), which was attributable to a rise in papillary thyroid carcinoma. The percentage increase in the annual incidence rate between 1992 and 2001 was 57% in women and 33% in men, mainly due to an increased rate of diagnosis of papillary carcinoma (Fig. 3).

The reason for the rise in incidence of differentiated thyroid cancer is currently a subject of active research and debate. Similar findings have been reported throughout

Table 2. Deaths due to Thyroid Cancer among 53,856 Patients Treated Between 1985 and 1995. in the USA*.

	Number of patients	% of all thyroid cancers	10-year Relative Survival	Number of cancer deaths	Deaths due to tumor type
Papillary	42686	79%	93%	2988	53%
Follicular	6764	13%	85%	1015	18%
Hürthle	1585	2%	76%	380	7%
Medullary	1928	4%	75%	482	9%
Anaplastic	893	2%	14%	768	14%

* Data from Hundahl et al. Cancer 1998; 83:2638–2648.

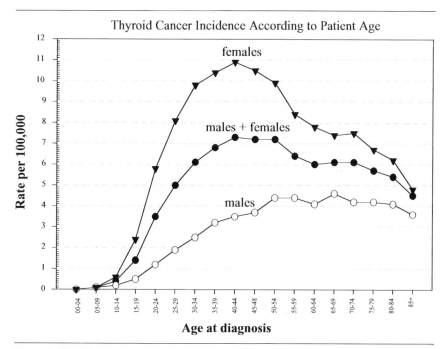

Figure 1. Thyroid cancer incidence based on age and gender. Data for this plot are from the Surveillance, Epidemiology, and End Results (SEER) Program (www.seer.cancer.gov) SEER*Stat Database: Incidence—SEER 9 Regs Public-Use, Nov 2003 Sub (1973–2001), National Cancer Institute, DCCPS, Surveillance Research Program, Cancer Statistics Branch, released April 2004, based on the November 2003 submission. Tumors with only one primary and microscopically confirmed.

Europe and in other but not all counties around the world. Possible explanations for the dramatic rise in papillary carcinoma in recent years include: exposure to ionizing radiation—especially radioiodine from nuclear weapons testing, the addition of iodine to common food products, changes in the histological criteria for the diagnosis of cancer versus benign thyroid neoplasia, and the widespread use of imaging studies for symptoms unrelated to the thyroid that demonstrate thyroid nodules as an incidental finding. A study by Leenhardt (2004) suggests that incidental detection is the main reason for the increase in the incidence of DTC.

PREVALENCE (PEOPLE LIVING WITH THE DIAGNOSIS AT A GIVEN POINT IN TIME)

With an indolent disease like DTC, disease prevalence is one of the most powerful ways to evaluate the impact of the disease on society. Prevalence represents the number of people alive on a certain day who were previously diagnosed with thyroid cancer, regardless of

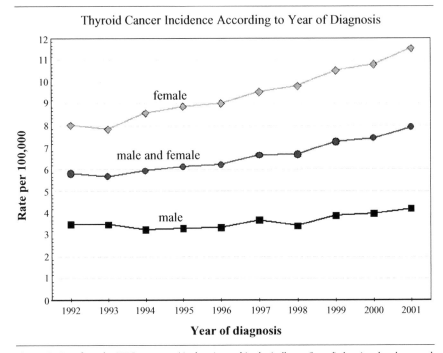

Figure 2. Data from the SEER program (single primary, histologically confirmed) showing that the annual incidence of differentiated thyroid cancer has increased in recent years. Specifically, the percentage increase in annual incidence between 1992 and 2001 was 57% in women and 33% in men. All incidence values are Age-Adjusted (2000 US Standard Population).

disease status. Using data from the SEER project (2004) we estimate that on January 1, 2001 there were almost 300,000 people in the United States who were living with a diagnosis of thyroid cancer, mostly differentiated thyroid carcinoma, approximately 75% of which were women. To put these numbers in perspective compared to cancers that usually result in death within a few years of diagnosis, the prevalence of differentiated thyroid cancer is three times higher than the prevalence of brain tumors and similar to the prevalence of lung cancer.

THE PROBLEM OF CANCER RECURRENCE

At the heart of many of the major controversies in thyroid cancer management is disagreement about the study endpoint. Analyses that focus on overall survival suggest that DTC is a benign disease in most subgroups. Overall survival is important but it is not the whole story when describing the outcome of a disease like DTC where tumor recurrence is common and patients often live for decades with residual cancer. The finding of residual or recurrent cancer is psychologically devastating to most patients and usually initiates diagnostic studies and therapeutic interventions that involve discomfort and risk.

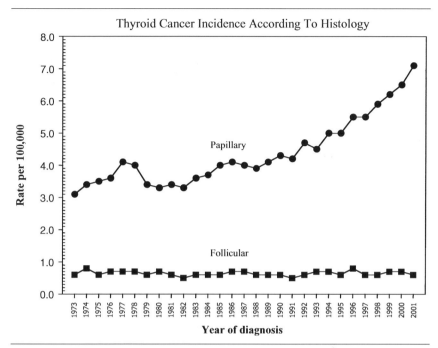

Figure 3. Data from the SEER program (single primary, histologically confirmed) showing that the increase in incidence of differentiated thyroid cancer is due exclusively to an increase in the incidence of papillary carcinoma. All incidence values are Age-Adjusted (2000 US Standard Population).

For this reason the rate of cancer recurrence is an important indicator of the morbidity of DTC.

The article by Mazzaferri and Jhiang (1994) is one of the few series in the literature that reports cancer-related mortality and the rate of tumor recurrence in a large number of patients with long-term follow-up. Figure 4 is constructed from the data in this study. The take-home message from these data is that cancer recurrence is a frequent event in patients with DTC. In this series, the cumulative rate of tumor recurrence at 30 years was 30% based on a positive imaging study or biopsy. The recurrence rate would be much higher if the calculation included patients in whom an elevated serum thyroglobulin level was the only evidence of cancer. This analysis did not report recurrence rate based on elevated serum thyroglobulin (scan negative) because many of the patients in this series where managed in the pre-thyroglobulin era. Prognostic factors in patients with DTC are the subject of the next chapter.

TIME TO DETECTION OF CANCER RECURRENCE

The time from initial diagnosis to detection of tumor recurrence is shown in Fig. 5. The data for these plots comes from Fig. 1 in the article by Mazzaferri and Kloos (2001).

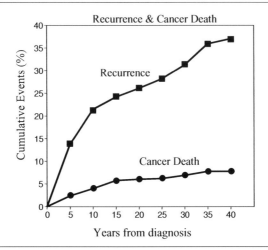

Figure 4. The rate of death from cancer and tumor recurrence in 1,533 patients with papillary or follicular thyroid cancer using data from the series reported by Mazzaferri and Jhiang (1994). At 30 years the cumulative rate of cancer recurrence is 30% based on a positive imaging study or biopsy. We predict that the recurrence rate would be much higher if the calculation included patients in whom an elevated serum thyroglobulin level was the only evidence of cancer.

Recurrent tumor was documented by a positive scan or biopsy in all cases. Seventy percent of recurrences were limited to the neck or upper mediastinum (local recurrence) and the remaining 30% were either in distant sites with no evidence of local recurrence (87% of patients with distant recurrence) or presented simultaneously in both local and distant sites (15% of patients with distant recurrence).

The take-home message from the plots in Fig. 5 is that it takes long-term follow-up to accurately evaluate the outcome of treatment of DTC. In these studies, just over half (53%) of all recurrences presented within five years of diagnosis, about three quarters (77%) were found within 10 years, and 16% of recurrences required more than 15 years of follow-up to detect. These data do not include patients with recurrent disease based only on an elevated serum thyroglobulin level (scan negative) because many of the patients in this series were treated in the prior to the routine measurement of thyroglobulin. Time to recurrence detection will likely be much shorter in future studies that use thyroglobulin level alone to diagnoses recurrent cancer.

DEATH FROM DIFFERENTIATED THYROID CANCER

A measure of the impact of a disease on society is the absolute number of patients who die from the disease over a period of time. Table 2 summarizes data on the incidence and mortality among 53,856 cases of thyroid cancer treated in the US between 1985 and 1995 from the National Cancer Data Base (Hundahl 1998). Approximately 4000 people died of papillary or follicular thyroid cancer during the ten-year period ending in 1995. Papillary carcinoma caused the great majority of deaths from thyroid

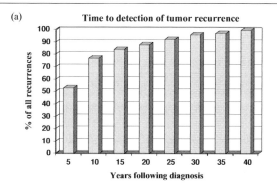

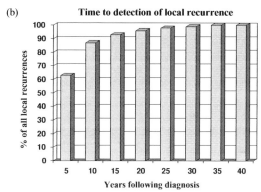

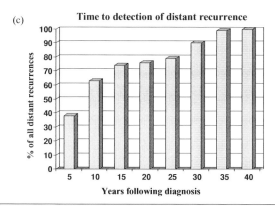

Figure 5. Time to detection of recurrence in patients with DTC. The data for these plots comes from Fig. 1 in the paper by Mazzaferri and Kloos (2001). Recurrent tumor was documented by a positive scan or biopsy in all cases. Local recurrence is cervical or mediastinal. Patients who presented simultaneously with local and distant recurrence (27 patients) are shown as distant recurrences. (A) All sites of recurrence (386 patients = 100%), (B) Local recurrence (272 patients = 70%), (C) Distant recurrence (114 patients = 30%). Just over half (53%) of all recurrences present within five years of diagnosis, about three quarters (77%) present with 10 years, and 16% of recurrences require more than 15 years of follow-up to detect.

cancer (53%), a finding explained by the fact that the prevalence of papillary carcinoma is much higher than that of other histologies.

REFERENCES

Hundahl, SA, ID Fleming, AM Fremgen, and HR Menck. 1998. A National Cancer Data Base report on 53,856 cases of thyroid carcinoma treated in the US, 1985–1995. Cancer **83**:2638–2648.

Leenhardt, L, MO Bernier, MH Boin-Pineau, DB Conte, R Marechaud, P Niccoli-Sire, M Nocaudie, J Orgiazzi, M Schlumberger, JL Wemeau, L Cherie-Challine, and F De Vathaire. 2004. Advances in diagnostic practices affect thyroid cancer incidence in France. Eur J Endocrinol **150**:133–139.

Mazzaferri, EL, and SM Jhiang. 1994. Differentiated thyroid cancer long-term impact of initial therapy. Trans Am Clin Climatol Assoc **106**:151–168.

Mazzaferri, EL, and RT Kloos. 2001. Current approaches to primary therapy for papillary and follicular thyroid cancer. J Clin Endocrinol Metab **86**:1447–1463.

Surveillance, Epidemiology, and End Results (SEER) Program (www.seer.cancer.gov) SEER Stat Database: Incidence—SEER 9 Regs Public-Use, Nov 2003 Sub (1973–2001), National Cancer Institute, DCCPS, Surveillance Research Program, Cancer Statistics Branch, released April 2004, based on the November 2003 submission. Tumors with only one primary and microscopically confirmed. National Cancer Institute, Bethesda, MD, 11-24-2004.

3.2. FACTORS THAT PREDICT CANCER RECURRENCE AND DEATH FROM DIFFERENTIATED THYROID CANCER

ROBERT J. AMDUR, MD AND ERNEST L. MAZZAFERRI, MD, MACP

The purpose of this chapter is to present an overview of the variables that predict cancer recurrence and death from cancer in patients with DTC. This information compliments the discussion in the chapter on long-term recurrence and mortality rates and the discussion of the AJCC staging system. Table 1 is modified from the National Comprehensive Cancer Network guidelines on the diagnosis and treatment of thyroid cancer. Table 2 summarizes the results of Cox regression analysis on a large group of patients with reliable long-term follow-up.

PROGNOSTIC VARIABLES

It is important for the treating physician to have a full understanding of the prognostic variables that affect outcome, for it is here that misjudgments concerning therapy are often made. There are important subtleties and exceptions that determine the patient's outcome. Perhaps the best example is how tumor size tends to change the course of papillary thyroid carcinoma: small tumors rarely cause morbidity or mortality, but there are major exceptions to this rule. Here we discuss selected variables that have a major impact on prognosis. The prognosis of various histologic types of thyroid cancer is discussed in a separate chapter.

YOUNG CHILDREN AND OLDER ADULTS HAVE A POOR PROGNOSIS

Nearly all thyroid cancer staging systems include age as a powerful prognostic variable. The problem with these staging systems, is that they often treat age as a binary variable

Table 1. Risk Stratification of Variables that Influence Cancer Recurrence and Cancer Death in Patients with DTC.

Factors predictive of high risk	Factors predictive of moderate-to-low risk
Age <15 yr or >45 yr	Age 15–45 yr
Male sex	Female sex
Family history of thyroid cancer	No family history of thyroid cancer
Tumor >4 cm in diameter	Tumor <4 cm in diameter
Bilateral disease	Unilateral disease
Extrathyroidal extension	No extrathyroidal extension
Vascular Invasion (both papillary and follicular thyroid cancer)	Absence of vascular invasion
Cervical, or mediastinal lymph node metastases	No lymph node metastases
Certain tumor subtypes: Hürthle cell, tall cell, columnar cell, diffuse sclerosis, insular variants	Encapsulated papillary thyroid carcinoma, papillary microcarcinoma, cystic papillary thyroid carcinoma
Marked nuclear atypia, tumor necrosis, and vascular invasion (*i.e.* histologic grade)	Absence of nuclear atypia, tumor necrosis, and vascular invasion
Tumors or metastases that concentrate radioiodine poorly or not at all	Tumors or metastases that concentrate radioiodine well
Distant metastases	No distant metastases

Modified from the National Comprehensive Cancer Network guidelines (http://www.nccn.org/professionals/physician_gls/PDF/thyroid.pdf).

where patients have a favorable prognosis if they are younger than 40 or 45 years old. There is now a large body of evidence that demonstrates children less than 15 years old have a pattern of tumor recurrence and distant metastases that is similar to that of adults of age >60 years. Figure 1 shows the shape of the outcome curves based on age, and shows that the risk of cancer death increases with each decade of life, dramatically rising after age 60 years. Children commonly present with more advanced tumor stage than adults and have more cancer recurrences after therapy, but often live for many years after recurrence (Borson-Chazot F 2004). Some experts believe that young age has such a favorable influence upon survival that it overshadows the prognosis predicted by the tumor characteristics. The majority of physicians, however, believe that the tumor stage and histologic differentiation are as important as the patient's age in determining prognosis and management (Mazzaferri & Jhiang 1994; Miccoli 1998; Mazzaferri 1999b; Hung & Sarlis 2002). Most physicians now recommend that children with thyroid carcinoma be treated in the same way as adults, with total thyroidectomy, I-131 remnant ablation, and aggressive management of distant metastases (Thompson 2004; Jarzab 2000; Landau 2000; Brink JS 2000; Haveman 2003).

DISTANT METASTASES

About 10% of patients with papillary carcinoma and up to 25% of those with follicular carcinoma develop distant metastases; half are present at the time of diagnosis and the others often are first recognized decades after the cancer was fist identified. They occur more often (35%) with Hürthle cell carcinoma and after the age of 40 years (Lopez-Penabad 2003). Among 1, 231 patients reported in 13 studies, 49% of the metastases were to

Table 2. Cox Regression Analysis of Prognostic Factors in Patients with DTC[#].

	Hazard ratio	P value
All Cancer Recurrence		
Age*	1.0	0.2
Local tumor invasion	1.4	.01
Lymph node metastases †	1.3	.01
Follicular histology	0.8	.012
Tumor size ‡	1.2	.0001
Thyroid remnant I-131 ablation ¶	0.8	.016
Therapy with I-131 ¶	0.5	.0001
Surgery more than lobectomy §	0.7	.0001
Distant Metastasis Recurrence		
Age*	1.0	.0001
Follicular histology	1.0	.864
Lymph node metastases †	1.6	.002
Local tumor invasion	1.6	.927
Tumor size ‡	1.2	.001
Thyroid remnant I-131 ablation ¶	0.6	.002
Therapy with I-131 ¶	0.4	.0001
Surgery more than lobectomy §	0.8	.379
Age*	1.0	.0001
Cancer Mortality		
Age*	9.5	.0001
Time to treatment **	2.4	.0001
Follicular histology	1.4	.003
Lymph node metastases †	2.0	.006
Tumor size ‡	1.2	.025
Local tumor invasion	1.1	.002
Female (versus male)	0.6	.046
Thyroid remnant I-131 ablation ¶	0.5	.0001
Surgery more than lobectomy §	0.5	.0001
Therapy with I-131 ¶	0.4	.010

Mazzaferri, E. L. and Kloos, R. T. Current approaches to primary therapy for papillary and follicular thyroid cancer. J.Clin.Endocrinol.Metab 86(4), 1447–1463. 2001. Note: Data on unfavorable subtype histology (e.g., tall cell, Hurthle cell) was not available for this analysys.
* Age stratified as <40 versus ≥40 years for cancer mortality, and by decade for recurrences and distant recurrences.
** Time to treatment ≤12 versus >12 months
† Lymph node metastases present versus absent
‡ Tumor diameter stratified into 1 cm increments from tumors <1 to >5 cm
¶ Remnant ablation is the use of I-131 I in patients with uptake only in the thyroid bed and no evidence of residual tumor; Therapy with I-131 is postoperative treatment of patients with known residual disease
§ Bilateral thyroid surgery versus lobectomy with or without isthmusectomy

lung, 25% to bone, 15% to both lung and bone and 10% to the central nervous system or other soft tissues (Mazzaferri 1993). The outcome is influenced mainly by the patient's age, the tumor's metastatic site(s), ability to concentrate I-131, and tumor bulk. Although some patients survive for decades, especially younger patients, about half die within five years regardless of tumor histology (Mazzaferri 1993). In a study from France, survival rates with distant metastases were 53% at 5 years, 38% at 10 years and 30% at 15 years (Schlumberger 1986). Survival is longest with diffuse microscopic lung metastases seen only on posttreatment I-131 imaging and not by x-ray. The prognosis is much worse when the metastases do not concentrate I-131 or appear as large lung

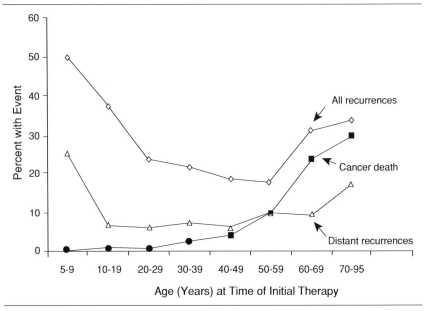

Figure 1. Age stratified by decade at the time of initial treatment as it affects the percentage of patients with tumor recurrence, distant recurrence and cancer deaths. The prognosis of children <15 years of age is similar to that of older adults. (From Mazzaferri EL and Kloos. J Clin Endocrinol Metab 2001. Reproduced with permission of the Endocrine Society).

nodules and is intermediate when the tumors are small nodules on x-ray that concentrate I-131.

DELAY IN DIAGNOSIS AND TREATMENT COMPROMISES OUTCOME

Several studies demonstrate that a delay in the diagnosis and treatment of DTC compromises outcome. Figure 2 plots a data set in which delay of treatment for 12 months was associated with a doubling of cancer mortality (Mazzaferri & Jhiang 1994). These data emphasize the importance of referring patients with a thyroid nodule promptly to a physician with expertise in the diagnosis and treatment of thyroid cancer. Delay in performing completion thyroidectomy also poses problems. In one study (Scheumann 1996), multivariate analysis by Cox's proportional hazards model showed that patients who underwent completion thyroidectomy within six months of the primary operation had significantly fewer recurrences, fewer lymph node metastases, fewer hematogenous metastases and survived significantly longer than those in whom the second operation was delayed for longer than six months. The authors of this study concluded that completion thyroidectomy as soon as possible after incomplete resection of the tumor may

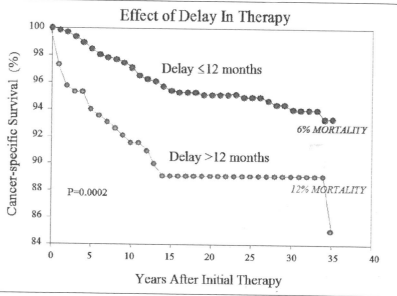

Figure 2. The effect of treatment delay on death from cancer. A delay of greater than 12 months was associated with a doubling of cancer-related mortality. The data for this plot is from Mazzaferri EL, Jhiang SM. Long-term impact of initial surgical and medical therapy on papillary and follicular thyroid cancer. Drawn from the data in Mazzaferri and Jhiang in Am J Med 1994; 97:418–428.

improve prognosis of DTC when the stage is worse than pT1 (5th AJCC classification in which T1 = 1 cm) or in patients whose recurrent tumor is diagnosed at follow-up.

MALE GENDER IS A POOR PROGNOSTIC FACTOR

Multiple studies demonstrate that the prognosis of differentiated thyroid cancer is worse for men than women. Figure 3 is a plot of data from the Surveillance, Epidemiology, and End Results (SEER)(2004) Program on the effect of gender on the rate of death from DTC (cancer-specific survival) ten years after diagnosis. Men typically present at a considerably older age than women. The peak age at the time thyroid cancer is diagnosed is about 20 years later in men than in women. Men have more than twice the frequency of distant metastases and about 30% more regional metastases at the time of diagnosis as compared with women. These differences have been largely attributed to how men and women access the health care systems, with men simply appearing at a later age and with more advanced stage tumors.

TUMOR SIZE DOES NOT ALWAYS PREDICT PROGNOSIS.

There is a linear relationship between tumor size and cancer recurrence and mortality for both papillary and follicular carcinomas (Mazzaferri & Jhiang 1994). Papillary

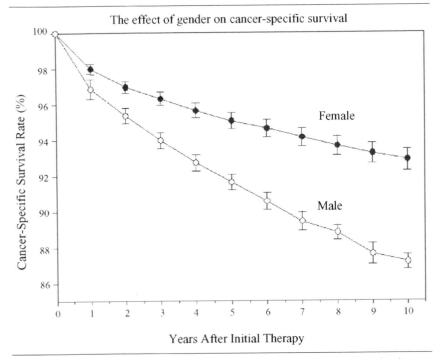

Figure 3. Relative survival curves for papillary and follicular thyroid carcinoma in patients with only one tumor that was microscopically confirmed Surveillance, Epidemiology, and End Results (SEER) Program (www.seer.cancer.gov) SEER*Stat Database: Incidence—SEER 9 Regs Public-Use, Nov 2003 Sub (1973–2001), National Cancer Institute, DCCPS, Surveillance Research Program, Cancer Statistics Branch, released April 2004, based on the November 2003 submission.

carcinomas 1 cm or smaller, termed microcarcinomas by the World Health Organization classification of thyroid tumors, are often found unexpectedly during surgery for benign thyroid conditions and usually pose no threat to survival and require no further surgery. The recurrence and cancer-specific mortality rates for microcarcinoma are near zero (Moosa 1997; Baudin 1998). Still, about 20% are multifocal and up to 60% have cervical lymph node metastases, and some with these features develop lung metastases, which are the only microcarcinomas with significant morbidity and mortality. An important study (Chow 2003) of patients with papillary microcarcinomas found the cause specific survival, locoregional failure-free survival and distant metastases failure-free survival rates at 10 years were 100%, 92.1%, and 97.1%, respectively. Five patients developed lung metastases and 2 died of their metastases. Locoregional recurrences were highly responsive to a combination of surgery, I-131 therapy, and external beam radiotherapy. The risk of cervical lymph node recurrence increased about 6-fold when nodal metastases or multifocal disease was present at the initial diagnosis, but thyroid remnant ablation reduced the lymph node recurrence rate significantly. Of great importance, lymph node metastasis increased the rate of distant metastasis about 11-fold, and age was not a significant factor in predicting recurrence or survival, although no patient with tumors smaller than 5 mm died of cancer. Thus, despite the overall excellent prognosis for patients with papillary microcarcinoma, a few of these tumors are associated with lymph node recurrence, distant metastasis and disease-related mortality.

MULTIPLE INTRATHYROIDAL TUMORS.

Multicentric tumors are found in about 20% of patients with papillary carcinoma when the thyroid is examined routinely and in up to 80% if the thyroid is examined with great care (Mazzaferri & Kloos 2001). Regarded as intrathyroidal metastases in the past, multiple distinct RET/PTC gene rearrangements found in the majority of multifocal papillary carcinomas indicates that they are individual tumors that arise independently in a background of genetic or environmental susceptibility thyroid tissue (Sugg 1998). Their presence in the contralateral thyroid lobe cannot be predicted on the basis of clinical risk stratification (Pacini 2001) and is thus not apparent until the final histologic sections of the entire thyroid gland have been studied. This has a bearing upon the need to surgically excise the contralateral lobe and to ablate the thyroid remnant with I-131. About half the patients undergoing routine completion thyroidectomy for presumed unilateral papillary thyroid carcinoma have tumor in the contralateral lobe (Scheumann 1996; Mazzaferri & Kloos 2001; Pacini 2001); however, when multifocal disease is present in the thyroid lobe first excised, or when the tumor has recurred in any site, bilateral multifocal tumor is almost always found (Pasieka 1992). Recurrence rates range from 5% to 20% in large thyroid remnants and lung metastases occur more frequently after subtotal than total thyroidectomy has been performed (Massin 1984; Mazzaferri 1997; Taylor 1998). Patients with multiple intrathyroidal tumors have almost twice the incidence of nodal metastases and three times the rate of pulmonary and other distant metastases than those with single tumors and the likelihood of persistent disease is two to three times more likely in those with multiple tumors (Massin 1984).

LOCAL TUMOR INVASION

About 5% to 10% of tumors grow directly into the surrounding neck tissues, increasing both morbidity and mortality. Local invasion, which can occur with both papillary and follicular carcinoma, ranges from microscopic to gross tumor invasion (Mazzaferri & Jhiang 1994). The most commonly invaded structures are the neck muscles and vessels, recurrent laryngeal nerves, larynx, pharynx, and esophagus, but tumor can extend into the spinal cord and brachial plexus.

The symptoms are usually hoarseness due to vocal cord paralysis, cough, dysphagia, hemoptysis and stridor or neurological dysfunction. Tumor invasion is a key risk factor that leads to lymph node and distant metastasis (Machens 2003). Tumor was locally invasive in 115 of our patients (8% of papillary and 12% of follicular carcinomas), whose 10-year recurrence rates were 1.5-times and cancer-specific death rates were 5 times those of patients without local tumor invasion. Nearly all who died with tumor invasion did so within the first decade after it was identified (Mazzaferri & Jhiang 1994).

Microscopic tumor invasion into surrounding tissues has a much better prognosis than does macroscopic tumor invading contiguous structures.

LYMPH NODE METASTASES

The first sign of thyroid carcinoma may be an enlarged cervical lymph node. When this occurs, multiple nodal metastases are usually found at surgery. About 33% of metastatic lymph nodes from papillary carcinoma are partly cystic (Wunderbaldinger 2002). The incidence and location of lymph node metastases varies with the tumor type, patient age and the extent of lymph node surgery. Gross lymph node metastases are found in about 36% of adults and in up to 80% of children with papillary carcinoma, and in about 17% with follicular carcinoma (Mazzaferri 1993; Hung 2002). Micrometastases occur even more often, being found in about 60% of cases, almost half of which are bilateral (Mirallie 1999; Qubain 2002). Tumors located in the upper third of the thyroid metastasize in the direction of upward lymphatic flow, whereas tumors located in the lower third or isthmus tend to metastasize inferiorly (Qubain 2002).

The prognostic importance of regional lymph node metastases is controversial, yet an increasingly larger number of studies find nodal metastases are a risk factor for local tumor recurrence, distant metastasis, and cancer-specific mortality, especially if they are bilateral cervical or mediastinal lymph node metastases or if tumor invades through the lymph node capsule (DeGroot 1990; Mazzaferri & Jhiang 1994; Yamashita 1997; Bernier 2001; Voutilainen 2001; Chow 2003). For example, in one study 15% of patients with and 0% without cervical node metastases died of disease (Sellers 1992). Another study of patients with distantly metastatic papillary carcinoma found that 80% had mediastinal node metastases at presentation (Lindegaard 1988). Our patients with papillary or follicular carcinoma who had cervical or mediastinal lymph node metastases had significantly higher 30-year cancer mortality rates than those without them (10% vs. 6%, P < 0.01). (Mazzaferri & Jhiang 1994)

REFERENCES

Baudin, E, JP Travagli, J Ropers, F Mancusi, G Bruno-Bossio, B Caillou, AF Cailleux, JD Lumbroso, C Parmentier, and M Schlumberger. 1998. Microcarcinoma of the thyroid gland—The Gustave-Roussy Institute Experience. Cancer **83**:553–559.

Bernier, MO, L Leenhardt, C Hoang, A Aurengo, JY Mary, F Menegaux, E Enkaoua, G Turpin, J Chiras, G Saillant, and G Hejblum. 2001. Survival and therapeutic modalities in patients with bone metastases of differentiated thyroid carcinoma. J Clin Endocrinol Metab **86**:1568–1573.

Borson-Chazot, F, S Causeret, JC Lifante, M Augros, N Berger, and JL Peix. 2004. Predictive factors for recurrence from a series of 74 children and adolescents with differentiated thyroid cancer. World J Surg.

Brink, JS, JA van Heerden, B McIver, DR Salomao, DR Farley, CS Grant, GB Thompson, D Zimmerman, and ID Hay. 2000. Papillary thyroid cancer with pulmonary metastases in children: long-term prognosis. Surgery **128**:881–887.

Chow, SM, SC Law, JK Chan, SK Au, S Yau, and WH Lau. 2003. Papillary microcarcinoma of the thyroid-Prognostic significance of lymph node metastasis and multifocality. Cancer **98**:31–40.

DeGroot, LJ, EL Kaplan, M McCormick, and FH Straus. 1990. Natural history, treatment, and course of papillary thyroid carcinoma. J Clin Endocrinol Metab **71**:414–424.

Haveman, JW, KM Van Tol, CW Rouwe, dA Piers, and JT Plukker. 2003. Surgical experience in children with differentiated thyroid carcinoma. Ann Surg Oncol **10**:15–20.

Hung, W, and NJ Sarlis. 2002. Current controversies in the management of pediatric patients with well-differentiated non-medullary thyroid cancer: a review. Thyroid **12**:683–702.

Jarzab, B, JD Handkiewicz, J Wloch, B Kalemba, J Roskosz, A Kukulska, and Z Puch. 2000. Multivariate analysis of prognostic factors for differentiated thyroid carcinoma in children. Eur J Nucl Med **27**:833–841.

Landau, D, L Vini, R A'Hern, and C Harmer. 2000. Thyroid cancer in children: the Royal Marsden Hospital experience. Eur J Cancer **36**:214–220.

Lindegaard, MW, E Paus, J Hie, G Kullman, and AE Stenwig. 1988. Thyroglobulin radioimmunoassay and ^{131}I scintigraphy in patients with differentiated thyroid carcinoma. Acta Chir Scand **154**:141–115.

Lopez-Penabad, L, AC Chiu, AO Hoff, P Schultz, S Gaztambide, NG Ordonez, and SI Sherman. 2003. Prognostic factors in patients with Hurthle cell neoplasms of the thyroid. Cancer **97**:1186–1194.

Machens, A, HJ Holzhausen, C Lautenschlager, PN Thanh, and H Dralle. 2003. Enhancement of lymph node metastasis and distant metastasis of thyroid carcinoma. Cancer **98**:712–719.

Massin, JP, JC Savoie, H Garnier, G Guiraudon, FA Leger, and F Bacourt. 1984. Pulmonary metastases in differentiated thyroid carcinoma. Study of 58 cases with implications for the primary tumor treatment. Cancer **53**:982–992.

Mazzaferri, EL. 1993. Thyroid carcinoma: papillary and follicular. In: Endocrine Tumors. Cambridge: Blackwell Scientific Publications Inc. (Mazzaferri EL, Samaan N, eds.) 278–333.

Mazzaferri, EL. 1997. Thyroid remnant ^{131}I ablation for papillary and follicular thyroid carcinoma. Thyroid **7**:265–271.

Mazzaferri, EL. 1999a. NCCN Thyroid Cancer Practice Guidelines. Oncology **13(Suppl. 11A)**. NCCN Proceedings http://www.nccn.org/physician_gls/f_guidelines.html.

Mazzaferri, EL. 1999b. NCCN Thyroid Carcinoma Practice Guidelines. Oncology **13(Suppl. 11A)**. NCCN Proceedings http://www.nccn.org/physician_gls/f_guidelines.html, 391–442.

Mazzaferri, EL, and SM Jhiang. 1994. Long-term impact of initial surgical and medical therapy on papillary and follicular thyroid cancer. Am J Med **97**:418–428.

Mazzaferri, EL, and RT Kloos. 2001. Current approaches to primary therapy for papillary and follicular thyroid cancer. J Clin Endocrinol Metab **86**:1447–1463.

Miccoli, P, A Antonelli, C Spinelli, M Ferdeghini, P Fallahi, and L Baschieri. 1998. Completion total thyroidectomy in children with thyroid cancer secondary to the Chernobyl accident. Arch Surg **133**:89–93.

Mirallie, E, J Visset, C Sagan, A Hamy, MF Le Bodic, and J Paineau. 1999. Localization of cervical node metastasis of papillary thyroid carcinoma. World J Surg **23**:970–973.

Moosa, M, and EL Mazzaferri. 1997. Occult thyroid carcinoma. Cancer J **10**:180–188.

Pacini, F, R Elisei, M Capezzone, P Miccoli, E Molinaro, F Basolo, L Agate, V Bottici, M Raffaelli, and A Pinchera. 2001. Contralateral papillary thyroid cancer is frequent at completion thyroidectomy with no difference in low- and high-risk patients. Thyroid **11**:877–881.

Pasieka, JL, NW Thompson, MK McLeod, RE Burney, and M Macha. 1992. The incidence of bilateral well-differentiated thyroid cancer found at completion thyroidectomy. World J Surg **16**:711–716.

Qubain, SW, S Nakano, M Baba, S Takao, and T Aikou. 2002. Distribution of lymph node micrometastasis in pN0 well-differentiated thyroid carcinoma. Surgery **131**:249–256. Ref Type: Electronic Citation

Scheumann, GFW, H Seeliger, TJ Musholt, O Gimm, G Wegener, H Dralle, H Hundeshagen, and R Pichlmayr. 1996. Completion thyroidectomy in 131 patients with differentiated thyroid carcinoma. Acta Chir. Eur J Surg **162**:677–684.

Schlumberger, M, M. Tubiana, F De Vathaire, C Hill, P Gardet, JP Travagli, P Fragu, J Lumbroso, B Caillou, and C Parmentier. 1986. Long-term results of treatment of 283 patients with lung and bone metastases from differentiated thyroid cancer. J Clin Endocrinol Metab **63**:960–967.

Sellers, M, S Beenken, A Blankenship, S Soong, E Turbat-Herrera, M Urist, and W Maddox. 1992. Prognostic significance of cervical lymph node metastases in differentiated thyroid cancer. Am J Surg **164**:578–581.

Sugg, SL, S Ezzat, IB Rosen, JL Freeman, and SL Asa. 1998. Distinct multiple *RET/PTC* gene rearrangements in multifocal papillary thyroid neoplasia. J Clin Endocrinol Metab **83**:4116–4122.

Surveillance, Epidemiology, and End Results (SEER) Program (www.seer.cancer.gov) SEER Stat Database: Incidence—SEER 9 Regs Public-Use, Nov 2003 Sub (1973–2001), National Cancer Institute, DCCPS, Surveillance Research Program, Cancer Statistics Branch, released April 2004, based on the November 2003 submission. Tumors with only one primary and microscopically confirmed. National Cancer Institute, Bethesda, MD, 11-24-2004.

Taylor, T, B Specker, J Robbins, M Sperling, M Ho, K Ain, ST Bigos, J Brierley, D Cooper, B Haugen, I Hay, V Hertzberg, I Klein, H Klein, P Ladenson, R Nishiyama, D Ross, S Sherman, and HR Maxon. 1998. Outcome after treatment of high-risk papillary and non-Hurthle-cell follicular thyroid carcinoma. Ann Intern Med **129**:622–627.

Thompson, GB, and ID Hay. 2004. Current strategies for surgical management and adjuvant treatment of childhood papillary thyroid carcinoma. World J Surg **28**:1187–1198.

Voutilainen, PE, MM Multanen, AK Leppaniemi, CH Haglund, RK Haapiainen, and KO Franssila. 2001. Prognosis after lymph node recurrence in papillary thyroid carcinoma depends on age. Thyroid **11**:953–957.

Wunderbaldinger, P, MG Harisinghani, PF Hahn, GH Daniels, K Turetschek, J Simeone, MJ O'Neill, and PR Mueller. 2002. Cystic lymph node metastases in papillary thyroid carcinoma. AJR Am J Roentgenol **178**:693–697.

Yamashita, H, S Noguchi, N Murakami, H Kawamoto, and S Watanabe. 1997. Extracapsular invasion of lymph node metastasis is an indicator of distant metastasis and poor prognosis in patients with thyroid papillary carcinoma. Cancer **80**:2268–2272.

PART 4. SURGICAL THERAPY OF DIFFERENTIATED THYROID CANCER

4.1. A TOTAL THYROIDECTOMY RARELY REMOVES ALL THYROID TISSUE

DOUGLAS B. VILLARET, MD, ROBERT J. AMDUR, MD
AND ERNEST L. MAZZAFERRI, MD, MACP

The presence of residual thyroid tissue following thyroid cancer surgery has major implications for post thyroidectomy treatment and testing (Maxon 1990). It is therefore important for physicians who manage patients with thyroid cancer to understand that the recommendations presented in this book are based on the assumption that there is probably no such thing as a "total" thyroidectomy. By this we mean that the standard thyroidectomy procedure almost always leaves a small amount of thyroid tissue in the neck.

Surgeons who object to the suggestion that their resection is in some way incomplete misunderstand that a small volume of residual thyroid tissue is the expected outcome. When it is necessary to make it clear that everyone in the conversation understands that there is almost certainly residual thyroid tissue we suggest that the term near-total thyroidectomy be used instead of total thyroidectomy. Throughout this book we use these terms interchangeably with the assumption that the reader understands that a total thyroidectomy does not remove every thyroid follicular cell. With medullary thyroid carcinoma, however, there is an attempt to do a more complete thyroid resection, including removal of the posterior thyroid capsule.

DOCUMENTATION THAT THERE IS RESIDUAL TISSUE FOLLOWING THYROIDECTOMY

The most straightforward evidence that the thyroidectomy procedure rarely removes all thyroid tissue comes from the iodine scans that are routinely done after thyroidectomy. With this type of study any concentration of radioactive iodine in the neck indicates

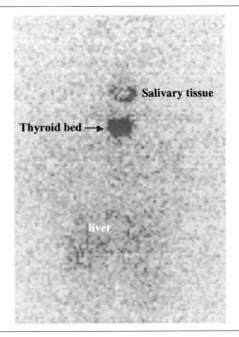

Figure 1. Total body I-131 scan following "total" thyroidectomy. This scan shows the pattern of uptake that is typically seen following gross total removal of the thyroid gland. This scan shows iodine uptake diffusely throughout the thyroid bed. In some cases the intensity of uptake is less that what is shown in this scan but the finding of some degree of iodine uptake in the thyroid bed, indicating residual thyroid tissue or cancer, is a common finding regardless of the perceived thoroughness of the surgical procedure.

residual thyroid tissue or thyroid cancer. Regardless of the perceived thoroughness of the resection at the time of surgery, iodine scans almost always demonstrate some degree of increased uptake in the region of the thyroid bed (Fig. 1).

The distinction between a radioiodine scan and a thyroid uptake study is discussed in an earlier chapter. The reason to mention it here is to remind readers that the pattern of uptake on the radioiodine scan may not correlate with the results of a thyroid uptake study. In other words, there can be clear evidence of radioiodine concentration in the thyroid bed in a patient with an extremely low (<1%) thyroid uptake value especially with uptake in the thyroglossal duct area.

THE REASON A TOTAL THYROIDECTOMY LEAVES RESIDUAL TISSUE

The thyroidectomy procedure usually leaves some normal thyroid tissue in the neck for two reasons. Berry's ligament connects the posterior surface of the thyroid to the trachea. Microscopic nests of thyroid tissue exist in this plane and are incompletely resected with total thyroidectomy.

The second place where thyroid tissue is usually not removed is at the point in the cricothyroid membrane where the recurrent laryngeal nerve enters the larynx. At this point the nerve is usually imbedded in thyroid tissue, or so close to the surface of the gland that it is not possible to remove all thyroid tissue without a high chance of nerve damage.

REFERENCE

Maxon III, HR, and HS Smith. 1990. Radioiodine-131 in the diagnosis and treatment of metastatic well differentiated thyroid cancer. Endocrinol Metab Clin North Am **19**:685–718.

4.2. NECK DISSECTIONS TO REMOVE MALIGNANT LYMPH NODES

DOUGLAS B. VILLARET, MD, ROBERT J. AMDUR, MD AND
ERNEST L. MAZZAFERRI, MD, MACP

Based on anatomic location and the pattern of cancer spread, the lymphatics of the neck have been organized into seven main levels (Robbins 1998, Som 1999). The boundaries of each node level correspond to landmarks that are identifiable at the time of surgery. These levels are illustrated in Fig. 1 and the boundaries of each level are described in Table 1.

ELECTIVE NECK DISSECTIONS ARE NOT ROUTINELY DONE FOR THYROID CANCER

The terms "elective neck dissection" and "prophylactic neck dissection" mean the same thing and refer to the removal of nodes from an area of the neck that has no evidence of adenopathy on clinical examination—meaning that there is no palpable lymph node enlargement and no abnormal lymph nodes on CT scan, MR scan, or ultrasound examination if any of these studies are done. Elective neck dissections are common practice with most kinds of head and neck cancer where surgical removal of subclinical disease in the regional lymphatics may increase the chance of cancer cure or determine the need for radiation or chemotherapy.

From the surgical standpoint, a factor that distinguishes thyroid cancer from other head and neck malignancies is that elective neck dissections are not routinely done in patients with differentiated thyroid cancer. The idea behind this is that identifying microscopic disease in the regional nodes will not affect the need for additional therapy, especially thyroid remnant ablation after surgery, nor will removal of lymph nodes with subclinical metastases affect prognosis (Bononi 2004, Noguchi 1990). Considering all

Table 1. Lymph Node Levels in the Neck.

Level I:	Contains the nodes of the submental and submandibular triangles, defined inferiorly by the digastric muscles.
Level II:	Contains the upper jugular nodes from the base of the skull to the hyoid bone.
Level III:	Contains the middle jugular nodes from the hyoid bone to the inferior edge of the cricoid cartilage.
Level IV:	Contains the low jugular nodes from the cricoid cartilage to the clavicle.
Level V:	Contains the nodes of the posterior triangle that is bounded anteriorly by the sternocleidomastoid muscle and posteriorly by the trapezius.
Level VI:	Contains the nodes of the anterior central compartment from the hyoid bone to the manubrium with lateral boundaries being the carotid arteries
Level VII:	Contains the superior mediastinal nodes from the level of the superior edge of the manubrium to the innominate vein.

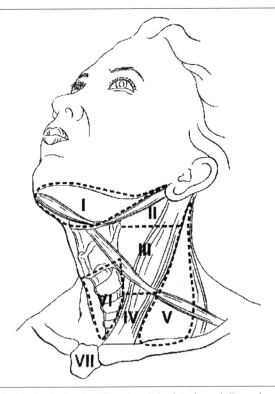

Figure 1. Schematic showing the location of lymph node levels in the neck (Reproduced from page 29 of the 6th edition of the AJCC Cancer Staging Handbook. Springer-Verlag, 2002). The boundaries of each level are described in the text.

Table 2. Summary of Principles Related to Neck Dissection for Differentiated Thyroid Cancer (DTC).

1.	Elective (prophylactic) dissection of the lateral neck compartments (Levels II, III, or IV) are not done in DTC
2.	The only indication for compartmental dissection is a clinically positive lymph node
3.	The jugular lymph nodes (Level II-IV) are dissected in an all or none fashion when one or more of the compartments contain malignant lymph nodes
4.	The posterior cervical nodes (Level V) are dissected only when there is a clinically positive level V lymph node or when there is extensive adenopathy in Level II, III, or IV
5.	The superior mediastinal lymph nodes (Level VII) are dissected only when there is a clinically positive level VII lymph node or when there is extensive adenopathy in Level IV or VI
6.	There is almost no indication for a thoracotomy to resect mediastinal adenopathy from DTC
7.	A neck dissection extends the surgical scar up the side of the neck

forms of thyroid cancer, the only one in which a lymph node compartment is electively dissected is medullary carcinoma where the nodes of the anterior central compartment (Level VI) are removed. The main principles regarding neck dissection in patients with differentiated thyroid cancer are explained in the remainder of this chapter and summarized in Table 2.

A CLINICALLY POSITIVE NODE IS THE INDICATION FOR NECK NODE COMPARTMENT DISSECTION

Dissection of a neck node compartment is performed whenever there is a clinically positive or highly suspicious lymph node. In our center this means finding a lymph node that is palpably abnormal prior to or during the thyroidectomy. We do not routinely obtain CT or MR preoperatively but do perform a careful ultrasound examination of the neck to detect abnormal cervical lymph nodes prior to surgery.

LEVELS II-IV ARE DISSECTED IN AN ALL OR NONE FASHION

The options are to remove only the nodes that are palpably abnormal (i.e., a node "pluck") or to systematically remove all the lymph nodes in a lymph node compartment that contains a positive lymph node (Noguchi 1998). Our policy is to dissect levels II, III, and IV (selective neck dissection) in an all or none fashion, meaning if one area needs to have all the lymph nodes removed on the basis of finding one or more positive lymph nodes, then lymph nodes in all three levels are resected.

DISSECTION OF NODES IN LEVEL I, V OR VII

Our policy is to *not* dissect compartment levels I or V for thyroid cancer unless lymph nodes in these levels are suspicious or have been preoperatively identified as malignant or the volume of adenopathy in level II–IV is extensive (Qubain 2002; Wada 2003). We do not dissect level VII lymph nodes, which are those in the superior mediastinum, unless they are clinically positive or suspicious. In some cases a preoperative MR or CT scan (without intravenous contrast) is done to evaluate the extent of mediastinal disease. When dissecting level VII nodes, the approach is transcervical and guided by dissection along the adventitia of each carotid artery until the lymph nodes approach the arch of the aorta. Care must be taken not to damage the innominate vein in this location.

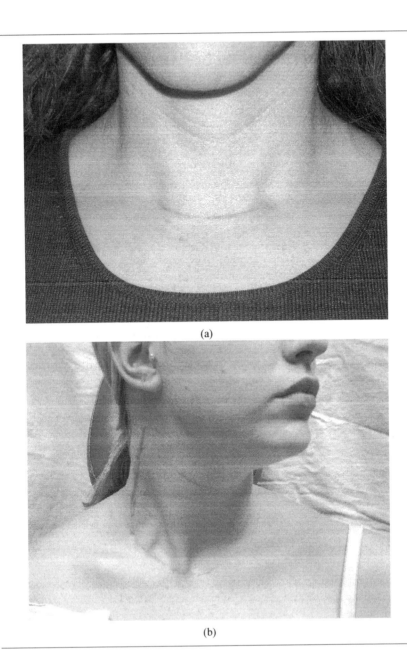

(a)

(b)

Figure 2. Neck scar with and without dissection of the level II–IV nodes. A thyroidectomy results in a relatively small scar that eventually blends in with the skin folds (A). Dissection of the jugular lymphatics (Level II–IV) +/− Level V results in a scar that extends up the neck to the angle of the mandible (B). If bilateral neck dissections are done, there will be a scar and the associated subcutaneous fibrosis on both sides of the neck.

In our opinion there is almost no indication for a thoracotomy to remove mediastinal nodes in thyroid cancer. We rely on radiotherapy and radioiodine therapy to control mediastinal disease that can not be removed with a transcervical dissection. Exceptions to this are massive mediastinal adenopathy especially if the trachea or large vessels are being invaded by tumor or are seriously compressed by lymph node metastases.

THE IMPLICATION OF A NECK DISSECTION FOR THE PATIENT

The risks of thyroid cancer surgery are the subject of the next chapter. The result of adding a neck dissection to the thyroidectomy procedure is a longer surgical scar and an increased risk of complications. In this chapter we will focus on the difference in the length of the surgical scar, as this is a factor that affects all patients who undergo dissection of the jugular nodes (level II–IV).

A thyroidectomy and level VI dissection, with or without a level VII (mediastinal) lymph node dissection can usually be done through a relatively small incision that is limited to the region of the thoracic inslet (Fig. 2A). This kind of incision usually blends with the normal skin folds and after a year is barely noticeable.

Dissection of the lateral or posterior neck compartments (levels II, III, IV, or V) requires enlarging the incision such that the patient will have a scar extending down the side of the neck (Fig. 2B). The superior extent of the neck dissection incision that includes level II is usually near the mastoid tip. If bilateral level II–IV neck dissections are done, the patient will have scars on both sides of the neck.

Extending the neck dissection to include levels II, III, IV, or V means that the patient will live with the cosmetic consequences of a long neck scar. There is always some degree of subcutaneous fibrosis around a surgical incision. Most patients who undergo a level II, III, IV, or V dissection have a degree of stiffness and discomfort in their neck that is not seen in patients who have only a thyroidectomy and level VI dissection. We do not recommend elective node dissection in patients with differentiated thyroid cancer for these reasons and because there is no evidence that prophylactic lateral compartment dissection is more efficacious than treatment with I-131 alone, when microscopic lymph nodes metastases are present.

REFERENCES

Bononi, M, A Tocchi, V Cangemi, A Vecchione, MR Giovagnoli, A De Cesare, et al. 2004. Lymph node dissection in papillary or follicular thyroid carcinoma. Anticancer Res **24(4):**2439–2442.

Noguchi, M, T Kumaki, T Taniya, M Segawa, T Nakano, N Ohta, et al. 1990. Impact of neck dissection on survival in well-differentiated thyroid cancer: a multivariate analysis of 218 cases. Int Surg **75:**220–224.

Noguchi, S, N Murakami, H Yamashita, M Toda, and H Kawamoto. 1998. Papillary thyroid carcinoma— modified radical neck dissection improves prognosis. Arch Surg **133:**276–280.

Randolph, G (ed). 2002. Surgery of the Thyroid and Parathyroid Glands, 1st ed. W.B. Saunders Company.

Wada, N, QY Duh, K Sugino, H Iwasaki, K Kameyama, T Mimura, et al. 2003. Lymph node metastasis from 259 papillary thyroid microcarcinomas: frequency, pattern of occurrence and recurrence, and optimal strategy for neck dissection. Ann Surg **237(3):**399–407.

4.3. POTENTIAL COMPLICATIONS OF THYROID CANCER SURGERY

DOUGLAS B. VILLARET, MD, ROBERT J. AMDUR, MD AND
ERNEST L. MAZZAFERRI, MD, MACP

The close proximity of important normal structures makes removal of the thyroid a technically demanding operation in the best of circumstances (Fig. 1). When tumor extends beyond the thyroid gland, cancer removal may require resection of normal structures in a way that is sure to result in permanent functional loss (Weissler 1995; Zarnegar 2003). In our opinion, a gross total tumor resection is such an important goal in thyroid cancer that predictable functional problems should be viewed as expected outcomes rather than unexpected complications in patients with locally advanced disease. The location of the thyroid gland explains the problems that may develop as a result of thyroid cancer surgery (Table 1).

THE RECURRENT LARYNGEAL NERVE

The most common complication of thyroidectomy is damage to the recurrent laryngeal nerve. Temporary weakness in a recurrent laryngeal nerve is common. The chance of permanent damage to the nerve is approximately 2%.

It is easy to damage the recurrent laryngeal nerve during a thyroidectomy because the nerve lies against the posterior surface of the gland and close to the inferior thyroid artery (Fig. 2). The thyroidectomy procedure requires ligation of the inferior thyroid artery, removal of as much thyroid tissue as possible, and separation of the parathyroid glands from the posterior surface of the thyroid. To accomplish these goals the surgeon must dissect the tissues immediately surrounding the thyroid gland to identify the recurrent laryngeal nerve. The nerve is then traced to its distal end where it penetrates the area behind the cricothyroid joint. The gland is then pulled medially away from the nerve.

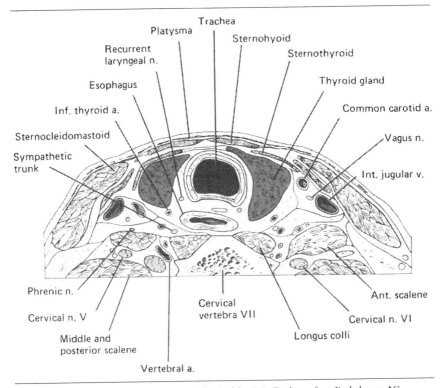

Figure 1. Axial section through the neck at the level of the C-7. (Redrawn from Eycleshymer AC, Schoemaker DM: A cross-section anatomy. New York, D. Appleton-Century, 1938:55).

Retraction injury of the nerve usually causes temporary loss in vocal cord mobility that may take months to resolve. Transection of the nerve or a severe compression injury causes permanent and complete vocal cord paralysis. The literature is still controversial, but it seems that re-aligning the severed ends of the nerve prevents atrophy of the vocalis muscle thereby preserving voice quality.

Loss of function of one recurrent laryngeal nerve results in a breathy voice. In the immediate post-operative period, there may also be a risk of aspiration. Over time, the patient's voice may improve by the compensatory over-rotation of the functional vocal cord. Should this not occur, the paralyzed cord could be physically pushed into place with a second surgery (Thyroplasty or injection augmentation), which generally results in a near-normal voice.

Loss of function of both recurrent laryngeal nerves increases the risk of aspiration even though the vocal cords usually end up opposed to one another. This configuration may easily confuse the clinician as the voice may sound normal due to the juxtaposition of the anterior vocal cords. Unfortunately, this also severely limits the area for respiration,

Table 1. Potential Complications of Thyroid Cancer Surgery.

Structure Injured	Incidence of Symptomatic Problems*
All Possible	No adenopathy or extrathyroidal tumor extension: Temporary: 10% Permanent: 2% Extensive adenopathy or extrathyroidal tumor extention: Temporary: 75% Permanent: 20%
Recurrent Laryngeal Nerve	Hoarseness Temporary: 30% Permanent: 2%
Parathyroid Glands	Hypoparathyroidism Temporary: 5% Permanent: 0.5%
Spinal Accessory Nerve	Shoulder weakness +/− pain Only with Level II/V dissection Rare with negative level II or V nodes. With clinically positive level II or V nodes: Temporary: 50% Permanent: 25%
Superior Laryngeal Nerve	Change in voice capability Incidence unknown. Usually symptomatic only in professional voice users
Vagus Nerve	Permanent Hoarseness: 0.5% (higher with extrathyroid tumor extension)
Trachea	Rare in the absence of extensive invasion by tumor
Esophagus	Rare in the absence of extensive invasion by tumor
Carotid Artery	Rare in the absence of invasion by tumor
Thoracic Duct	Rare in the absence of dissection of level IV, VI, or VII

* These incidence values are generalizations that may be major underestimates in specific situations.

resulting in a critical airway with the least amount of swelling. A tracheostomy can be avoided by widening the posterior glottis with laser surgery.

THE PARATHYROID GLANDS

Hypoparathyroidism is the second most common complication of thyroidectomy. The risk of temporary hypoparathyroidism following routine thyroidectomy is approximately 5%. The risk of permanent hypoparathyroidism is approximately 0.5%.

The parathyroid glands produce parathyroid hormone which stimulates the release of calcium from the bones, the reabsorption of calcium in the kidneys and the synthesis of vitamin D. The number and exact location of the parathyroid glands are variable. Most people have 4–6 glands that are either imbedded in the posterior surface of the thyroid or in the connective tissue immediately adjacent to the posterior surface of the gland (Fig. 3).

A potential complication of thyroidectomy is hypoparathyroidism because removing the thyroid may require removal of the parathyroid glands (intrathyroidal parathyroids) or interruption of the blood supply to the parathyroids that remain in place. The blood supply of most parathyroids is through the inferior thyroid artery. Indelicate

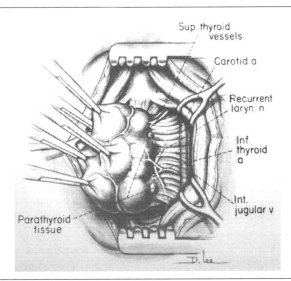

Figure 2. Artist illustration of the relationship of the recurrent laryngeal nerve to the posterior surface of the thyroid, the parathyroid glands, and the inferior thyroid artery. (From Dozois RR, Beahrs OH: Surgical anatomy and technique of the thyroid and parathyroid surgery. Surg Clin North Am 57:647–661, 1977. Reproduced with permission from Elsevier, Inc.)

handling of the terminal branches of this artery may compromise the vascularity of all the parathyroid glands. When the surgeon knows that a parathyroid has been separated from its blood supply the gland is minced and implanted into either the sternocleidomastoid or brachioradialis muscle. The gland pieces, now with a higher surface area to volume ratio, usually develop a secondary blood supply and resume hormone production in 3 months.

The Superior Laryngeal Nerve

The frequency of damage of the superior laryngeal nerve during thyroidectomy is probably higher than what is reported in the literature or realized in general clinical practice. Descending from the inferior vagal ganglion and passing deep to the carotid artery, the superior laryngeal nerve joins the superior thyroid artery in its course to the larynx. The internal branch then travels through the thyrohyoid membrane to supply sensation to the supraglottic larynx. The external branch passes in close proximity to the superior pole of the thyroid gland before supplying the motor innervation to the cricothyroid muscle. It is at the superior pole that the external branch is most susceptible to damage. The cricothyroid is a tensor of the larynx and its dysfunction is usually only noted in professional voice users who notice a decrease in their ability to reach higher pitches.

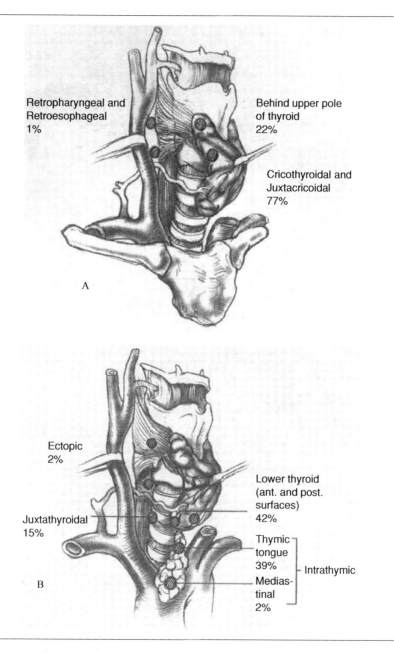

Figure 3. Usual locations of the superior (A) and inferior (B) parathyroid glands. (Fig. 14–1 in Weissler MC and Pillsbury HC, Editors. Complications of head and neck surgery. Thieme Medical Publishers, Inc, 1995. Reproduce with permission from Thieme Medical Publishers, Inc.).

The Vagus Nerve

The vagus nerve lies in the connective tissue between the internal jugular vein and carotid artery (Fig. 1). Damage to this nerve may occur if the cervical nodes need to be dissected or when there is direct extension of thyroid cancer into the tissues surrounding the nerve. Damage to the vagus nerve results in hoarseness. Tachycardia and gastroparesis do not develop unless there is damage to both vagus nerves.

THE SPINAL ACCESSORY NERVE (CRANIAL NERVE XI)

Spinal accessory nerve damage is rare in thyroid cancer surgery because most patients do not have adenopathy in the most superior portion of the level II or V node stations (neck dissection issues are the subject of the previous chapter). When adenopathy in these regions is present the surgeon must retract or cut the spinal accessory nerve. The spinal accessory nerve innervates the trapezius muscle that is required to lift the arm above the horizontal plane. Damage to the spinal accessory nerve results in two problems: inability to lift the arm above the shoulder and shoulder pain. The mechanism of the pain that accompanies spinal accessory nerve damage is not well understood but it is often quite severe. When the spinal accessory nerve is stretched it is not unusual for patients to have shoulder pain and weakness for 1–6 months following the procedure. When the nerve must be resected, weakness and discomfort are likely to be permanent problems.

The Trachea

The posterior surface of the thyroid gland lies against the anterior surface of the trachea (Fig. 1). When thyroid cancer involves the posterior aspect of the gland it is not unusual for tumor to be adherent to, or directly invade, the tracheal wall. When this is the case the surgeon must resect a portion of the trachea. There are a variety of procedures for repairing tracheal defects. If the area of resection is small (≤ 1 cm) tracheal stenosis or other problems are rare. If the defect is larger, or if an entire segment of trachea must be resected, then the chance of airway complications increases. Multiple surgical reconstructions are possible, but recurrent laryngeal nerve damage and tracheal stenosis present a very real possibility.

The Esophagus

The lateral portions of the thyroid wrap posteriorly around the trachea and come close to the lateral surface of the esophagus (Fig. 1). There is usually connective tissue separating the thyroid from the esophagus such that esophageal damage is rare unless tumor extends beyond the thyroid capsule in this area. When tumor involves the esophagus a portion or segment of the esophagus is resected and the area reconstructed. As with the trachea, the functional outcome depends of the extent of the esophagus that must be removed.

The Carotid Artery

The carotid artery is almost never involved with thyroid cancer, either by direct invasion of the primary tumor or by extracapsular spread of metastatic tumors in lymph nodes.

Unless tumor completely encases the carotid artery it is possible to resect all gross tumor with a low (~1%) chance of a carotid laceration or thrombosis. When encasement of the carotid artery is extensive an aggressive resection is associated with a substantial risk of carotid damage.

The Thoracic Duct

The thoracic duct is rarely injured in performing a total thyroidectomy. It originates in the mediastinum, passes posterior to the arch of the aorta and the venous drainage, and generally empties into the junction of the internal jugular and brachiocephalic vein. This occurs on the left side of the neck. The right side also has lymphatic ducts from the mediastinum, but they are of lesser caliber. When performing a low neck dissection for thyroid cancer, the thoracic duct may be injured in either level IV or level VI. When noticed intraoperatively, it may be found and ligated. If it persists, the patient must have pressure dressings and be placed on a medium chain triglyceride diet until the leak resolves. Occasionally, the patient must return to the operating room for exploration.

Thyroid Hormone Replacement and Wound Healing

Some surgeons feel strongly that patients should be maintained on thyroid hormone replacement for at least a month following thyroidectomy to promote wound healing. This policy extends the time between surgery and radioiodine therapy and increases the complexity of the overall treatment package when the patient is to be prepared for I-131 therapy by withdrawing thyroid hormone. Data on the effect of hypothyroidism on wound healing in this setting are scarce. Experimental work performed in animal models has shown delayed wound healing in the hypothyroid state due to decreased levels of collagen type IV and hydroxyproline in the proliferative phase as well as a delay or imbalance in the synthesis of proteins involved in the assembly of sarcomeres. Human data comes from patients made hypothyroid in the treatment of head and neck cancer where surgery involves resection of portions of the upper aerodigestive track. In this setting it has been shown that wound complication rates can double when the patients are hypothyroid.

In our opinion delaying thyroid hormone replacement for a few months following surgery does not increase the rate of wound complications. When we plan to use levothyroxine (T4) deprivation to prepare a patient for I-131 therapy we start patients on T3 immediately postoperatively but we do not put patients on T4. Our preference is to refer patients for I-131 therapy no sooner than 4 weeks after surgery. If the patient is going to be prepared for radioiodine therapy by depriving them of thyroid hormone then thyroid hormone replacement will not be started until a few days after radioiodine therapy (usually 6–8 weeks after surgery). If the patient is going to be prepared for radioiodine therapy with recombinant human thyroid stimulating hormone (Thyrogen®) then the patient is started on T4 replacement soon after surgery. If the decision to use Thyrogen was made preoperatively, T4 replacement is started on the first postoperative day. Otherwise T4 replacement is started after I-131 therapy (usually 2–4 weeks after surgery).

REFERENCE

Weissler, MC, and HC Pillsbury (eds). 1995. Complications of Head and Neck Surgery. Thieme Medical Publishers Inc.

PART 5. MEDICAL THERAPY OF DIFFERENTIATED THYROID CANCER

PART 5A. BACKGROUND INFORMATION AND PROCESS ADMINISTRATION

5A.1. HALF-LIFE AND EMISSION PRODUCTS OF I-131

ROBERT J. AMDUR, MD AND ERNEST L. MAZZAFERRI, MD, MACP

THE HALF-LIFE OF I-131

The half-life of a radioactive isotope is the time it takes for the isotope to decrease in activity by 50%. There are three kinds of half-life that should be considered when radioactive iodine is used to study or treat a patient with thyroid cancer. The Physical Half-life is the time it takes for the amount of radioiodine to decrease by 50% purely as a result of radioactive decay. The Biologic Half-life is the time it takes for the amount of radioiodine in a person's body to decrease by 50% purely as a result of the excretion of iodine in the sweat, saliva, feces, and urine. In the thyroid gland or in thyroid cancers the Biologic Half-life is mainly determined by the time that the isotope remains in the normal or malignant follicular cell. The Effective Half-Life is the combination of the effects of radioactive decay and physiologic excretion. How the three types of half-lives interact to provide a therapeutic effect of I-131 in patients with differentiated thyroid carcinoma is shown in Fig. 1A. A short Effective half-life of I-131 in the thyroid follicular cell or thyroid tumor cell is the main reason for failure of I-131 therapy (Maxon 1983). This can be altered by lithium (Fig. 1B).

Table 1 presents the physical, biologic, and effective half-life of I-131. The values for biologic and effective half-life are different for the thyroid and extrathyroidal compartment because thyroid follicle cells normally concentrate iodine to a much greater degree than many other tissues (Kreiakes 1980). We will discuss several of these numbers

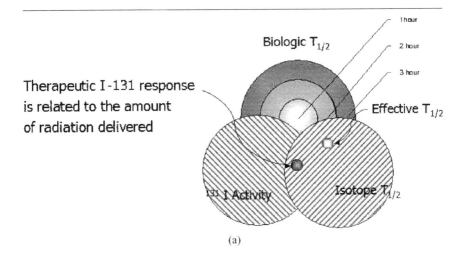

Therapeutic I-131 response
is related to the amount
of radiation delivered

(a)

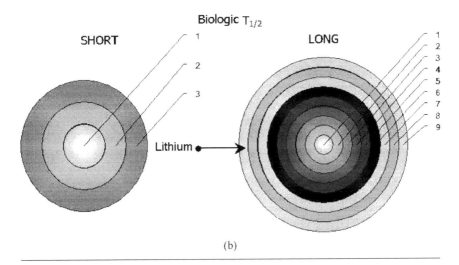

(b)

Figure 1. The interaction between the biologic half-life, effective half-life and isotope half-life in the I-131 treatment of differentiated thyroid carcinoma (A). Alteration of the biologic half-life by lithium (B).

Table 1. Half-Life of I-131.

	I-131 Biologic half-life		I-131 Effective half-life	
I-131 Physical Half-life	Normal Thyroid compartment	Extrathyroidal compartment	Thyroid compartment	Extrathyroidal compartment
8 days	80 days	12 days	7.3 days	8 hours

in more detail in subsequent chapters. They are presented here because it is useful to have a reference where all the relevant half-lives are presented in the same table.

RADIOACTIVE DECAY PRODUCTS OF I-131

The particles that are emitted as a result of radioactive decay of an isotope determine the potential usefulness of that isotope in the diagnosis and treatment of disease. Figure 2 presents the decay scheme for I-131, which is produced by the fission of uranium atoms during operation of nuclear reactors or during detonation of a nuclear bomb. I-131 decays to Xenon-131 (ICRP 1987). The mechanism of transformation is called "beta decay" because a neutron is converted to a proton and an electron. For readers that are not familiar with this subject, "electron" and "beta particle" are synonyms.

The first emission product is an electron with a range in energy between 250–800 keV. It is this product that makes I-131 useful for ablating normal thyroid tissue and treating differentiated thyroid cancers. Electrons in this energy range usually travel less than a millimeter before depositing their energy and causing an ionization event. This means that most of the damage from the electrons produced from the decay of I-131 occurs in the cells in which the I-131 is concentrated. This is exactly what we want to happen when we use I-131 to treat thyroid disease.

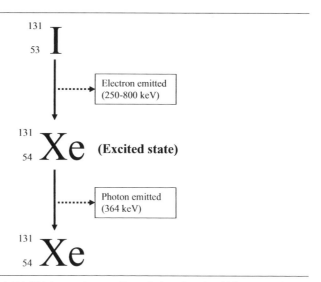

Figure 2. Decay scheme for I-131. This isotope decays to Xenon by beta decay in which a neutron is converted to a proton and an electron. The electron that is produced in this process is the primary mechanism by which I-131 damages residual thyroid tissue and thyroid cancer. Transition from an excited to the ground state of Xenon produces a 364 keV photon. It is this process that is the basis for the use of I-131 to image residual thyroid tissue and thyroid cancer.

The second decay product of I-131 is a moderate energy photon (364 keV). From the standpoint of treating thyroid disease this emission product is undesirable because it travels far from its source before depositing its energy and thus increases total body dose with relatively little impact on thyroid tissue. The value of the 364 keV photon emitted from the decay of I-131 is that it makes I-131 useful for diagnostic studies. In an iodine scan or uptake study it is the photons that are not attenuated by the patients body that are being counted or processed into diagnostic images.

5A.2. CHOOSING THE ACTIVITY OF I-131 FOR THERAPY

ROBERT J. AMDUR, MD AND ERNEST L. MAZZAFERRI, MD, MACP

The purpose of this chapter is to explain the three basic approaches that have been described to select the dose of I-131 for therapy. Table 1 summarizes the major points from this chapter.

Three dosimetry methods are available to treat patients with differentiated thyroid carcinoma, the fixed dose method that administers empiric fixed amounts of I-131 for different tumor stages, a dosimetry-guided technique that calculates the upper limits of a safe blood and whole body level of irradiation from I-131, and a dosimetry approach that calculates the radiation delivered by I-131 to a tumor site.

FIXED-DOSE EMPIRIC I-131 DOSIMETRY

The empiric fixed dose method is the most widely used and simplest to administer because of the technical and logistic problems associated with the other approaches. Thus most centers in the USA and Europe have adapted the fixed-dose or standard-dose technique for I-131 therapy.

The distinguishing feature of a fixed-dose regimen is that the amount of I-131 given for therapy is not based on individual measurements of radioiodine uptake or dosimetry studies. With this approach, an empiric amount of I-131 is administered regardless of the percentage I-131 uptake on diagnostic whole body scintigraphy or the percentage uptake of I-131 by the thyroid remnant or metastatic lesion. Although hospitalization was required in the United States in the past to administer I-131 activities larger than 30 mCi, it is no longer necessary as long as the exposure to the public is calculated to be less than 5.0 mSv (Brierley 1998). We use a fixed-dose

Table 1. Summary of the Four Main Approaches to Specifying Dose for Radioiodine Therapy.

Fixed-dose
The most common approach used in both academic and private practices
All patients with a given clinical situation get the same dose
Many different prescription programs are in common usage. Examples:
*   Use the same dose (usually 100 or 150 mCi) for all situations
*   Escalate the dose based on perceived risk: 30–50 mCi for low-risk remnant ablation, 150–175 mCi for recurrent tumor in the neck, 200 mCi for lung metastases

Quantitative Blood or Whole Body Dosimetry
Prescribes the dose that will result in the maximum acceptable level of toxicity
Focuses only on the acute tolerance of the bone marrow to a single administration
Measures total body counts 2, 24, 48, and 72 hours after a diagnostic dose of I-131
Whole blood limit set at 200 cGy with total body retention <120 mCi at 48 hours (48 hour retention required to be <80 mCi with diffuse pulmonary disease)
These dose limits ignore the effect of prior radioiodine administrations
Complex to measure to the point that it is only used at a few large medical centers

Quantitative Tumor Dosimetry
Prescribes the dose that delivers a set minimum absorbed dose to target tissue
Technique as for whole blood dosimetry with the addition of focal measurements
Target dose: 30,000 cGy to the thyroid remnant (80% success rate)
              8,000–12,000 cGy to nodal or soft tissue metastases (80% control rate).
Extreme complexity and questionable accuracy limit current use to a few institutions

Using RAIU to select the dose for remnant ablation
Uses Becker's formula to calculate the mCi of I-131 needed to deliver 30,000 cGy to the thyroid remnant
Requires an estimate of remnant size in addition to RAIU value
Outcome data limited and based on large remnants (hemithyroidectomy)
Results similar to fixed-dose prescription (∼100 mCi) following near total thyroidectomy

approach for the full range of clinical situations that one encounters in managing patients with thyroid cancer. Table 2 summarizes our approach to choosing I-131 activities for therapy.

THYROID REMNANT ABLATION

Remnant ablation can be achieved by either administering an empiric fixed amount of I-131 or by using dosimetry-guided techniques; however, because of the nature of the target tissue and the technical and logistic problems, most centers have adapted the fixed-dose or standard-dose technique for I-131 remnant ablation.

Multiple studies have compared the efficacy of various amounts of I-131 given to ablate a thyroid remnant (Table 3). A meta-analysis by (Doi 2000) that compared the efficacy of remnant ablation following a single low dose (29 to 30 mCi versus high dose (75–100 mCi) of I-131 found that the average failure rate of a single low dose was twice as high (46%) as that of a single high dose (27%). They estimated that for every seven patients treated, one more patient would have a successful ablation if given a high rather than a low dose Also, a significantly greater proportion of patients had successful ablation after a single high or low dose if they underwent near-total rather than subtotal thyroidectomy. However, the definitions of successful ablation differed among the studies.

Table 2. I-131 Dose Prescription Guidelines Following (near) Total Thyroidectomy.

For the first I-131 treatment following total thyroidectomy[1]:		
Low risk	Stage[2] T1N0M0	30–50 mCi
Standard risk	All situations that do not qualify as low or high-risk	150 mCi
High risk	Stage[2] T4 or M1 or any situation where there is known residual disease (e.g., a positive margin or a residual positive node by imaging)	200 mCi
When there has been at least one prior I-131 treatment:		
No visible disease	Elevated thyroglobulin is the only evidence of disease	150 mCi
Gross disease, positive margin, or distant metastasis	Positive surgical margin or disease that is visible on imaging	200 mCi

Lithium Carbonate[3]:
Lithium is used in all patients unless there is a specific contraindication

Preparation with rhTSH instead of T4 deprivation[3]:
We prefer to use rhTSH in all situations except: children, lack of insurance coverage, or patient preference for T4 deprivation

I-131 therapy in children[3]:
Dose prescriptions are not standardized to the degree that they are in adults. In children who are well below adult size and stage of development we usually prescribe an amount of I-131 adjusted by the child's total body surface area that makes it comparable to that given to an adult (see chapter on treatment of lung metastases)
As with adults, we use lithium in all cases unless there are specific contraindications to its use
We do not use rhTSH in children unless there are major contraindications to making the patient hypothyroid

---

[1] This includes situations where the goal is to ablate the thyroid remnant.
[2] 6th edition of the AJCC staging system.
[3] Seperate chapters are devoted to these topics.

In the prospective study by (Zidan 2004), 238 patients with papillary or follicular carcinoma were treated with I-131 based on the percentage of neck uptake in the postoperative thyroid scans. Complete ablation, defined as absent uptake on neck I-131 scintigraphy at follow-up, was observed in 92% to 96% of patients receiving between 30 and 85 mCi.

In another randomized prospective study in 63 patients, Johansen et al. were unable to demonstrate a difference in the efficacy of low- and high-dose I-131 (29 mCi vs 100 mCi) for remnant ablation using neck scintigraphic uptake as the endpoint. However, thyroglobulin levels were elevated in 40% of the patients who had achieved successful ablation with low I-131 doses and in 44% treated with high doses.

In the prospective randomized study by Bal et al. (1996), 149 patients were divided into four groups treated with incremental amounts of I-131 ranging from 25 to 200 mCi. Six months to 1 year after treatment, successful ablation was defined as the absence of thyroid bed activity on a 5 mCi diagnostic whole body scan, along with neck uptake of <0.2% and a thyroglobulin value of <10 ng/mL. Complete ablation was achieved in 63% of the 30 mCi group and approximately 78% in all of the higher dose groups, indicating that an amount of I-131 between 25 and 50 mCi was optimal for remnant ablation.

Table 3. Studies Comparing Different Amounts of I-131 to Ablate the Thyroid Remnant.

Author	I-131 Dose (mCi)	Patients (n)	Successful Ablation (%)	Criteria for Ablation
McCowen 1976	30	36	NA*	I-131 scintigraphy
	80–100	28	NA*	
DeGroot 1982	26–30	18	83	I-131 scintigraphy
	47–53	21	100	
	60	9	100	
Ramacciotti 1982	30	20	40	I-131 scintigraphy
	50	10	30	
	75	14	71	
Johansen 1991	29	36	81	I-131 scintigraphy
	100	37	84	
Mazzaferri & Jhiang 1994	29–59	59	NA†	NA†
	51–100	79	NA†	NA†
Hodgson 1998	29	20	80	I-131 scintigraphy
	50	5	80	
	75	1	100	
	100	1	0	
Bal 1996	30	27	63	I-131 scintigraphy
	51	54	78	RAIU‡ Tg
	87	38	74	
	155	30	78	
Bal 2004	15	47	60	I-131 scintigraphy
	20	55	63	RAIU‡ Tg
	25	70	81	
	30	73	84	
	35	63	79	
	40	60	78	
	45	64	84	
	50	77	82	
Zidan 2004	85	43	92	I-131 scintigraphy
	80	33	94	
	60	41	95	
	50	55	93	
	30	39	94	
			96	

* No data concerning successful ablation rate, relapse-free and actuarial survival rates equal in both groups.
† No data concerning ablation rate, but recurrence rates equal in both groups.
‡ RAIU is thyroidal I-131 uptake.

A subsequent study by Bal et al. (2004, Table 3) randomized 565 patients into eight groups and administered I-131 in 5 mCi increments between 15 and 50 mCi. This study found that after 6 months to 1 year, using the same criteria for complete remnant ablation as employed previously, remnant ablation was achieved by one dose of I-131 in almost 78% of the patients. The ablation rate was statistically lower (62%) in patients receiving less than 25 mCi of 131-I compared with those receiving at least 25 mCi (82%). There was no significant intergroup difference in outcome among patients receiving 25–50 mCi. Patients with small tumor size (≤5 cm), adequate surgery (total or near-total thyroidectomy), and radioiodine neck uptake of 10% or less had odds ratios of 2.4 [CI, 1.3–3.98], 2.6 (CI, 1.6–4.2), and 2.2 (CI, 1.4–3.5), respectively, for successful remnant ablation. Patients receiving at least 25 mCi of I-131 had a three times better chance of achieving successful remnant ablation than did patients receiving smaller doses. These studies suggest that an I-131 dose of 25–50 mCi is adequate to ablate the thyroid remnant after near total thyroidectomy. Still, these studies would be even more convincing had a 2 ng/mL Tg cutoff been used.

MAXIMUM RADIATION DOSE TO THE BLOOD AND BONE MARROW

The second approach to treating differentiated thyroid carcinoma with I-131 is to use quantitative dosimetry methods to deliver maximal radiation doses to the thyroid remnant or metastases while maintaining acceptable levels of whole body radiation to nontarget tissues, especially the bone marrow and lungs when there are diffuse metastases. With the technique for measuring whole body and blood dosimetry described by Benua et al. (1962), the dose of I-131 is based upon total body counts at 2, 24, 48, and 72 hours following the administration of a diagnostic dose of I-131. The I-131 dose is calculated to deliver a maximum of 200 rads (2 Gy) to the whole blood while keeping the whole body retention less than 120 mCi at 48 hours, or less than 80 mCi when there is diffuse pulmonary uptake or diffuse bone metastases. Some limit the maximum administered dose to 300 mCi (Benua 1962). In a more recent study (Dorn 2003) in which up to 300 rads (3 Gy) were delivered to the bone marrow, all patients developed transient bone marrow suppression that was severe enough in four to require hospitalization. Five patients with lung micrometastases had a Tg <1 ng/mL after treatment, but whether this could have been achieved with lower I-131 activities is uncertain.

MAXIMAL RADIATION DOSES TO TUMOR FOCI

The most comprehensive approach to using I-131 therapeutically is based on quantitative tumor dosimetry as described by Maxon et al. (1992). The procedure is the same as that used to measure blood dosimetry with the addition of cone down measurements of the thyroid remnant or individual tumor deposits. The calculation of the amount of I-131 to administer is based on a target dose of 30,000 cGy to the thyroid remnant (80% success rate) and 8,000-12,000 cGy to nodal or soft tissue metastases (80% control rate).

Lesional dosimetry is favored by some because radiation exposure from arbitrarily fixed doses of I-131 can vary considerably. If the calculated lesional dose is less than 3,500 rads (35 Gy) when reaching radiation limits in non-target tissues, it is unlikely that the tumor will respond to I-131 therapy (Maxon 1992; Brierley 1998). On the other hand, I-131 activities that will deliver 30,000 rads (300 Gy) to the residual thyroid remnant or 8,000 to 12,000 rads (80 to 120 Gy) to metastatic foci are likely to be effective. To make these calculations, however, it is necessary to estimate tumor size, which is difficult in many situations.

LIMITATIONS TO CHOOSING THE METHOD THAT DELIVERS THE OPTIMAL AMOUNT OF I-131 FOR THERAPY

Using fixed empiric amounts of I-131 is the easiest means of treating patients with differentiated thyroid carcinoma. Yet this is clearly the most arbitrary method of selecting therapy that has the potential to under treat some patients while over treating others.

It also assumes that we know the optimal empiric dose of I-131 to treat metastases in various locations. Empiric therapy is based on experience rather than careful therapeutic trials. Still, the general experience is that this method is safe when used by experts and does result in good therapeutic responses in patients with distant metastases.

Dosimetry is complicated and is performed in a limited number of large medical centers that have a dedicated team of physicists, nuclear medicine technologists and physicians with thyroid cancer expertise. It is often reserved for patients with distant metastases or unusual circumstances such as concurrent renal failure. Comparison of outcomes between empiric fixed dose methods and dosimetric approaches is difficult and unreliable. Moreover, prospective randomized trials to address the optimal therapeutic approach have not been done (Van Nostrand 2002). Those in favor of high dose therapy cite the positive relationship between the total I-131 uptake per tumor mass and outcome (Maxon 1983), but this has not been confirmed (Schlumberger 1998; Samuel 1998).

The other problem with dosimetry studies that deliver large amounts of I-131 is that acute bone marrow toxicity is not the only dose-limiting toxicity from radioiodine therapy. Severe damage to the salivary glands, lacrimal ducts, gonads, and other organs occur with the large single dose administrations that often result from quantitative dosimetry calculations. There is also the issue of cumulative damage from multiple radioiodine administrations, which is not taken into account in calculations based on a single administration limit of 200 cGy.

Our opinion of quantitative blood dosimetry is that it is an important approach that may be of value in certain situations where the risk of acute bone marrow suppression from conventional-dose radioiodine therapy is likely to be unusually high (e.g., a patient with compromised bone marrow reserve and renal insufficiency). However, we are not comfortable using the results from blood dosimetry measurements to escalate the dose of radioiodine. We use lithium to potentiate the effect of standard doses of I-131.

USING RAIU TO SELECT THE DOSE FOR REMNANT ABLATION

In the final section of this chapter we describe the use of the standard thyroid uptake measurement (also called Radioactive Iodine Uptake, RAIU) for determining the dose of radioiodine for remnant ablation. This is the approach described by Zidan et al. (2004) who used a mathematical model called "Becker's formula" to determine the activity of I-131 that would deliver 30,000 cGy to the thyroid remnant. The variables that are needed for this calculation include RAIU (measured prior to therapy), remnant weight (estimated from the operative note or scan (or better done by ultrasonography) at the time of RAIU, and effective half-life of radioiodine (standard values used). The authors report a >90% success rate for remnant ablations based on a negative diagnostic scan six months after therapy (Table 3).

Our opinion of this approach is that it warrants further study but we do not use it because the great majority of patients in the Zindan et al. study had large thyroid remnants (RAIU >10%), which we preferentially treat with completion thyroidectomy. The RAIU values that we typically see after a near total thyroidectomy are well below 5%, which would result in an I-131 activity of 80–100 mCi using Becker's formula. These values are similar to the doses used in many programs that empirically treat thyroid remnant or metastases with fixed I-131 activities. Another issue is the general problem of reaching conclusions about the efficacy of radioiodine therapy based on a negative nuclear medicine scan. An extremely low thyroglobulin level (probably <2 ng/mL) in the presence of a negative radioiodine scan and/or RAIU <0.2% is the ideal standard for evaluating the success of radioiodine therapy.

REFERENCES

Bal, CS, A Kumar, and GS Pant. 2004. Radioiodine dose for remnant ablation in differentiated thyroid carcinoma: a randomized clinical trial in 509 patients. J Clin Endocrinol Metab **89**:1666–1673.

Bal, C, AK Padhy, S Jana, GS Pant, and AK Basu. 1996. Prospective randomized clinical trial to evaluate the optimal dose of ^{131}I for remnant ablation in patients with differentiated thyroid carcinoma. Cancer **77**:2574–2580.

Benua, RS, NR Cicale, M Sonenberg, et al. 1962. The relation of radioiodine dosimetry to results and complications in the treatment of metastatic thyroid cancer. AJR **87**:171–178.

Brierley, J, and HR Maxon. 1998. Radioiodine and external radiation therapy. In: Thyroid Cancer. Boston/Dordrecht/London: Kluwer Academic Publishers (Fagin JA, ed) 285–317.

DeGroot, LJ, and M Reilly. 1982. Comparison of 30- and 50-mCi doses of iodine-131 for thyroid ablation. Ann Intern Med **96**:51–53.

Doi, SA, and NJ Woodhouse. 2000. Ablation of the thyroid remnant and ^{131}I dose in differentiated thyroid cancer. Clin Endocrinol (Oxford) **52**:765–773.

Dorn, R, J Kopp, H Vogt, P Heidenreich, RG Carroll, and SA Gulec. 2003. Dosimetry-guided radioactive iodine treatment in patients with metastatic differentiated thyroid cancer: largest safe dose using a risk-adapted approach. J Nucl Med **44**:451–456.

Hodgson, DC, JD Brierley, RW Tsang, and T Panzarella. 1998. Prescribing [131]iodine based on neck uptake produces effective thyroid ablation and reduced hospital stay. Radiother Oncol **47**:325–330.

Johansen, K, NJ Woodhouse, and O Odugbesan. 1991. Comparison of 1073 MBq and 3700 MBq iodine-131 in postoperative ablation of residual thyroid tissue in patients with differentiated thyroid cancer. J Nucl Med **32**:252–254.

Maxon, HR, EE Englaro, SR Thomas, VS Hertzberg, JD Hinnefeld, LS Chen, H Smith, D Cummings, and MD Aden. 1992. Radioiodine-131 therapy for well-differentiated thyroid cancer—a quantitative radiation dosimetric approach: outcome and validation in 85 patients. J Nucl Med **33**:1132–1136.

Maxon, HR, SR Thomas, VS Hertzberg, JG Kereiakes, IW Chen, MI Sperling, and EL Saenger. 1983. Relation between effective radiation dose and outcome of radioiodine therapy for thyroid cancer. N Engl J Med **309**:937–941.

Mazzaferri, EL, and SM Jhiang. 1994. Long-term impact of initial surgical and medical therapy on papillary and follicular thyroid cancer. Am J Med **97**:418–428.

McCowen, KD, RA Adler, N Ghaed, T Verdon, and FD Hofeldt. 1976. Low dose radioiodine thyroid ablation in postsurgical patients with thyroid cancer. Am J Med **61**:52–58.

Ramacciotti, C, HT Pretorius, BR Line, JM Goldman, and J Robbins. 1982. Ablation of nonmalignant thyroid remnants with low doses of radioactive iodine: concise communication. J Nucl Med **23**:483–489.

Samuel, AM, B Rajashekharrao, and DH Shah. 1998. Pulmonary metastases in children and adolescents with well-differentiated thyroid cancer. J Nucl Med **39**:1531–1536.

Schlumberger, MJ. 1998. Medical progress—papillary and follicular thyroid carcinoma. N Engl J Med **338**:297–306.

Van Nostrand, D, F Atkins, F Yeganeh, E Acio, R Bursaw, and L Wartofsky. 2002. Dosimetrically determined doses of radioiodine for the treatment of metastatic thyroid carcinoma. Thyroid **12**:121–134.

Zidan, J, E Hefer, G Iosilevski, K Drumea, ME Stein, A Kuten, and O Israel. 2004. Efficacy of I131 ablation therapy using different doses as determined by postoperative thyroid scan uptake in patients with differentiated thyroid cancer. Int J Radiat Oncol Biol Phys **59**:1330–1336.

5A.3. REQUIREMENTS FOR OUTPATIENT RELEASE FOLLOWING I-131 THERAPY

ROBERT J. AMDUR, MD, GEORGE SNYDER,
AND ERNEST L. MAZZAFERRI, MD, MACP

In May 1997, the United States Nuclear Regulatory Commission (NRC) regulations were revised in a way that permits outpatient I-131 therapy for cancer in most situations (NRC 1997). The purpose of this chapter is to explain the NRC release regulations in a way that is directly applicable to clinicians who manage patients with thyroid cancer.

CURRENT NRC REGULATIONS (REVISED IN MAY 1997)

Currently applicable NRC regulations related to the release of patients following I-131 administration are described in the NRC Regulatory Guide 8.39 (April 1997). A copy of this document may be found on the NRC web site. The current link to the actual document is included in the reference list at the end of this chapter.

The major change is that the 1997 revised regulations permit patients to be released from the control of the licensee (usually a hospital) if the Total Effective Dose Equivalent (TEDE) to any person as a result of contact with the treated individual is likely to be no greater than 500 mR. The innovative thing about the TEDE approach is that it takes into account the precautions that patients plan to take during the first few days following I-131 administration (Grigsby 2000). These regulations permit individuals who can isolate themselves from other people to be treated as an outpatient with doses of I-131 that would have required inpatient confinement prior to 1997.

THREE ABSOLUTE CONTRAINDICATIONS TO OUTPATIENT I-131 THERAPY

In our program we find it useful to establish release standards that are not mentioned in NRC regulations. Regardless of TEDE, or patient specific measurements, we do not deliver outpatient I-131 therapy in any of the following situations:

- The patient is unable to care for themselves
- The patient lives in a nursing home or communal living facility
- The patient prefers not to be released after taking I-131

CALCULATING TOTAL EFFECTIVE DOSE EQUIVALENT (TEDE)

NRC regulations permit patients to be released after receiving I-131 if the TEDE to other people is likely to be no greater than 500 mR. To determine if this condition will be met Regulatory Guide 8.39 presents an equation to calculate the expected TEDE to people who may come in contact with the person who has received I-131. The TEDE equation has three variables: The activity of I-131 that will be administered to the patient, the result of a thyroid uptake study, and a factor called the "occupancy factor", which takes into account the amount of time the treated individual will spend around other people during the first few days after receiving I-131.

Administered I-131 activity: This is the mCi of I-131 administered to the patient. Typical doses for cancer therapy are 50–250 mCi.

Thyroid uptake study: This study is described in a previous chapter. Basically, the patient is given a diagnostic dose of either I-123 or I-131 and then the percent of the activity that is retained in the thyroid bed is recorded at 2–24 hours after radioiodine administration. A typical result following near total thyroidectomy is 0.5–5%.

Occupancy factor: NRC regulations set the occupancy factor as either 0.25 or 0.75. The value to use is determined by how much contact the patient will have with other people during the first two days after receiving I-131. Basically, the occupancy factor is 0.25 when these five requirements are met for 2 days after the patient receives I-131:

- The patient will not use public transportation
- A pregnant woman or a child will not enter the patient's home
- The patient will not leave their home
- The patient will not touch another person or spend more than a few minutes in the same room with another person
- The patient will have sole use of a bathroom

If it is likely that any one of these requirements will not be met for 2 days after receiving I-131, then the TEDE must be calculated with an occupancy factor of 0.75.

To facilitate and document the evaluation of a patients eligibility for outpatient therapy we fill out a standardized questionnaire at the time of the clinic visit when we discuss the details of I-131 therapy. A version of our questionnaire is included below.

Table 1. Thyroid Uptake Values and I-131 Doses that Meet NRC Requirements for Outpatient Management*.

	Occupancy Factor 0.25	Occupancy Factor 0.75
Thyroid uptake	I-131 dose	I-131 dose
0.5%	295 mCi	165 mCi
1%	285 mCi	155 mCi
2%	265 mCi	138 mCi
3%	245 mCi	125 mCi
4%	230 mCi	113 mCi
5%	220 mCi	105 mCi
6%	208 mCi	97 mCi
7%	197 mCi	90 mCi
8%	187 mCi	84 mCi
9%	178 mCi	79 mCi
10%	171 mCi	74 mCi
11%	163 mCi	70 mCi
12%	157 mCi	67 mCi
13%	151 mCi	63 mCi
14%	145 mCi	60 mCi
15%	140 mCi	57 mCi

* These uptake-dose combinations result in a Total Effective Dose Equivalent of ≤ 500 mR based on the equation presented in NRC Regulatory Guide 8.39.

A TABLE SHOWING THE I-131 DOSES THAT CAN BE DELIVERED AS AN OUTPATIENT

Well in advance of the date of I-131 administration the physician must specify the dose of I-131 and determine if the patient will be treated as an outpatient. To make these decisions it is useful to have a table that shows the combinations of I-131 dose, thyroid uptake value, and occupancy factor that result in a TEDE of ≤ 500 mR using the equation described in NRC Regulatory Guide 8.39. Table 1 provides this information.

WE DO NOT PERMIT A PATIENT TO STAY IN A HOTEL FOR 3 DAYS AFTER RECEIVING I-131

In our practice we encounter the situation were a patient would like to stay in a hotel to meet the requirements for outpatient I-131 therapy. We prohibit patients from staying in a hotel for 3 days after receiving I-131 because it is difficult to control or monitor the people who may come in contact with the linen and objects that may have been contaminated with I-131.

THE REQUIREMENT TO GIVE THE PATIENT RADIATION SAFETY INSTRUCTIONS

NRC regulations require that a patient who is released following I-131 therapy be given written instructions on how to limit the dose to other individuals. The instructions that we send patients home with are included below.

YOUR HOSPITAL'S RELEASE REQUIREMENTS MAY BE STRICTER THAN NRC REGULATIONS

The final point to make is that the requirements that we explain in this chapter reflect only the standards presented in the NRC regulations. State governments and local institutions (hospitals) may establish standards that are more restrictive than those of the NRC. The relationship between these three entities is hierarchical- meaning that state regulations must be at least as restrictive as those of the NRC and local policy must be at least as restrictive as both federal and state regulations. For example, NRC regulations currently permit a patient who has received 150 mCi of I-131 to be released from the hospital when the TEDE to other people is likely to be ≤ 500 mR. Some state governments are uncomfortable with the TEDE approach and have established state regulations that prohibit the release of a patient whose total body I-131 activity is > 30 mCi or when the exposure at 1 meter from a patient is > 5 mR/hour. Similarly, some hospitals go beyond the "or" standard by establishing policy that requires that both of these requirements be met to release a patient following I-131 administration. The bottom line is that physicians who deliver I-131 need to know what the release policy is at the institution in which they deliver I-131 because such policy may be more restrictive than NRC or state government regulations.

A related issue that is confusing to people who are not familiar with the regulation of radioactive material is the role of state government in the process. A state may elect to take responsibility for regulating the use of radioactive material or it may leave this responsibility with the NRC. There are political and financial reasons that a state would want to take responsibility for this activity. To regulate the use of radioactive material a state must establish a formal relationship with the NRC in which the state agrees to apply regulations that are at least as restrictive as those of the NRC. States that establish this agreement, and thus regulation the use of I-131 through a state government agency, are called "Agreement States". Currently there are approximately 33 Agreement States.

QUESTIONNAIRE TO EVALUATE ELIGIBILITY FOR OUTPATIENT I-131 THERAPY

Patient's Name_____Today's Date _____

Physician prescribing I-131:_____Treatment Date _____

Dose: _____mCi of I-131   Thyroid Uptake value _____%

1. Do you need someone else to help you dress, eat, or go to the bathroom?   Y* N
2. Do you live in a nursing home or other communal living facility?   Y* N
3. a) Do you live with a pregnant woman?   Y N
   b) If yes, can she and you live in separate homes for 2 days after
      you receive I-131   Y N#
4. a) Are there children (< 19 years old) living with you?   Y N
   b) If yes, can you and the children live in separate homes for 2 days
      after receiving I-131?   Y N#
5. Can you get home after receiving I-131 without using public
   transportation?   Y N#
6. Are you able and willing to go straight home and not leave your home
   for 2 days after receiving I-131?   Y N#
7. Are you able and willing to make it so children and pregnant women
   do not enter the home that you will stay in for 2 days after you
   receive I-131?   Y N#
8. Are you able and willing to isolate yourself in your home so that you
   spend almost no time in the same room with another person and
   do not touch another person for 2 days after receiving I-131?   Y N#
9. Are you able and willing to arrange things so that you have sole use
   of a bathroom for 2 days after you receive I-131?   Y N#
10. Do you prefer to be admitted to the hospital for a few days after
    taking I-131?   Y* N

Patient signature _____ Date _____

---

* If the answer is YES to any of these questions, the patient may not be released until the I-131 activity has dropped below 30 millicuries or the dose rate at 1 meter is less than 500 mR/hr.

If the answer to all of these questions is YES, the Occupancy Factor used to calculate Total Effective Dose Equivalent is 0.25. If the answer to any of these questions is NO, the Occupancy Factor must be 0.75 and it may be appropriate to require inpatient confinement regardless of the TEDE calculation.

RADIATION EXPOSURE TO OTHER PEOPLE AFTER I-131 THERAPY

Patient name:_____Todays Date: _____

Date of I-131 administration:_____Dose of I-131 administered:_____

You have received I-131 for treatment of a medical condition. Show this document to anyone who is concerned about your radioactive exposure to other people. For questions contact: Dr. XXXXXXX or the doctor on-call, Phone XXX-XXX-XXXX

NO RADIATION SAFETY PRECAUTIONS ARE NECESSARY AFTER:

_____, 20_____

- Children and pregnant women should not enter your home for _____days
- Do not leave your home for _____days
- Isolate yourself in your home so that you spend almost no time in the same room with another person for _____days
- Try not to do anything that could transfer your saliva to another person, such as kissing or sharing food, for _____days
- Use disposable eating utensils for _____days
- Wash your bedding, towels, and laundry separately for _____days
- Do not work or volunteer outside the house for _____days
- Do not take public transportation for _____days
- Arrange things so that you have sole use of a bathroom for _____days
- Dispose of all tissues in the toilet for _____days.
- Flush the toilet twice after each use for _____days.
- Do not sleep with, or lay or sit next to, another person for _____days
- Do not have sexual relations with anyone for at least _____days
- Do not get pregnant or get someone pregnant for at least 1 year

REFERENCE

U.S. Nuclear Regulatory Commission Regulatory Guide 8.39. April 1997. Release of Patients Administered Radioactive Materials. This document may be accessed at: http://www.nrc.gov/reading-rm/doc-collections/reg-guides/occupational-health/active/8-39/08-039.pdf.

5A.4. A CHECKLIST OF THINGS TO DO AT THE CLINIC VISIT PRIOR TO I-131 THERAPY

ROBERT J. AMDUR, MD AND ERNEST L. MAZZAFERRI, MD, MACP

Optimal therapy with I-131 requires that the patient and managing physician accomplish a long list of tasks on a specific timeline. The rationale and details of specific tests, medications, and procedures are the subject of other chapters in this book. The purpose of this chapter is to summarize the list of things that the physician is responsible for doing weeks before the date of I-131 administration. In our program we schedule a separate clinic visit with the patient specifically to explain the I-131 protocol. At the time of this clinic visit we use the checklist shown in Table 1 to help us remember the main tasks that we need to accomplish to make the program work properly.

TASKS REQUIRED FOR ALL PATIENTS

Schedule a neck ultrasound if there is a question about the extent of thyroidectomy: The presence of a large thyroid remnant (>2 grams) or, gross deposits of thyroid cancer, changes management decisions. Our policy is to resect all gross thyroid tissue, and thyroid cancer (including malignant lymph nodes) whenever resection can be done without unacceptable morbidity. In our program we perform a neck ultrasound on all patients following thyroidectomy to be sure that we are not attempting to treat gross tumor, or a large volume of residual normal thyroid remnant tissue, with I-131.

Confirm NO history of Iodinated intravenous contrast in the past 6 months: Referring physicians may forget to mention or determine if the patient has recently undergone a radiographic study involving intravenous contrast containing iodine. A history of intravenous iodinated contrast means that the patient will need to wait at least 6 months before receiving I-131. The procedure for determining when a patient has metabolized

Table 1. Checklist of tasks to prepare the patient for I-131 therapy.

These tasks are required in all cases:
☐ If there is a question about the extent of thyroidectomy, schedule neck ultrasound
☐ Confirm NO history of Iodinated intravenous contrast in the past 6 months
☐ Explain potential complications and have the patient sign the consent document
☐ Record an order for the I-131 dose to be used in this patient
☐ Determine if inpatient confinement after I-131 is preferred or required
☐ If applicable, give the patient a prescription for blood draw for beta HCG
☐ Give the patient a prescription for Promethazine 25 mg PO q 6hr, #6
☐ Give the patient a prescription for Pilocarpine 5 mg PO TID, #15
☐ Instruct the patient to start the low-iodine diet 2 weeks prior to receiving I-131
☐ Give the patient information about where to report for the I-131
☐ Instruct the patient not to eat anything 4 hours before and 2 hours after taking I-131
☐ Explain and schedule the Total Body Scan, usually 5–7 days after administering I-131
☐ Schedule a clinic visit the day of, or a few days after, the Total Body Scan
☐ Schedule a follow-up appointment for 6 weeks after I-131 administration

If using lithium carbonate:
☐ Give the patient a prescription for lithium carbonate, usually 300 mg TID, #21
☐ Give the patient a prescription for, or schedule, a blood draw for lithium level

When using rhTSH to elevate TSH:
☐ Explain and record the dates of the two rhTSH injections
☐ Instruct the patient to stop taking T4 three days prior to receiving I-131

When using T4 deprivation to elevate TSH:
☐ Instruct the patient to stop T4 six weeks prior to recieving I-131
☐ Give the patient a prescription for Cytomel (T3), usually 25 MCG PO BID #42
☐ Give the patient a prescription for, blood draw for TSH PO 1 week before I-131 adminstration

When the patient will NOT be admitted to the hospital after receiving I-131:
☐ Schedule a visit with the radiation safety officer to approve outpatient precautions
☐ Schedule the thyroid uptake study ~1 week or 1 day before I-131 administration

When the patient will be admitted to the hospital after I-131:
☐ Schedule inpatient admission for the day of I-131 administration

the iodine received in an intravenous contrast study is the subject of a separate chapter.

Explain potential complications and have the patient sign the consent document: We find it useful to read through the consent document with the patient as part of the discussion about receiving I-131 therapy. Our consent document discusses both acute side-effects and potential long-term complications and includes instructions for how to minimize the risk of problems. The chart that is made up for the clinic visit contains two copies of the consent document. We give an unsigned copy to the patient to take home and keep a signed copy for our records.

Record an order for the I-131 dose to be used in this patient: The factors that determine the I-131 dose are discussed in other chapters. In our program the physician records the dose of I-131 as part of the paperwork that is initiated on the day the patient is seen in the clinic to explain I-131 therapy. The I-131 is scheduled to arrive a few days before the date of administration.

Determine if inpatient confinement after I-131 is preferred or required: The requirements for outpatient I-131 therapy are discussed in another chapter. We encourage patients to be treated as an outpatient whenever their living situation permits them to isolate themselves from other people for at least 2 days. We prefer to admit patients when young children or pregnant women will be in the house during the 2 days after I-131 administration even if the patient says that they will not have contact with them. Some patients prefer to be admitted even if they could comply with all required precautions. Since we do not perform a thyroid uptake study in patients who will be admitted after I-131 has been administered, and the radiation safety department needs lead time to prepare a hospital room, it is useful make the inpatient/outpatient decision early in the planning process.

If applicable, give the patient a prescription for blood draw for beta HCG: We require a pregnancy test (serum beta HCG) the week prior to I-131 administration in all women who have the potential to become pregnant.

Give the patient a prescription for an antiemetic, usually Promethazine 25 mg PO q 6hr, #6: Some patients become nauseated 2-24 hours after taking I-131, occasionally with vomiting. At the clinic visit when we explain I-131 therapy, we give patients a prescription for an antiemetic and ask them to fill it prior to the date that they will receive I-131. We instruct most patients to take the antiemetic on a p.r.n. basis but recommend using it prophylactically during the first day when the I-131 dose will be >150 mCi.

Give the patient a prescription for Pilocarpine 5 mg PO TID, #15: Pilocarpine is a cholinergic that stimulates salivary flow and thereby decreases the transit time of I-131 through the salivary glands and the concentration of I-131 in the saliva. We start the patient on Pilocarpine two days prior to I-131 and continue for two days after the administration. Narrow angle glaucoma is a relative contraindication to pilocarpine but in our experience the short duration of the use of this medication does not cause problems. Some patients develop nausea, sweating, or diarrhea with pilocarpine. If there is any question that the patient is developing toxicity from pilocarpine, we decrease the dose to 5 mg BID or discontinue it completely.

Instruct the patient to start the low-iodine diet 2 weeks prior to receiving I-131: A strict low-iodine diet for two weeks prior to, and one days after, I-131 administration improves the efficacy of therapy. We use a one page summary of guidelines for a low-iodine diet and refer patients to a source of more detailed information.

Give the patient information about where to report to receive I-131: We include this on our checklist because we currently explain the I-131 procedure in either the endocrinology or radiation oncology clinic but deliver the I-131 in the nuclear medicine department. It is helpful to use the clinic visit as a time to remind patients were to go for pretreatment testing and where they need to report to receive the I-131. Written directions and maps are helpful.

Remind the patient not to consume anything but water 4 hours prior to, and for 2 hours after, taking I-131: A variety of foods may decrease the absorption of I-131. For this reason, it is best to have the patient take I-131 with an empty stomach. We instruct patients not to eat or drink anything but water during the 4 hours before, and 2 hours after taking I-131.

Explain the post treatment total body scan and schedule it for 5–7 days after I-131 administration: Patients are often confused about the reason for doing the post treatment total body scan and they need to plan ahead for the visit that is required to do this study. We find it useful to explain the timing and details of the post treatment total body scan as part of the discussion of the overall plan for I-131 therapy.

Schedule a clinic visit the day of, or a few days after, the post treatment Total Body Scan: Our policy is to have the patient come for a clinic visit immediately after completing the post treatment Total Body Scan. The purpose of this clinic visit is to review the results of the Total Body Scan with the patient, confirm that they are taking T4 medication, evaluate any residual side-effects from I-131, and confirm that they have an appointment for endocrinology follow-up in approximately 6 weeks. Many patients are anxious about the results of the whole body scan and we find it reassures them to know that they will get a chance to discuss these results with a physician soon after the study. Confirming that the patient is taking T4 replacement is important because some patients forget to resume their medication as directed.

Schedule a follow-up appointment for 6 weeks after I-131 administration: Our policy is to evaluate the patient 6 weeks after I-131 therapy. The purpose of this visit is to check for recurrent tumor with a neck ultrasound and to check a serum TSH level to determine if the dose of T4 replacement is correct. In our program an endocrinologist directs these evaluations.

TASKS REQUIRED WHEN THE PATIENT WILL BE TAKING LITHIUM CARBONATE

Give the patient a prescription for lithium carbonate: The use of lithium carbonate to increase the potency of I-131 therapy is discussed in a separate chapter. We currently use lithium carbonate in all patients who are likely to tolerate it. During the clinic visit prior to I-131 therapy we give the patient a prescription for lithium, and explain the purpose of lithium in this setting, the importance of taking it as directed, and the side-effects that suggest toxicity to the point that they should stop taking this medication. The dose of lithium is 10 mg per kilogram of body weight. The usual lithium carbonate prescription is for 300 mg po TID, #21 but in small patients or patients with borderline cardiac or renal function we write for 300 mg BID, #14.

If needed, give the patient a prescription for, or schedule, blood draw for lithium level: It is currently our policy to arrange for the patient to have a serum lithium level checked on the 4th and 5th day of taking lithium (2 and 1 day before the patient receives I-131). We discontinue lithium as soon as the patient develops palpitations, chest pain, shortness of breath, moderate nausea, confusion, ataxia, or dysarthria.

WHEN USING rhTSH TO ELEVATE TSH

Explain and record the dates of the two rhTSH injections: Explaining the reason for, and schedule of, rhTSH injections will decrease patient anxiety and increase the chance that the patient will report for the injections at the appropriate time. We schedule the two rhTSH injections in the morning of days one and two prior to I-131 administration.

Scheduling the injections in the morning leaves the afternoon to schedule the thyroid uptake study that is required when the patient is going be treated as an outpatient. *Instruct the patient to stop taking T4 three days prior to receiving I-131:* As explained in another chapter, thyroid hormone contains iodine that may compete with I-131 for uptake in target cells. Our policy is to stop thyroid hormone replacement for a total of 4 days, beginning 3 days prior to I-131 administration.

WHEN USING T4 DEPRIVATION TO ELEVATE TSH

Instruct the patient to stop T4 six weeks prior to receiving I-131: The serum half-life of T4 is relatively long (~7 days) such that a patient usually has to be deprived of T4 for 4–6 weeks before serum TSH will rise above 30 µU/mL. It creates problems for the patient and our department to have to reschedule the I-131 administration on short notice so we set the date for I-131 to be 6 weeks after stopping T4.

Give the patient a prescription for Cytomel (T3), usually 25 mcg PO BID #42: The period of time that the patient will experience symptoms of hypothyroidism is decreased by using T3 for the first three weeks that the patient is off T4. We instruct the patient to begin taking T3 on the day that they stop taking T4. The serum half-life of T3 is approximately 1.5 days. In many patients the TSH will rise above 30 µU/mL one week after stopping T3 but we prefer to stop T3 two weeks before I-131 administration to minimize the chance that we will have to change the date of I-131 administration.

Give the patient a prescription for blood draw for TSH and thyroglobuln, approximately 1 week before I-131 administration: In our system it takes a few days to get the results from of a serum TSH test. Our policy is to send blood for a TSH level the week prior to I-131 administration so that we get the results back in time to cancel the order for I-131 if need be. With our preparatory program we expect the serum TSH level to be at least 30 µU/mL seven days prior to I-131 administration.

WHEN THE PATIENT WILL NOT BE ADMITTED TO THE HOSPITAL AFTER RECEIVING I-131

Schedule a visit with the radiation safety officer to approve outpatient precautions: To send the patient home after administering I-131, state regulations require that the radiation safety officer determine that the patient is capable of complying with all necessary radiation safety precautions. Most radiation safety officers prefer to meet with the patient well before they plan to receive I-131 to discuss the requirements. In our program the radiation safety officer meets with the patient as part of the clinic visit with the physician to discuss all aspects of I-131 therapy.

Schedule the thyroid uptake study, usually during the week prior to I-131 administration: Federal regulations require the measurement of thyroid uptake to make the calculation that determines if it is permissible to send the patient home after giving them I-131. When the patient is being prepared for I-131 by thyroid hormone deprivation, we schedule the thyroid uptake study during the week prior to I-131 administration; on the same day as the blood draw for TSH. When the patient is prepared for I-131 with rhTSH we schedule the thyroid uptake study on the afternoon of the day that they receive the second rhTSH injection (the day prior to I-131 administration). We perform the thyroid uptake study after the second rhTSH injection in an attempt to estimate the conditions that will exist when the patient goes home after receiving I-131.

WHEN THE PATIENT WILL BE ADMITTED TO THE HOSPITAL AFTER I-131

Schedule inpatient admission for the day of I-131 administration: The radiation safety officer and hospital administration need lead time to prepare a room for a patient who has been treated with I-131. Our policy is to choose the date for the admission (and I-131 administration) on the day of the clinic visit to discuss I-131 therapy.

5A.5. A CHECKLIST OF THINGS TO DO ON THE DAY OF I-131 ADMINISTRATION

ROBERT J. AMDUR, MD AND ERNEST L. MAZZAFERRI, MD, MACP

The previous chapter lists the things that the physician should do at the time of initial consultation for I-131 therapy. The purpose of this chapter is to list the things that the physician needs to do on the day of I-131 administration (Table 1).

TASKS REQUIRED IN ALL PATIENTS

Confirm the patient's identity: For many reasons it is important to confirm the identity of the patient prior to administering I-131. We do this by asking the patient to state their full name and confirming that this name matches that on the paperwork related to the consultation for I-131 therapy.

Review the history to confirm that the ordered dose is correct for this patient: This will be the last chance the physician has to catch an error that was made in the dose of I-131 that was ordered for this particular patient. It may be a major problem to reschedule the I-131 administration but this is better than giving the patient a dose of I-131 that is substantially lower or higher than their situation warrants.

Confirm the dose of I-131 in the capsules that will be given to this patient: Our policy is for the physician who will be administering the I-131 to observe the well-counter readout to confirm that the pharmacy delivered the correct dose of I-131.

If a pregnancy test was to be done, confirm a negative result: Obviously it is desirable to discover problems before the day of I-131 administration but we include the confirmation of all critical tests on this last minute checklist as the final opportunity to avoid a major mistake.

Table 1. Checklist of Tasks to be Done at the Time of I-131 Administration.

These tasks are required in all patients:
☐ Confirm the patient's identity
☐ Review the history to confirm that the ordered dose is correct for this patient
☐ Confirm the dose of I-131 in the tablets that will be given to this patient
☐ If a pregnancy test was to be done, confirm a negative result
☐ Confirm that the patient has an appointment for a Total Body Scan in 5–7 days
☐ Confirm that the patient has a clinic appointment soon after the Total Body Scan
☐ Confirm that the patient has a clinic appointment ~6 weeks from now
☐ Remind the patient to resume taking T4 "tomorrow"
☐ Remind the patient to maintain a low-iodine diet for the next two days
☐ Remind the patient about the things to do to decrease the chance of I-131 toxicity

If using lithium carbonate:
☐ Confirm that there are no signs or symptoms of lithium toxicity
☐ If a lithium level was to be checked, confirm that it is <1.2
☐ Remind the patient to stop taking lithium after tomorrow
☐ If the patient is an inpatient, confirm that the orders include lithium carbonate

When the patient will NOT be admitted to the hospital after receiving I-131:
☐ Confirm that the patient understands the precautions to follow as an outpatient
☐ Give the patient written instructions regarding radiation safety precautions

When the patient will be admitted to the hospital after I-131:
☐ Write appropriate admission orders

Confirm that the patient has an appointment for a whole body scan in 5–7 days: Confirming this appointment at the time of the I-131 administration decreases the chance of a scheduling error and decreases the chance that the patient will forget to come at the scheduled time.

Confirm that the patient has a clinic appointment soon after the whole body scan: We see the patient in clinic within a few hours after the whole body scan has been completed.

Confirm that the patient has a clinic appointment ~6 weeks from now: The purpose of seeing the patient in clinic approximately 6 weeks after I-131 is to rule out gross recurrence with a neck ultrasound and to optimize the dose of thyroid replacement by check serum TSH level. As noted above, confirming this appointment at the time of I-131 administration decreases the chance of a scheduling error and decreases the chance that the patient will forget to come at the scheduled time.

Remind the patient to resume taking levothroxine (T_4) tomorrow (the day after receiving I-131): In view of all the things patients have to think about as they prepare for I-131 therapy, it is not surprising that we have had patients forget to resume T4 replacement after receiving I-131. Verbally reminding them to resume T4 "tomorrow", and then confirming that this was done at the time of the clinic visit soon after the Total Body Scan, will eliminate the chance of prolonged hypothyroidism due to confusion about when to resume medication.

Remind the patient to maintain a low-iodine diet for the next two days: Our patients want to resume their regular diet as soon as possible. We find it useful to remind both inpatients and outpatients that they need to continue the low iodine diet for two days after receiving I-131. This means that if they take I-131 on a Friday that they can resume their regular diet on Sunday morning.

Remind the patient about the things to do to decrease the chance of I-131 toxicity: Just prior to giving the patient I-131 we find it useful to review the instructions that we previously gave them regarding things to do to decrease the chance of discomfort and complications following I-131 therapy. In addition to the standard radiation precautions to avoid exposure to other people, we tell patients that, for the next 3 days, they must stay well hydrated, have a bowel movement at least once-a-day, not wear contact lenses, and continue to take Pilocarpine (if they are tolerating it).

IF USING LITHIUM CARBONATE

Confirm that there are no signs or symptoms of lithium toxicity: Regardless of the serum lithium level, we discontinue lithium if there is any sign of toxicity, or if the patient is tolerating it poorly. Just prior to administering I-131 we observe the patient and ask them about nausea, confusion, ataxia, chest pain, palpitation, and dyspnea. If there is any question of lithium toxicity we tell them to not take any more lithium and to discard the remainder of their lithium supply. We have never had a patient develop side-effects from lithium to the point that we have had to cancel the I-131 administration.

If a lithium level was to be checked, confirm that it is < 1.2 mEq/L: If lithium levels were to be checked the day prior to I-131 administration it is best to try to arrange to get this result by the time of I-131 administration. We discontinue lithium therapy with a serum level of 1.2 mEq/L or greater, regardless of symptoms.

Remind the patient to stop taking lithium after tomorrow: The goal is to have the patient take lithium for 7 total days with the 6th day being the day of I-131 administration. This means that, in the absence of signs of toxicity, patients continue taking lithium the day of, and the day after, they receive I-131. There should be no way a patient can continue taking lithium beyond this point because the initial prescription should be for a nonrefillable 7 day supply of tables. But mistakes in writing or filling prescriptions happen and it is reassuring to the patient to know that running out of lithium tablets the day after receiving I-131 is what should happen.

If the patient is an inpatient, confirm that the orders include lithium carbonate: In our experience it is easy to forget to write for a low-iodine diet and lithium carbonate. Standardized admission orders for patients who are admitted for radiation safety reasons following I-131 are included in the next chapter.

WHEN THE PATIENT WILL NOT BE ADMITTED TO THE HOSPITAL AFTER RECEIVING I-131

Confirm that the patient understands the precautions to follow as an outpatient: In our program a radiation safety officer is present at the time of I-131 administration and takes responsibility for confirming that the patient understands, and is able to comply with, the required radiation safety precautions after receiving I-131. Many patients have questions that pertain to their specific situation at home or work and this is a good time to clarify instructions with them. The instructions that we give patients related to outpatient precautions following I-131 therapy are included in the next chapter.

Give the patient written instructions regarding radiation safety precautions: Federal regulations require that the patient be given written instructions on how to limit radiation exposure to other people. The instruction form that we send home with the patient is included in the next chapter.

WHEN THE PATIENT WILL BE ADMITTED TO THE HOSPITAL AFTER I-131

Write appropriate admission orders: Standardized admission orders for patients who are admitted following I-131 are included in the next chapter.

5A.6. DOCUMENTS THAT FACILITATE I-131 SCHEDULING AND PATIENT EDUCATION

ROBERT J. AMDUR, MD AND ERNEST L. MAZZAFERRI, MD, MACP

Previous chapters reviewed the things the physician needs to do at the time of initial consultation for I-131 therapy and on the day that I-131 is administered. The purpose of this chapter is to present the forms and documents that we use to accomplish these tasks. A summary of the contents of this chapter is presented in Table 1.

Table 1. Documents included in this chapter.

Documents used at the initial consultation for I-131 therapy:
Event Schedule For Patients Who Are Prepared For I-131 With rhTSH
Event Schedule For Patients Who Are Prepared For I-131 With T4 Deprivation
Low-iodine Diet
Consent For I-131 Therapy For Thyroid Cancer

Documents used on the day of I-131 administration:
Handout for the patient: Things To Remember To Do After I-131 Therapy For Cancer
Hospital admission orders for patients admitted for I-131 therapy
Limiting Radiation Exposure To Other People After Receiving I-131 (as an out patient)
Limiting Radiation Exposure To Other People After Leaving The Hospital

---

SCHEDULE FOR I-131 THERAPY: RHTSH (THYROGEN)

Patient Name_____ Phone#_____

MR#_____ D.O.B. _____

2 weeks before taking I-131: Start low-iodine diet _____

1 week before taking I-131: Get blood drawn for pregnancy test _____

5 days before taking I-131: Start lithium _____

(3 pills per day for 7 days)

3 days before taking I-131: Stop Synthoid or Levoxyl _____

2 days and *1 day* before taking I-131: Get blood drawn for lithium level:____ and __

(Less than 1.2 is OK) (Have results faxed to Dr. XXXX, XXX-XXX-XXXX)

2 days before taking I-131: Start Salagen (1 pill three times-a-day):_____

2 days before taking I-131: Thyrogen #1 Injection _____

Location and time: XXXXXX

1 day before taking I-131: Thyrogen #2 Injection _____

Same Location and time

1 day before taking I-131: Go to XXX Nuclear Medicine Dept. to take the I-123 pill
for The Thyroid Uptake Study. (Scan 2–4 hours later)._____

At this time on this day: Go to XXX Nuclear Medicine Dept. to take I-131:_____

- Do not eat or drink anything but water 4 hours before, and 2 hours after, taking I-31
- Continue taking lithium until the tablets are gone (the day after taking I-131)
- Continue taking Salagen until the tablets are gone (2 days after taking I-131)
- Resume taking your Synthroid (or Levoxyl) the day after you take I-131
- Stay on the low-iodine diet for 2 days after you take I-131
- You will be given an appointment to return to XXX 5–7 days after taking I-131 for a Total Body Scan. When you finish the total body scan come to XXX to meet with Dr. XXX to go over the results of the scan
- You will receive an appointment to see Dr. XXX approximately 6 weeks after you take I-131

SCHEDULE FOR I-131 THERAPY: THYROID HORMONE (T4) DEPRIVATION

Patient Name_____ Phone#_____
MR#_____ D.O.B. _____

6 weeks before taking I-131: Stop Synthroid and start Cytomel 25 mcg
twice-a-day_____
3 weeks before taking I-131: Stop Cytomel_____
2 weeks before taking I-131: Start low-iodine diet_____
1 week before taking I-131: Go to XXX lab for Blood Draw_____
(TSH, Thyroglobulin, Pregnancy)
5 days before taking I-131: Start lithium _____
(3 pills per day for 7 days)
2 days before taking I-131: Start Salagen (1 pill three times-a-day):_____
2 days and *1 day* before taking I-131: Get blood drawn for lithium level:___ and ___
(Less than 1.2 is OK) (Have results faxed to Dr. XXX, XXX-XXX-XXXX)

1 day before taking I-131: Go to XXX Nuclear Medicine Dept. to take the I-123 pill
for The Thyroid Uptake Study. (Scan 2–4 hours later)._____

(same day as Blood Draw)

At this time on this day: Go to XXX Nuclear Medicine Dept. to take I-131:_____

- Do not eat or drink anything but water for 4 hours before, and 2 hours after, taking
  I-31
- Continue taking lithium until the tablets are gone (the day after taking I-131)
- Continue taking Salagen until the tablets are gone (2 days after taking I-131)
- Resume taking your Synthroid (or Levoxyl) the day after you take I-131
- Stay on the low-iodine diet for 2 days after you take I-131
- You will be given an appointment to return to XXX 5–7 days after taking I-131
  for a Total Body Scan. When you finish the total body scan come to XXX to meet
  with Dr. XXX to go over the results of the scan
- You will receive an appointment to see Dr. XXX approximately 6 weeks after you
  take I-131

LOW-IODINE DIET

It is important that you follow a low-iodine diet for at least 2 weeks before receiving I-131. Continue the diet for two days after you receive I-131.

DO NOT EAT THESE FOODS:

Iodized salt and foods containing iodized salt: Do not eat iodized salt or sea salt. Non-iodized salt (such as Kosher salt) is OK.

Restaurant food: Avoid restaurant foods as most use iodized salt.

Processed food: Most commercially prepared food contain iodized salt

Seafood: Fish, shell fish, sea weed, and kelp are usually high in iodine

Dairy products: The milk from farm animals is high in iodine. Do not drink milk or eat ice cream, yogurt and butter or eat margarine because it usually contains iodized salt.

Commercial bakery products: Commercial bakery products like bread, cakes, muffins, and pastries often contain iodized salt or iodine dough conditioners. Homemade bread without iodized salt or iodine conditioners is OK.

Chocolate: Chocolate that contains milk is off limits. Milk-free chocolate is OK

Egg yolk: Egg yolk contains iodine. Egg whites are OK on this diet.

The following additives contain iodine: Carrageen, agar, algin, alginates.

Cured, corned or spicy meats, including most meat cold cuts: Bacon, ham, sausage, salami, lox, corned beef, etc. contain salt with iodine. Fresh meat is OK.

Vitamins and food supplements: Most vitamin preparations contain iodine. Check the label and ingredients and do not take vitamins or supplements that contain iodine.

Red, orange or brown food, pills, and capsules: Many red, red-orange, and brown food dyes contain iodine. FD&C Red Dye #3 contains iodine.

Other foods that may contain iodine dyes and preservatives: Soy products (soy sauce, tofu, soy milk), molasses, instant coffee and tea, canned fruits and vegetables often contain additives with iodine. Avoid these foods.

WHAT CAN YOU EAT? Unprocessed (fresh or frozen) fruits, vegetables, egg whites, and meat (other than seafood) are OK. Non Iodized or Kosher salt, unsalted nuts, unsalted peanut butter, and bread made without salt or iodine are OK. Fresh ground (not instant) coffee or tea is OK. Beer, wine, and hard liquors are OK. More information and specific menus and recipes are listed on the web at http://www.thyca.org/ThyCa%20Cookbook%20011804.pdf

---

CONSENT FOR I-131 THERAPY FOR THYROID CANCER

Name_____ #_____ Date_____

Swelling of the saliva glands or neck: It is not unusual to experience mild pain and swelling of the saliva glands or neck after taking I-131. This is a temporary condition that usually goes away in 5 days.

Taste change: It is not unusual to experience a change in the way food tastes. In most patients taste returns to normal 3 weeks after taking I-131.

Nausea: It is not unusual to feel nauseated 2–24 hours after taking I-131. Take the nausea medication that we give you as often as you need it.

I-131 can cause cancer: We will try to estimate the risk of cancer from I-131 in your situation. To decrease the chance that you will get cancer in the future you should do these things:

Stay well hydrated for 3 days after taking I-131: Drink enough fluid so that you need to urinate every few hours. This will decrease radiation exposure to your saliva glands, bladder and other organs.

Have at least one bowel movement each day for 3 days after taking I-131: Bowel movements will decrease radiation exposure to your bowels. Eat prunes or take a laxative, as needed.

I-131 can cause dry mouth and tooth decay (cavities): I-131 may permanently decrease saliva that effects taste, mouth comfort, and dental status. Inform your dentist of this so they can clean your teeth more frequently if needed. To decrease damage to the saliva glands from I-131 you should stay well hydrated for at least 3 days (explained above), suck on sour candy every few hours, and take the Pilocarpine medication as directed if this is prescribed for you.

Do not wear contact lenses for 5 days after receiving I-131.

I-131 can damage your testicles or ovaries: I-131 therapy can weaken your testicles or ovaries so they do not make enough male or female hormones. This can cause irregular periods or early menopause if you are a woman and impotence and other problems if you are a man. The chance that you could get these problems depends on your age and dose of I-131.

Some studies suggest that I-131 therapy may decrease your fertility or ability to produce a normal baby. You should definitely not get pregnant if you are a woman, or get a woman pregnant if you are a man, for 12 months after I-131 therapy. If you are a man and you think you might want to conceive a child in the future, we recommend that you bank a sperm sample before I-131 therapy.

_____   _____
Physician Obtaining Consent   Patient or Surrogate Decisionmaker

Hospital Admission Orders

Date of admission:
Patient name:

1. Admit to PRIVATE ROOM
2. Physician: Dr. XXXXXX, Contact number XXXXX
3. Diagnosis: Admitted to limit radiation exposure to the public following I-131
   therapy for thyroid cancer
4. Condition: Stable
5. Allergies:
6. Vital signs: once on admission but no routine checking thereafter to limit
   radiation exposure to hospital staff
7. Activity: Unrestricted but confined to room
8. Diet: Low-iodine diet (no salt, processed foods, or dairy products)
9. Medications: If taking lithium: lithium 300 mg PO BID or TID
   Pilocarpine 5 mg PO TID
   Acetomenophen 650 mg PO Q 6 hours PRN pain
   Antacid of Choice, 30 cc PO Q 4–6 hours PRN dyspepsia
   Temazepam 15–30 mg PO, Q HS PRN insomnia
   Promethazine 25 mg PO or IM Q 6hr PRN nausea
   Biscodyl 15 mg PO q 8 hours PRN constipation
   Other medications the patient takes regularly:
10. Call Physician for: Vomiting
   Temperature Elevation > 101 F
   Blood Pressure Systolic > 180 or < 90 mmHg
   Blood Pressure Diastolic > 100 or < 40 mmHg
   Heart Rate > 140 bpm

Physician signature:

Things To Remember To Do After I-131 Therapy For Cancer

(Physician contact: Dr. XXX or the physician on-call at XXX-XXX-XXXX)

For 3 days after taking I-131 (the day you take I-131 and two days thereafter):

• Drink lots of water so that you urinate every few hours
• Have a bowel movement at least once a day. Take a laxative if needed.
• Do not wear contact lenses

The day after taking I-131:

• Start taking thyroid hormone pills (Synthroid, Levoxyl)

On the 3rd day after taking I-131:

• Resume your regular diet

For 7 days after taking I-131:

• Follow the instructions given to you on a separate piece of paper that explain how you should limit your contact with other people when you go home

For at least 12 months after taking I-131:

• Do not get pregnant if you are a woman, or get a woman pregnant if you are a man

Return appointments:

• **About 1 week after taking I-131:** Appointment for a Whole Body Scan and discussion with Dr. XXXX
• **About 6 weeks after taking I-131:** Clinic appointment with Dr. XXXX

Limiting Radiation Exposure To Other People After Receiving I-131

Patient name: _____ Todays Date: _____
Date of I-131 administration:_____ Dose of I-131 administered:_____

You have received I-131 for treatment of a medical condition. Show this document to anyone who is concerned about radiation exposure to other people. For questions contact: Dr. XXXXXXX or the doctor on-call, Phone XXX-XXX-XXXX

NO RADIATION SAFETY PRECAUTIONS ARE NECESSARY AFTER:
_____, 20_____

The drive home:
Children and pregnant women are not permitted to be in the car with you
If someone else is with you, one person should be in the back seat on the passenger side
Do not get out of the car on the trip home unless you need to use a bathroom. Do not go into a restaurant. If you use a toilet, wipe down the seat after you use it
Your sweat contains radioactivity. After the trip wipe down any part of the car that your skin touched

For 72 hours after you take I-131:
Isolate yourself so that you have no contact with another person. If other people live with you then you should stay in your room except when using the bathroom
Nobody else can use the bathroom that you use
Do not touch objects (furniture, computers, eating utensils, etc) that other people may touch before all sweat or saliva from your body can be removed from them
Do not kiss your dog or cat or let them lick your mouth

At the end of 72 hours after taking I-131:
Wash your bed linen, and the clothes that you have worn, and the towels that you have used since taking I-131 separate from other items
Place all disposable paper waste that can not be flushed down the toilet in a garbage bag and dispose of it as you normally do with the rest of your garbage

During days 3–7 after taking I-131:
Do not sleep in the same bed with, or transfer saliva to, anyone. Do not have sex or kiss people on the mouth. Use only disposable eating utensils, plates, and cups
Avoid contact with any woman who is pregnant

For at least 6 months after taking I-131:
Do not get pregnant if you are a woman, or get a woman pregnant if you are a man

---

An Alternate Form for Radiation Safety Precautions Following I-131 Therapy

Patient name: _____ Todays Date: _____
Date of I-131 administration:_____ Dose of I-131 administered:_____

You have received I-131 for treatment of a medical condition. Show this document to anyone who is concerned about your radiation exposure to other people. For questions contact: Dr. XXXXXXX or the doctor on-call, Phone XXX-XXX-XXXX

NO RADIATION SAFETY PRECAUTIONS ARE NECESSARY AFTER:
_____, 20 _____

- Children and pregnant women should not enter your home for _____ days
- Do not leave your home for _____ days
- Isolate yourself in your home so that you spend almost no time in the same room with another person for_____ days
- Try not to do anything that could transfer your saliva to another person, such as kissing or sharing food, for _____ days
- Use disposable eating utensils for _____ days
- Wash your bedding, towels, and laundry separately for _____ days
- Do not work or volunteer outside the house for _____ days
- Do not take public transportation for _____ days
- Arrange things so that you have sole use of a bathroom for _____ days
- Dispose of all tissues in the toilet for _____ days.
- Flush the toilet twice after each use for_____ days.
- Do not sleep with, or lay or sit next to, another person for_____ days
- Do not have sexual relations with anyone for at least _____ days
- Do not get pregnant or get someone pregnant for at least 6 months

PART 5B. PREPARING PATIENTS FOR I–131 THERAPY

5B.1. THE LOW-IODINE DIET

ROBERT J. AMDUR, MD AND ERNEST L. MAZZAFERRI, MD, MACP

Following the introduction of iodized salt and iodine in other foods, iodine deficiency was eliminated in the United States and eventually dietary iodine and urine iodine excretion were well above the range (<100 μg/day) associated with iodine deficiency. However, The National Health and Nutrition Surveys (NHANES) III (1988–1994), and NHANES I (1971–1974) found that the median urinary iodine (UI) concentration decreased from 320 μg/L to 145 μg/L over the 20 years of the two reports (Hollowell 1998). Nonetheless, the usual diet provides sufficient iodine to compete with the radioiodine for uptake in thyroid tissue or thyroid cancer during cancer therapy or diagnostic scanning. To increase the uptake of radioiodine in target tissues, it is standard procedure to place the patient on a diet that is low in iodine for 2 weeks before, and 1–2 days after, radioiodine administration. The purpose of this chapter is to review the issues that clinicians should consider when prescribing a low-iodine diet in the management of thyroid cancer patients. Table 1 summarizes the main points from this chapter.

A LOW-IODINE DIET IS AN IODINE INTAKE OF ≤ 50 μg/day

The recommended daily intake of iodine in the United States is 150 μg/day for adults. The major source of dietary iodine for most people is iodized salt, bread made with iodized conditioners and dairy products that are high in iodine because it is a component of animal foods and medications.

Table 1. Summary of Information about the Low-Iodine Diet.

---

* It is important that all patients go on a low-iodine diet in preparation for radioiodine therapy or diagnostic scans
* A low-iodine diet means an iodine intake of ≤ 50 μg/day
* Forced diuresis is unnecessary
* Measuring iodine levels to evaluate compliance is not done in most patients
* The usual role of iodine measurements is to evaluate the status of patients who have received intravenous iodinated contrast compounds
* We recommend starting the low-iodine diet 2 weeks prior to radioiodine administration and continuing it for 2 days after the administration
* We explain the importance and basic details of the low-iodine diet to the patient and then provide a one page document that lists prohibited foods

---

EFFICACY OF A LOW-IODINE DIET

The purpose of a low-iodine diet is to deplete the total body iodine stores to a degree that maximizes the uptake of radioiodine by thyroid tissue and thyroid cancer. The lower the iodine in the diet the better, but the amount that appears to balance the need for iodine depletion against the difficulty of eliminating iodine from the diet is an iodine intake of approximately 50 μg/day. Studies (Maxon 1983) demonstrate that this degree of iodine restriction approximately doubles the absorbed radiation dose to the thyroid remnant and produces a major increase in the sensitivity of diagnostic radioiodine scans. Nonetheless, some have questioned the benefit of a low-iodine diet.

A retrospective study by (Morris 2001) of 44 patients placed on a low-iodine diet (LID) and 50 patients on a regular diet found a 68% successful remnant ablation rate (defined as absent uptake on diagnostic whole body scan) for LID patients and a 62.% rate for those on a regular diet, a difference that was not statistically significant. However, all the patients in this study had relatively high urine iodine levels at the time of treatment: 174 μg/L in the LID patients and 381 μg/L in the patients on a regular diet, which are not in the acceptable range for patients undergoing I-131 treatment. Moreover, the ablation rates in this study were substantially lower than the average rates of about 85% found in most large studies (Bal 2004), particularly when I-131 scintigraphy alone is the endpoint for successful ablation.

In anther study by Pluijmen et al. (2003), two groups of patients who had received either a standard diet or a LID during thyroid remnant ablation were retrospectively studied. The 24 hour urine iodide level decreased to 27 μg in the LID group compared with 159 μg in controls. The 24 hour I-131 uptake was significantly higher in the LID group than in the controls and I-131 uptake by thyroid remnants increased by 65% over baseline in the LID group in which 65% had a successful ablation (defined by absent neck uptake and serum thyroglobulin < 2 ng/mL) compared with 48% in the control group. In a subgroup of T1-3, N0 patients, 8% of the LID group had a thyroglobulin higher than 2 ng/mL compared with 32% of the control group, and successful ablation was achieved in 71% of patients in the LID group versus 45% in the control group. All the differences mentioned were statistically significant and underscore the salutary effects on I-131 treatment with a low-iodine diet.

FORCED DIURESIS

Studies in the 1960s demonstrated increased radioiodine uptake following a combination of forced diuresis and an iodine restricted diet. Since this observation, diuretics have been used in some patients prior to radioiodine therapy or scanning. However, the potential benefit of forced diuresis does not outweigh the risks and discomforts in the great majority of patients. In addition to the usual risks of diuretics, forced diuresis decreases iodine clearance by a variety of mechanisms, which results in a major increase in the total body dose from a given activity of radioiodine.

The incremental benefit from forced diuresis is likely to be small if other aspects of the preparatory regimen are done correctly. Today, it is difficult to find an expert that uses forced diuresis in any setting. We do not use forced diuresis in our practice.

MEASURING TOTAL BODY IODINE

Several methods have been described for measuring a patient's iodine status in preparation for radioiodine therapy or scanning. Iodine measurement is unnecessary unless there is some reason to suspect that a patient has not complied with the prescribed diet or has received an excessive amount of iodine. Urine iodine measurement is discussed in the next chapter.

THE DURATION OF THE LOW-IODINE DIET

Most physicians put patients on an iodine restricted diet for two weeks prior to radioiodine therapy or a diagnostic scan but there are some who claim good results with a one-week diet. This issue was recently evaluated by Park and Hennessey (2004) in patients who were prepared for diagnostic scanning with rhTSH. This study shows that a two week low-iodine diet (Fig. 1) was much more likely than a one week diet (Fig. 2) respectively, 71% versus 41%, to produce a urine iodine level that the authors considered adequate for diagnostic scanning (urine iodine < 100 µg/mg Cr.

We recommend an iodine-restricted diet for two weeks in all patients prior to therapy or diagnostic scanning with radioiodine. The duration to continue iodine restriction after the administration of radioiodine has not been well studied. We continue the low-iodine diet for two days following radioiodine administration (the day of and the day after the day of administration).

INSTRUCTIONS FOR THE LOW-IODINE DIET

A variety of diets have been used to achieve a low-iodine diet to increase radioiodine uptake. All of them are unpleasant for patients. To improve compliance, some centers have a dietician monitor each patient's eating habits. In other centers each patient is supplied with prepackaged meals. This degree of structure is unworkable in most practices. We emphasize the importance of the low-iodine diet with each patient during a face-to-face clinic visit and give each patient a document that lists the foods that are prohibited on the diet. In our experience, patients prefer that diet instructions be limited

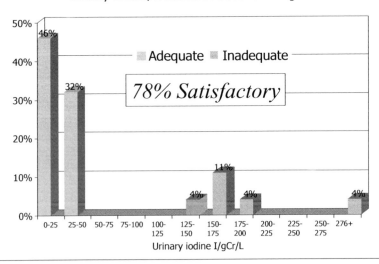

Figure 1. The effect of a 2 week low-iodine diet (LID) on urinary iodine levels. Drawn from the data of Park, J.T. & Hennessey, J.V. (2004) *Thyroid*. **14**, 57–63.

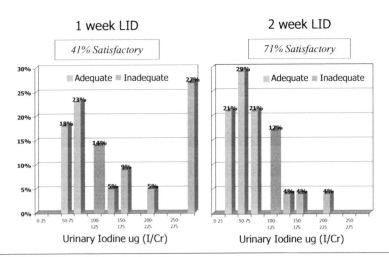

Figure 2. Urine iodine after (A) 1 week of a low-iodine diet (LID) on thyroid hormone and (B) 2 weeks of a low-iodine diet (LID) off thyroid hormone. Drawn from the data of Park, J.T. & Hennessey, J.V. (2004) *Thyroid*. **14**, 57–63.

to one page and want advice about a web site were they can seek further information. The handout that we use is reproduced below.

REFERENCES

Bal, CS, A Kumar, and GS Pant. 2004. Radioiodine dose for remnant ablation in differentiated thyroid carcinoma: a randomized clinical trial in 509 patients. J Clin Endocrinol Metab **89**:1666–1673.

Hollowell, JG, NW Staehling, WH Hannon, DW Flanders, EW Gunter, GF Maberly, LE Braverman, S Pino, DT Miller, PL Garbe, DM DeLozier, and RJ Jackson. 1998. Iodine nutrition in the United States. Trends and public health implications: Iodine excretion data from National Health and Nutrition Examination Surveys I and III (1971–1974 and 1988–1994). J Clin Endocrinol Metab **83**:3401–3408.

Maxon, HR, TA Boehringer, and J Drilling. 1983. Low iodine diet in I-131 ablation of thyroid remnants. Clin Nucl Med **8**:123–126.

Morris, LF, MS Wilder, AD Waxman, and GD Braunstein. 2001. Reevaluation of the impact of a stringent low-iodine diet on ablation rates in radioiodine treatment of thyroid carcinoma. Thyroid **11**:749–755.

Park, JT, and JV Hennessey. 2004. Two-week low iodine diet is necessary for adequate outpatient preparation for radioiodine rhTSH scanning in patients taking levothyroxine. Thyroid **14**:57–63.

Pluijmen, MJ, C Eustatia-Rutten, BM Goslings, MP Stokkel, AM Arias, M Diamant, JA Romijn, and JW Smit. 2003. Effects of low-iodide diet on postsurgical radioiodide ablation therapy in patients with differentiated thyroid carcinoma. Clin Endocrinol (Oxford) **58**:428–435.

5B.2. INTRAVENOUS IODINATED CONTRAST EFFECTS IODINE UPTAKE FOR MONTHS

ROBERT J. AMDUR, MD AND ERNEST L. MAZZAFERRI, MD, MACP

Radiographic studies such as Computerized Tomography (CT) scans and angiograms are commonly done with intravenous injection of contrast agents that contain organic iodine. The purpose of this chapter is to explain the implications of a history of exposure to iodinated contrast for the management of patients with differentiated thyroid cancer. Table 1 summarizes the main points.

IODINATED CONTRAST CONTAINS AN ENORMOUS AMOUNT OF IODINE

The quantity of iodine that a patient receives from injection with an iodinated contrast agent is enormous compared to the amount of iodine in the normal diet. For example, the typical chest CT study is done with a minimum of 100 ml of intravenous contrast material that contains at least 150 mg of iodine per ml of contrast. This means that a single contrast-enhanced chest CT scan gives and adult over one hundred thousand times the minimum daily allowance of dietary iodine (>15 grams versus 150 μg, respectively). When exposed to an iodine load of this magnitude, body stores of iodine in interstitial fluids, in colloid within the thyroid, and in virtually every organ in the body (Costa 1978) are expanded. This represents a major problem in thyroid cancer management because the body draws on iodine stores to prevent the iodine depletion that we are trying to achieve when preparing a patient for I-131 therapy or a radioiodine scan.

Table 1. Summary of Points About Iodinated Contrast.

- Iodinated contrast agents contain an enormous amount of iodine
- A single iodinated contrast exposure is likely to compromise radioiodine uptake for 3–12 months
- Do not use iodinated contrast in a patient with differentiated thyroid cancer
- Determine if the patient has received iodinated contrast within the past 6 months before scheduling radioiodine therapy or a radioiodine scan
- Measure a 24-hour urinary iodine level on day 7 of a low-iodine diet in any patient with a history of iodinated contrast exposure in the past 6 months*
- Do not begin the preparatory program for radioiodine administration unless the 24-hour urinary free iodine level is ≤ 100 micrograms*

---

* These recommendations are explained in more detail in the chapter "Measuring Urinary Iodine".

DURATION OF THE EFFECT OF INTRAVENOUS CONTRAST ON IODINE METABOLISM

The degree and duration of reduced I-131 uptake as a result of exposure to iodinated contrast has not been well studied. However, the available data suggests that giving a patient iodinated contrast agents substantially increases total body iodine stores for at least three months following contrast exposure, and in some cases as long as 2 years (Costa 1978). A study by Spate et al. (1998) measured iodine content in the toenails at monthly intervals following injection of iodinated contrast as part of a radiographic study done for medical purposes. They found that it took a minimum of 100 days (∼ 3 months) for the body iodine level to return to baseline following a single injection of iodinated contract and the time required to achieve this in most patients in their study was 200–300 days (∼6-10 months). The study by Costa et al. (1978) found that in some cases tissue levels of iodine remained high for as long as 2 years after administration of radiologic contrast material.

RECOMMENDATIONS

The data from the Spate and Costa studies suggest that iodinated contrast may compromise the uptake of radioiodine for many months following contrast administration. Based on this, we recommend that iodinated contrast not be given to patients who may need radioiodine therapy or radioiodine whole body scans over the next year. In our opinion, ultrasound, MR scan, PET scan, technetium bone scan, and noncontrast CT scan are more than adequate to evaluate thyroid cancer status. We attempt to educate our colleagues in other disciplines about the importance of not using iodinated contrast in patients with a history of differentiated thyroid cancer but find it more productive to remind the patient to call us before undergoing a radiographic study at the request of another physician. When we want to give radioiodine to a patient who has received iodinated contrast within the past 6 months we measure a 24-hour urinary iodine level on day seven of a low-iodine diet as described in the chapter "Measuring Urinary Iodine".

REFERENCES

Costa, A, OB Testori, C Cenderelli, G Giribone, and M Migliardi. 1978. Iodine content of human tissues after administration of iodine containing drugs or contrast media. J Endocrinol Invest **1**:221–225.

Spate, VL, JS Morris, TA Nichols, CK Baskett, MM Mason, TL Horsman, PL Horn-Ross, AC Shiau, and IR McDougall. 1998. Longitudinal study of iodine in toenails following IV administration of an iodine-containing contrast agent. J Radioanal Nucl Chem **236(1–2)**:71–76.

5B.3. MEASURING URINARY IODINE (UI)

ROBERT J. AMDUR, MD AND ERNEST L. MAZZAFERRI, MD, MACP

URINARY IODINE EXCRETION

The urinary iodine (UI) excretion level provides an accurate estimate of the dietary iodine status of the patient and is best determined from a 24-hour urine sample (Baloch 2003; National Academy of Clinical Biochemistry Web site 2005). Although differences in the dilution of spot urine specimens can be compensated for by expressing results normalized to urine creatinine as μg of iodine excreted/gram of creatinine, the diurnal and seasonal variations of iodine and creatinine urinary excretion are different enough that the ratio of iodine/creatinine can vary during the day or the time of year. UI has a diurnal variation, with values reaching a median in early morning or 8–12 hours after the last meal, suggesting that spot samples may not represent 24 hour UI (Als 2000a). Although recent reports (Knudsen 2000) suggest that the use of age and sex adjusted UI/Cr ratios in a fasting morning specimen comes close to the true 24 hour iodine excretion if nutrition is adequate, there is no ideal substitute for the accuracy of a 24-hour urine collection. For these reasons and to avoid errors introduced in the performance of different creatinine assays, the World Health Organization recommend that the excretion of UI be expressed as μg of iodine per volume (pg/dL or μg/L) of urine (i.e., a 24 hour urine sample) (Baloch 2003; National Academy of Clinical Biochemistry Web site 2005).

DIETARY IODINE

The recommended daily iodine intake is 90 μg/day for children, 150 μg/day for adults and 200 μg/day for pregnant or lactating mothers (Delange 1995). The suggested norms for UI excretion as an index of iodine intake expressed in μg/L are as follows: > 100 is no iodine deficiency, 50–99 is mild iodine deficiency, 20–49 is moderate iodine deficiency, and < 20 is severe iodine deficiency. (Baloch 2003; National Academy of Clinical Biochemistry Web site 2005).

EXCESSIVE IODINE INTAKE

Excessive iodine intake can lead to thyroid dysfunction, including the inhibition of thyroid hormone synthesis (the Wolff Chaikhoff effect, see physiology chapter) and can be of iatrogenic origin. Excessive iodine intake has been implicated in the increased prevalence of autoimmune thyroiditis and the increase in thyroglobulin antibody positivity following iodine prophylaxis, which may be due to increased antigenicity of more highly iodinated forms of thyroglobulin (Rose 1999; Premawardhana 2000). It is important to remember that organic iodine present in radiological contrast material can be taken up into body fat, and that the slow release of iodine from body fat stores has been associated with a high UI excretion rates that can persist for several months to years following the administration of radiographic contrast material. In a study by Costa et al. (1978) in which total iodine contents were determined in 209 biopsy or autopsy specimens of various extrathyroidal tissues, subjects with previous exposure to iodine containing drugs or x-ray contrast media showed increased iodine contents of various degree in all tissues examined, including adipose tissue, bone, brain, kidney, liver, lung, skeletal muscle, skin and spleen. Accumulation of iodine in adipose tissue was still demonstrable more than two years after cholecystography.

MEASURING UI IN PATIENTS WITH THYROID CANCER

The patient's iodine status should be measured when it is known or suspected that there has been a study in the past 6 months that involved intravenous iodinated contrast or when there is reason to suspect that the patient is consuming iodine rich foods in violation of the low-iodine diet instructions. As a practical matter, it is rarely necessary to do this for other reasons such as suspecting the patient has not been compliant with the low-iodine diet.

A patient is usually considered to be optimally prepared for radioiodine therapy or scanning when the 24-hour urine iodine level is no greater than 50 μg. However, the urine iodine level may remain around 100 μg even after the patient has been on a 2-week low-iodine diet, in which case we proceed with treatment. If the UI is elevated above 150 μg, obtain serial measurements every month or two until the level is low enough (usually around 100 μg) to begin the process of preparing the patient for I-131 therapy. In this case the level usually will be ≤ 50 μg by the time the patient completes the two-week low-iodine diet.

IODINE METHODOLOGY

Methodology for measuring UI is complex and is well beyond the scope of this chapter. However, the clinician should have some understanding of the methodologic problems. Methods that measure UI have traditionally relied on the conversion of organic iodinated compounds to inorganic iodine and the removal of potential interfering substances such as thiocyanate that can interfere with the colorimetric measurement of inorganic iodine.

The procedure involves a preliminary digestion step followed by the colorimetric estimation of iodine through its catalytic action in the Sandell-Kolthoff (SK) reaction that produces the color change (Baloch 2003). There are problems associated with the removal of interfering substances such as thiocyanate in the SK reaction, and a report comparing 6 methods for iodine analysis attributed much of these interferences with the SK reaction to inadequate digestion procedures (May 1990). Two major methods of sample digestion, dry ashing and wet ashing are routinely employed (Baloch 2003).

The following is an excerpt from the National Academy of Clinical Biochemistry (NACB) guidelines. (Baloch 2003; Kaplan, National Academy of Clinical Biochemistry Web site 2005)

- The Technicon AutoAnalyzer for measuring UI is generally no longer commercially available.
- Many simplified digestion methods incorporating SK colorimetry have been described.
- Inter and intra assay coefficient of variation (CV) should be < 10% and recovery of added iodide should be between 90 and 100%.
- Clinical laboratories are frequently requested to perform urinary iodide measurements to investigate iodide overload. One of the simplified methods or a semi-quantitative kit is the method of choice.
- To facilitate uniformity in concentration units used to report urinary iodide excretion, UI should be expressed as μg Iodide /L of urine (μg/L).

Several national laboratories measure UI accurately enough to be used in patients with thyroid cancer in whom contamination with radiologic contrast material is suspected.

ORDERING A URINE IODINE MEASUREMENT

Table 1 summarizes how to arrange a 24-hour urinary free iodine measurement. The laboratory that collects the specimen will give the patient instructions on how to collect

Table 1. Instructions for Arranging the Urinary Free Iodine Measurement.

Give the patient a prescription that reads:
24-Hour Urine for Free Iodine. CPT code 82190
Fax results to Dr. XXX at XXX-XXX-XXXX

Give the patient the Low-Iodine Diet handout:
Our Low-Iodine Diet handout is presented in the chapter "The Low-Iodine Diet"

Instruct the patient to collect urine on the 7th day of the low-iodine diet
Instruct the patient to not take thyroid hormone during the 3 days prior to, and the day of, urine collection
Optional: Specify the lab you want the specimen sent to, for example:
Mayo Medical Laboratory
phone for mailing and processing information: 800-533-1710
Test # 9549 (Urinary free iodine)
It usually takes 7–14 working days to get urinary iodine results

---

Table 2. Patient Instructions for the 24-Hour Urine Iodine Measurement.

Instructions For The 24-hour Urine Iodine Test

- We will give you a prescription for a urine iodine test
- Take this prescription to the facility where you have blood tests done
- The laboratory will give you a container for collecting urine during a 24-hour period
- Go on the low-iodine diet for seven days
- Collect your urine for 24-hours on the seventh day that you are on the low-iodine diet
- Do not take your thyroid medication (Synthroid or Levoxyl) for three days prior to, and the day of, urine collection. This means that you do not take thyroid medication for 4 total days
- Unless instructed otherwise, restart your thyroid medication as soon as you have completed the 24-hour urine collection
- Be sure to follow the directions that they will give you with the collection container for keeping the urine specimen on ice or in the refrigerator until you return it to the laboratory

and store a 24-hour urine sample and will provide the container, which needs to be refrigerated or stored on ice during the collection.

Table 2 summarizes the instructions that we give patients regarding the measurement of UI. In addition to the prescription for the urine iodine study, the patient must have material that explains the low-iodine diet along with instructions to follow the diet for seven total days with the urine collection to be done during the seventh day. We give the patient the single page "Low-Iodine Diet" (see previous chapters) handout with written instructions to follow the diet for 7 days with urine collection on day 7. It is also important to instruct the patient to discontinue thyroid hormone replacement for the three days before, and the day of, urine collection.

REFERENCES

Als, C, A Helbling, K Peter, M Haldimann, B Zimmerli, and H Gerber. 2000a. Urinary iodine concentration follows a circadian rhythm: a study with 3023 spot urine samples in adults and children. J Clin Endocrinol Metab **85:**1367–1369.

Als, C, A Helbling, K Peter, M Haldimann, B Zimmerli, and H Gerber. 2000b. Urinary iodine concentration follows a circadian rhythm: a study with 3023 spot urine samples in adults and children. J Clin Endocrinol Metab **85:**1367–1369.

Baloch, Z, P Carayon, B Conte-Devolx, LM Demers, U Feldt-Rasmussen, JF Henry, VA LiVosli, P Niccoli-Sire, R John, J Ruf, PP Smyth, CA Spencer, and JR Stockigt. 2003. Laboratory medicine practice guidelines. Laboratory support for the diagnosis and monitoring of thyroid disease. Thyroid **13:**3–126.

Costa, A, OB Testori, C Cenderelli, G Giribone, and M Migliardi. 1978. Iodine content of human tissues after administration of iodine containing drugs or contrast media. J Endocrinol Invest **1:**221–225.

Delange, F. 1995. Correction of iodine deficiency: benefits and possible side effects. Eur J Endocrinol **132:**542–543.

Kaplan, LA, and CT Sawin. 2005. National Academy of Clinical Biochemistry Website. Standards of Laboratory Practice: Laboratory Support for the Diagnosis & Monitoring of Thyroid Disease. http://www.nacb.org/lmpg/thyroid_lmpg_pub.stm. 1-20-2005.

Knudsen, N, E Christiansen, M Brandt-Christensen, B Nygaard, and H Perrild. 2000. Age- and sex-adjusted iodine/creatinine ratio. A new standard in epidemiological surveys? Evaluation of three different estimates of iodine excretion based on casual urine samples and comparison to 24 h values. Eur J Clin Nutr **54:**361–363.

May, W, D Wu, C Eastman, P Bourdoux, and G Maberly. 1990. Evaluation of automated urinary iodine methods: problems of interfering substances identified. Clin Chem **36:**865–869.

Premawardhana, LD, AB Parkes, PP Smyth, CN Wijeyaratne, A Jayasinghe, DG de Silva, and JH Lazarus. 2000. Increased prevalence of thyroglobulin antibodies in Sri Lankan schoolgirls—is iodine the cause? Eur J Endocrinol **143**:185–188.

Rose, NR, L Rasooly, AM Saboori, and CL Burek. 1999. Linking iodine with autoimmune thyroiditis. Environ Health Perspect **107**(Suppl. 5):749–752.

5B.4. USING LITHIUM CARBONATE TO INCREASE THE EFFECTIVENESS OF I-131

ROBERT J. AMDUR, MD AND ERNEST L. MAZZAFERRI, MD, MACP

THE EFFECT OF LITHIUM ON RADIOIODINE RETENTION TIME BY FOLLICULAR CELLS

Lithium is a monovalent cation similar to sodium and potassium. At the cellular level, lithium competes with sodium, potassium, calcium, and magnesium at protein binding sites and in transport channels. It causes a decrease in the formation of cellular products such as thyroglobulin and thyroid hormone that contain iodine but the exact mechanism of the lithium effect is not clear. It decreases the rate of radioiodine release from the follicular cell without interfering with iodine uptake by the cell. The net result is that lithium increases the time that radioiodine is retained in the normal thyroid or malignant follicular cell, thus increasing the biologic half-life (cellular retention) of I-131 in the cell.

THE RADIATION DOSE FROM I-131 TO NORMAL AND MALIGNANT FOLLICULAR CELLS

The radiation dose to a cell depends on the number of I-131 molecules that are taken up by the cell and the length of time it retains each I-131 molecule. Retention time (biologic half-life) is a major factor in determining the effectiveness of radioiodine therapy because it is generally shorter in tumors than in normal thyroid tissue. The biologic half-life of I-131 is approximately 10 days for differentiated thyroid cancers and 60 days for normal thyroid tissue.

In Maxon's study (1983), the effective I-131 half-life (biologic plus physical half-life) in tumors that responded to I-131 averaged 78.7 hours (equivalent to a biological half-life of 5.5 days), whereas in non-responders it was 45.8 hours (equivalent to a biological half-life of 2.5 days). This was the most important factor affecting the therapeutic response to I-131. One way to increase the retention time of radioiodine is to give lithium at doses that are commonly used to treat mood disorders (Maxon III 1990; Koong 1999; Sarlis 2001). Although the traditional emphasis in designing I-131 therapy has been on selecting the optimal amount of I-131 to administer, it is equally important to prolong the residence of I-131 in the tumor.

MAGNITUDE OF THE EFFECT OF LITHIUM IN FOLLICULAR CELLS

Lithium increases the biologic half-life of I-131 by as much as 50% in tumor deposits and 90% in the thyroid remnant. In the study by Koong et al. (1999), the increase in the accumulated I-131 and the lengthening of the effective half-life combined to increase the estimated I-131 radiation dose in metastatic tumors by about 2.3 fold. Lithium increases the total radiation dose by approximately 50% in tissue with an iodine biologic half-life of 10 days and approximately 200% in tissue with a biologic half-life of 2 days. In the study by Koong et al. (1999), the incremental change as a result of lithium was greater in tissues with intrinsically low-iodine retention times. This means that lithium will increase the efficacy of I-131 therapy more in a tumor deposit that eliminates radioiodine rapidly than in tumors that concentrate I-131 for longer periods. Since tumors with low-iodine retention times are likely to be the most difficult to eradicate, a more pronounced lithium effect in tissue with rapid iodine turnover is a desirable feature.

THE EFFECTS OF HYPOTHYROIDISM AND RECOMBINANT HUMAN TSH (rhTSH)

Renal clearance is the major means of eliminating I-131 from the body. During thyroid hormone withdrawal, renal I-131 clearance decreases as the patient becomes progressively more hypothyroid and may fall as much as 50%, an alteration that by serendipity serves to maintain high blood I-131 levels. This allows I-131 that has been rapidly released by the follicular cell to recirculate back into the cell, thus promoting the efficacy of I-131 therapy. When rhTSH has been given in preparation for I-131 therapy, however, renal I-131 clearance is normal and the chance that I-131 will recirculate back into the cell is low.

There are studies that show I-131 retention time is lower than usual when rhTSH has been given prior to therapy and that this results in a low biologic half-time for the isotope. For example, in the study by Menzel et al. (2003) the mean effective half-life of I-131 was 0.43 ± 0.11 days for patients after rhTSH stimulation and 0.54 ± 0.11 days after thyroid hormone withdrawal, a reduction of about 20% in the retention of I-131 that was attributable to rhTSH stimulation. Lithium thus is especially useful in patients who undergo I-131 therapy after preparation with recombinant rhTSH because lithium has its greatest effect when the retention times of I-131 in tumors are shortest. Koong et al. (1999) found that lithium increased the retention time as much as three-fold when the retention times were the shortest.

LITHIUM IN THE TREATMENT OF DIFFERENTIATED THYROID CARCINOMA

There are no studies directly showing that lithium therapy increases disease-free survival or lowers cancer-specific mortality rates. The drug is not widely used, mainly because it requires extra steps in the preparation of patients being treated with I-131 and it has potentially severe toxicities.

Nonetheless, lithium is likely to increase the efficacy of I-131 therapy to a degree that is clinically important in most patients. As lithium prolonged the effective half-life in over 70% of metastatic lesions in the study by Koong et al. (1999) and in at least one metastatic lesion in every patient with tumor, we believe that the data concerning the effects of lithium are consistent and show that the drug has a powerful impact on the cellular retention I-131 by normal and malignant follicular cells. We use lithium as an adjunct to I-131 therapy in all patients undergoing thyroid remnant ablation or treatment of metastases who are at low risk for serious problems from lithium toxicity. Background information and prescription guidelines are presented in the remainder of this chapter and summarized in Table 1.

REGULATORY STATUS OF THE USE OF LITHIUM TO AUGMENT I-131 THERAPY

Lithium is approved by the U.S. Food and Drug Administration (FDA) for the treatment of bipolar disorder. Lithium is not FDA approved to increase the effectiveness of I-131 therapy. Use of lithium in this setting is described as "off label use of an approved medication."

FORMULATIONS OF LITHIUM

Two different salts of lithium are used in commercial formulations. Lithium carbonate is used in tablets and capsules. Lithium citrate is used in oral solutions. The rate of absorption is 95–100% for both formulations. The citrate formulation is manufactured because some patients cannot take pills. lithium carbonate is preferred in most clinical situations because it has a longer shelf life and more lithium per weight of formulation.

Lithium carbonate is available in regular and extended-release formulations. The regular-release formulation is used when prescribing lithium with I-131 because the duration of therapy is short. Regular-release lithium preparations reach peak serum concentrations 0.5–3 hours after administration and absorption is complete within 6 hours. The presence of food does not affect the rate of lithium absorption to a meaningful degree. Lithium carbonate regular-release capsules are manufactured in strengths of 150 mg, 300 mg, and 600 mg.

THE DAILY DOSE OF LITHIUM

Lithium therapy is given in divided doses, 2–4 times per day. When using lithium with I-131 therapy the standard approach is to prescribe lithium three-times-a-day.

The recommended dose of regular-release lithium as maintenance therapy for bipolar disorder is 900–1800 mg/day in a normal sized adult and 15–20 mg/kg/day in children. In both children and adults, the dose schedule is adjusted as needed to achieve a

Table 1. Summary of Information Related to Using Lithium with I-131 Therapy.

Contraindications to using lithium in our program:
- psychiatric problems
- dementia
- seizure disorder
- cardiac arrhythmia
- renal insufficiency (90% of lithium elimination is through the kidneys)
- hepatic impairment (affect of hepatic dysfunction on lithium toxicity is not known)
- hypo or hyper natremia
- medications*: a diuretic, antidepressant, NSAID, seizure medication, or calcium channel blocker

Lithium prescription in a normal sized adult:
- Lithium 300 mg capsules
- Take one capsule by mouth each morning, noon, and night
- Dispense 21 capsules

Timing of lithium relative to the date of I-131 administration:
- Begin lithium 5 days prior to the day of I-131 administration.
- Continue lithium the day of, and one day after, the day of I-131 administration
- (7 total days of lithium therapy)

Measuring serum lithium levels (therapeutic range 0.6–1.2 mEq/L):
- Check a lithium level on days 4 and 5 of lithium therapy
- Schedule the blood draw early in the morning, before the first lithium dose that day

Side-effects of lithium: mild in severity and usually do not require a dose reduction:
- nausea, abdominal discomfort, diarrhea
- increased thirst and polyuria
- mood change characterized by a vague sense of depression or fatigue
- tremor
- psoriasis exacerbation

Toxicities for which we discontinue lithium:
- more severe manifestations of the symptoms listed above
- cardiac arrhythmia
- seizure
- confusion

* In cases where it can be done safely, we discontinue medications that would make lithium contraindicated. It is usually difficult to discontinue antidepressants. It is frequently safe to discontinue diuretics, NSAIDs, or calcium channel blockers 3 days prior to and 2 days after the 7 day course of lithium.

serum concentration of 0.6–1.2 mEq/L (0.8–1.2 is optimal) with a prescribing limit of 2400 mg/day.

There are publications on the use of lithium with I-131 that state that the usual adult dose of lithium is 400-800 mg/day (10 mg/kg) with the desirable serum concentration as stated for bipolar disorder. However, in our experience 800 mg/day frequently does not put the lithium level in the therapeutic range and the 900–1800 mg/day dose is likely to apply to most patients.

The psychiatry literature contains guidelines for reducing the dose of lithium in patients with impaired renal function or other conditions that effect lithium excretion. We do not use lithium in patients who are clearly at increased risk for lithium toxicity. Contraindications to lithium are discussed below.

In a normal sized adult with no history of conditions that are likely to increase the chance of lithium toxicity we start with 300 mg three-times-a-day (900 mg/day total

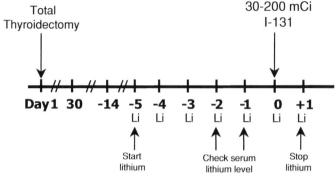

Figure 1. Schema for delivering lithium in preparation for I-131 therapy.

dose). In a patient who is over 70 years of age, or has any condition that suggests a potential for increased toxicity, we decrease the starting dose to 300 mg twice-a-day (600 mg/day total dose). In children or small adults we use a starting dose of 10 mg/ kg/day, usually divided into three daily doses.

THE TIMING OF LITHIUM RELATIVE TO THE DATE OF ADMINISTRATION OF I-131

The optimal duration of lithium therapy before and after the date of I-131 administration is not known. Some authorities start lithium approximately 7 days prior to the day of I-131 administration and continue it for approximately 7 days thereafter (14 total days). We start lithium 5 days before I-131 and continue it for a total of 7 total days (Fig. 1) as described by Koong et al. (1999).

MEASURING SERUM LEVELS OF LITHIUM

The chance of lithium toxicity increases rapidly as the serum concentration exceeds the upper limit of the therapeutic range (1.2 mEq/L). For this reason it is important to monitor the serum concentration of lithium even in patients who are taking lithium for only 7 days. Peak serum concentrations of regular-release lithium occur within 3 hours of a dose. Serum levels may fluctuate for 6–10 hours after a dosing, so it is ideal to use a 12-hour post-dose level for monitoring purposes.

It is not unreasonable to check the serum lithium level every day of lithium therapy. However, in our experience patients do not approach the upper limit (1.2 mEq/L) before day 4 at the earliest. For this reason we only check lithium levels on days 4 and 5 (two days, and one day, before I-131 administration). We do not check a lithium level after administering I-131 because this creates problems related to radiation safety precautions and because a lithium level result usually takes almost two days to process, at which time the patient has completed our lithium prescription.

ADVERSE REACTIONS FROM LITHIUM

Common side-effects of lithium at therapeutic doses include mild nausea, abdominal discomfort, diarrhea, increased thirst, polyuria, tremor, and/or a slight mood change characterized by a vague sense of depression or fatigue. Lithium may exacerbate psoriasis. We do not change the dose schedule as long as these symptoms are mild in severity.

Symptoms of lithium toxicity that require a decrease in dose, and possibly additional monitoring or interventions, include more severe manifestations of the symptoms listed above, cardiac arrhythmia, seizure, confusion or psychosis. Our threshold for discontinuing lithium because of concern about potential toxicity is low.

DRUG INTERACTIONS WITH LITHIUM

Any kind of diuretic increases the risk of lithium toxicity. Diuretics induce sodium loss, which decreases the renal clearance of lithium.

Nonsteroidal anti-inflammatory drugs (NSAIDs), including the selective COX-2 inhibitors, increase serum lithium concentrations by a variety of mechanisms.

Any type of medication that directly affects the central nervous system increases the risk of toxicity when combined with lithium. Unexpected central nervous system toxicity has been reported when lithium was used in combination with cyclic antidepressants, selective serotonin reuptake inhibitors (SSRIs), neuroleptic medications, and medications used to prevent seizure.

There are reports of the calcium channel blockers diltiazem and verapamil precipitating lithium neurotoxicity but this effect is variable and unpredictable.

CONTRAINDICATIONS TO USING LITHIUM TO AUGMENT I-131 THERAPY

Contraindications to using lithium to augment I-131 therapy will depend on the level of risk that the managing physician is willing to accept. We currently take a conservative approach to the use of lithium to augment I-131 therapy and err on the side of avoiding toxicity. In our program contraindications to the use of lithium include:

- psychiatric problems
- dementia
- seizure disorder
- cardiac arrhythmia
- renal insufficiency (90% of lithium elimination is through the kidneys)
- hepatic impairment (affect of hepatic dysfunction on lithium toxicity is not known)
- hypo or hyper natremia
- current use of a diuretic, selective serotonin reuptake inhibitor, cyclic antidepressant, nonsteroidal anti-inflammatory drug, anti seizure medication, or calcium channel blocker.

Prior to prescribing lithium we evaluate the patient's history, medication list, physical examination, electrolytes, renal function, and hepatic function with specific attention to the factors that could increase the risk of lithium toxicity. In cases where it can be done safely, we discontinue medications that would make lithium contraindicated. It is usually difficult to discontinue antidepressants. It is frequently safe to discontinue diuretics, NSAIDs, or calcium channel blockers 3 days prior to and 2 days after the 7 day course of lithium.

REFERENCES

Drug evaluation information related to lithium can be found on the web at http://cpip.gsm.com and then enter "Lithium" in the search window.

Koong, SS, JC Reynolds, EG Movius, AM Keenan, KB Ain, MC Lakshmanan, and J Robbins. 1999. Lithium as a potential adjuvant to ^{131}I therapy of metastatic, well differentiated thyroid carcinoma. J Clin Endocrinol Metab **84**:912–916.

Maxon III, H, and HS Smith. 1990. Radioiodine-131 in the diagnosis and treatment of metastatic well differentiated thyroid cancer. Endocrinol Metab Clin North Am **19**:685–718.

Maxon III, HR, SR Thomas, VS Hertzberg, et al. 1983. Relation between effective radiation dose and outcome of radioiodine therapy for thyroid cancer. N Engl J Med **309**:937–941.

Menzel, C, WT Kranert, N Dobert, M Diehl, T Fietz, N Hamscho, U Berner, and F Grunwald. 2003. rhTSH stimulation before radioiodine therapy in thyroid cancer reduces the effective half-life of (131)I. J Nucl Med **44**:1065–1068.

Sarlis, NJ. 2001. Metastatic thyroid cancer unresponsive to conventional therapies: novel management approaches through translational clinical research. Curr Drug Targets Immune Endocr Metab Disord **1**:103–115.

5B.5. THYROID HORMONE WITHDRAWAL TO ELEVATE TSH

ROBERT J. AMDUR, MD AND ERNEST L. MAZZAFERRI, MD, MACP

When treating or scanning a patient with radioiodine it is important to stimulate iodine uptake by elevating serum Thyroid Stimulating Hormone (TSH) levels prior to radioiodine administration. There are several ways to do this: deprive the patient of thyroid hormone or inject the patient with recombinant human TSH (rhTSH). The purpose of this chapter is to describe how to withdraw thyroid hormone in preparation for radioiodine therapy or scanning. The next chapter explains the use of rhTSH to prepare a patient for I-131 therapy.

ELEVATION OF TSH TO AT LEAST 30 μU/mL

Hypothyroidism is considered adequate to deliver radioiodine when the serum TSH level is ≥ 30 μU/mL. This standard is based on studies that suggest that this degree of hypothyroidism reliably produces radioiodine uptake in thyroid cancer metastases. It is not known if higher TSH levels produce a better rate of remnant ablation or cancer cure.

OUR THYROID HORMONE DEPRIVATION PROTOCOL

The protocol that we use when preparing patients for radioiodine by depriving them of T4 is summarized in Table 1. The serum half-lives of levothyroxine (T4) and triiodothyronine (T3) are approximately 7 days and 1.5 days, respectively. We stop T4 for 6 weeks to stimulate the TSH to rise above 30 μU/mL (Mazzaferri 2005). Discontinuing T4 for six weeks produces uncomfortable, and sometimes disabling, symptoms that last for months in some patients. To decrease the duration of symptoms of hypothyroidism we start T3 on the day that the patient stops T4. The patient takes T3 for 4 weeks, meaning

T3 is discontinued weeks prior to I-131 administration. TSH should be ≥30 mIu/L 2 weeks after stopping T3.

THE DOSE OF TRIIODOTHYRONINE (T3)

The generic name of L-triiodothyronine (T3) is Liothyronine. Cytomel is currently the only brand of Liothyronine that is marketed in the United States. It is manufactured in 5, 25, and 50 µg tablets. The recommended daily dose ranges from 50 to 100 µg/day (0.3 µg/pound/day) given in two divided doses. Our policy is to give young adults (<40 years old) 100 µg/day (50 µg twice-a-day) and older adults 50 µg/day (25 µg twice-a-day).

OTHER T4 WITHDRAWAL PROTOCOLS

In another protocol described by Serhal et al. (2004), T4 is discontinued without starting T3 and the serum TSH is serially measured 2 or 3 times a week until it reaches 30 mIU/L. Using this protocol, these investigators reported that a TSH elevation of 30 mIU/L was achieved 18 days after thyroidectomy and 22 days after T4 withdrawal in more than 95% of the patients. They noted minimal symptoms during this preparation, but did not formally quantify or test for symptoms attributable to hypothyroidism.

In another protocol described by Golger et al. (2003), patients simply underwent a 3-week T4 withdrawal period, before and after which TSH was measured. The TSH concentration rose to 45.2 mIU/L. A quality of life questionnaire [Short-Form 36 (SF-36)] was administered before withdrawal, at peak TSH concentration and after resumption of therapy. The overall degree of functional impairment was described as being not severe and did not result in loss of employment time, yet significant change in symptoms was observed from day 1 to day 22 in the Physical Function, Role-Physical, Vitality, Social Function, Role-Emotional and Mental Health categories of SF-36. Moreover, 17% of patients had a TSH <25 mIU/L at the end of three weeks. As a practical matter this poses a problem in scheduling I-131 therapy, low-iodine diets, lithium therapy.

In yet another withdrawal protocol, Guimaraes and DeGroot (1996) compared the efficacy of inducing moderate hypothyroidism by cutting replacement therapy in half, to a standard method using T3 described above. Moderate hypothyroidism induced by the half-dose protocol induced TSH elevations above the target level of 25–30 mIU/L at 5 weeks in most patients. Pulse, weight gain, and cholesterol were significantly different in the two protocols, and the patient's subjective evaluation of hypothyroid symptoms was significantly reduced in the half-dose arm. Still, patients did not undergo quantitative testing of symptomatology, and 15% of the total cohort did not achieve the serum TSH goal for withdrawal.

Any protocol that entails T4 withdrawal produces symptoms, albeit less in some of the studies than in others. The most difficult problem is that from 15% to 17% of the patients did not achieve a high enough TSH level after the shortened or half-dose T4 protocols to perform a radioiodine scan.

We have to test the TSH level at least five working days before the planned date of radioiodine administration because it takes a few days to get the result back and we have

Table 1. Protocol for Depriving Patients of Thyroid Hormone Prior to Radioiodine Administration.

6 weeks prior to radioiodine: stop T4 and start Cytomel* (on Cytomel for 4 weeks)
3 weeks before radioiodine: stop Cytomel
1 week before radioiodine: check serum TSH level (must be > 30 μU/mL)
The day after radioiodine administration: restart T4

* Cytomel dose: age < 40 years: 50 mcg PO BID, age > 40 years: 25 mcg PO BID.

to order the radioiodine a few days prior to the day of administration. If we stop T3 two weeks before the date of administration it means that the patient is off T3 for only one week when we check the TSH. If the TSH level is below 30 μU/mL at this time we must either assume that it will rise to an adequate level before the day of administration or to delay radioiodine administration for at least a week to document that the TSH level is above 30 μU/mL prior to administering radioiodine. This causes increased symptoms of hypothyroidism.

Both of these options are undesirable. We prefer to be sure that TSH elevation is adequate when we deliver radioiodine. Changing the I-131 administration date at the last minute causes major problems for most of our patients and for the team that schedules and administers the radioiodine. For these reasons, we often stop T3 three weeks before the planned date of radioiodine administration, which means that TSH is measured two full weeks after stopping T3 (five weeks after stopping T4), which is almost always sufficient to produce a TSH level above 30 μU/mL.

REFERENCES

Guimaraes, V, and LJ DeGroot. 1996. Moderate hypothyroidism in preparation for whole body ^{131}I scintiscans and thyroglobulin testing. Thyroid **6**:69–73.

Serhal, DI, MP Nasrallah, and BM Arafah. 2004. Rapid rise in serum thyrotropin concentrations after thyroidectomy or withdrawal of suppressive thyroxine therapy in preparation for radioactive iodine administration to patients with differentiated thyroid cancer. J Clin Endocrinol Metab **89**:3285–3289.

5B.6. RECOMBINANT HUMAN TSH: BACKGROUND INFORMATION AND STANDARD PROTOCOL

ROBERT J. AMDUR, MD AND ERNEST L. MAZZAFERRI, MD, MACP

When treating or scanning a patient with radioiodine it is important to stimulate iodine uptake by elevating Thyroid Stimulating Hormone (TSH) prior to radioiodine administration. There are two ways to do this: deprive the patient of thyroid hormone or inject the patient with recombinant human TSH (rhTSH). The protocols for withdrawing thyroid hormone are explained in another chapter. The purpose of this chapter is to provide background information and the standard protocol for prescribing rhTSH. The next chapter discusses indications for using rhTSH to prepare a patient for I-131 therapy.

DESCRIPTION OF THYROTROPIN ALFA

Thyrotropin alpha, which is the form of recombinant human TSH (rhTSH) used for medical purposes, is synthesized in a genetically modified Chinese hamster ovary cell line. Thyrogen® is the only brand of the drug marketed in the United States.

FDA APPROVED INDICATIONS FOR THYROTROPIN ALFA

Thyrotropin Alfa is approved by the Food and Drug Administration as an alternative to thyroid hormone withdrawal in preparation for diagnostic studies for thyroid cancer. The main indication for rhTSH is to avoid hypothyroidism when preparing thyroid cancer patients for radioiodine scans. The drug is also approved for thyroglobulin testing independent of diagnostic radioiodine scanning. Thyrotropin Alfa is not approved to prepare patients to ablate the thyroid remnant or treat cancer.

Table 1. The Standard Protocol for Using Recombinant Human TSH (Thyrotropin Alfa)*.

Day 1: Give Thyrotropin Alfa injection #1: 0.9 mg IM
Day 2: Give Thyrotropin Alfa injection #2: 0.9 mg IM
Day 3: Administer radioiodine
Day 4: Nothing
Day 5 or 7–10, depending on the reason for elevating TSH:
Day 5: Diagnostic whole body scan (DxWBS)** and/or serum thyroglobulin measurement
Day 7–10: Post-treatment whole body scan (RxWBS)**

* Days 1–5 refer to consecutive calendar days.
** Whole body scan: minimum scanning time: 30 minutes, minimum counts: 140,000.

USE OF THYROTROPIN ALFA IN CHILDREN

Safety and efficacy of Thyrotropin Alfa in children <16 years of age has not been studied.

DOSE, ROUTE OF ADMINISTRATION AND PHARMACOKINETICS

Thyrotropin Alfa is administered as a once–a–day intramuscular injection. Intravenous administration is contraindicated. The standard injection contains 0.9 mg of Thyrotropin Alfa in 1 ml total fluid volume. Following a 0.9 mg intramuscular injection the mean peak serum TSH concentration is 116 mIU/L, which occurs at a median of 10 hours following administration of one injection of 0.9 mg with a mean elimination half time of 22 hours (Fig. 1). To put this number in perspective it is useful to remember from the previous chapter that a TSH of > 30 µU/mL is considered to be adequate when preparing a patient for radioiodine by depriving them of thyroid hormone.

Recombinant human TSH is given as a 0.9 mg IM injection on two consecutive days, causing serum TSH levels to rise immediately and to peak about 24 hours after the injection, falling to normal levels within about 4 days and to baseline levels after about 6–7 days (Fig. 1). It is normally not necessary to measure TSH levels following rhTSH injection, although peak TSH levels are related to body surface area and weight, and may not reach valid stimulation range in morbidly obese patients (Vitale 2003).

CONTRAINDICATIONS AND PRECAUTIONS

Dose modifications of Thyrotropin Alfa are not necessary in patients with renal or hepatic insufficiency.

Cardiovascular disease: In patients with gross residual thyroid tissue or functional thyroid cancer, Thyrotropin Alfa may result in a significant and rapid rise in the level of thyroid hormone. For this reason Thyrotropin Alfa should be used with caution in patients with coronary artery disease or uncontrolled hypertension.

Brian or spinal cord metastases: In patients with CNS metastasis, Thyrotropin Alfa may result in acute edema, or growth leading to neurologic complications.

Paratracheal mass: Patients with large thyroid remnants or gross tumor near the trachea may experience airway compression due to the acute edema or growth after Thyrotropin Alfa injection.

RhTSH (Thyrogen®) Dosing Regimen

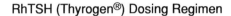

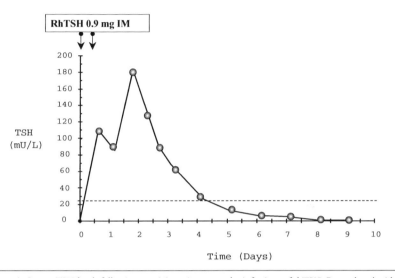

Figure 1. Serum TSH levels following two 0.9 mg intramuscular infections of rhTSH. Reproduced with permission from the Genzyme Corporation.

Coagulopathy: As Thyrotropin Alfa is administered as an intramuscular injection, this drug should be used with caution in patients with a coagulopathy such as hemophilia or thrombocytopenia.

SIDE-EFFECTS OF THYROTROPIN ALFA

The standard protocol is two 0.9 mg intramuscular injections of Thyrotropin Alfa. Most patients have no side-effects from this regimen. About 10% of patients report side-effects, most commonly symptoms of asthenia (the loss of strength and energy), mild headache, and/or nausea.

Patients with a large thyroid remnant or a large volume of function thyroid cancer may experience symptoms of hyperthyroidism after receiving Thyrotropin Alfa.

PROTOCOL FOR USE OF THYROTROPIN ALFA

Table 1 summarizes the standard protocol for preparing a patient with Thyrotropin Alpha for a diagnostic study (radioiodine scan or thyroglobulin measurement) or I-131 therapy. Figure 2 is a schematic of the protocol for using rhTSH to prepare a patient for I-131 therapy.

An injection is given on two consecutive days. Radioiodine is administered on Day 3 (approximately 72 hours after injection #1). When radioiodine is administered for diagnostic purposes, a scan is done and/or thyroglobulin level checked, two days later.

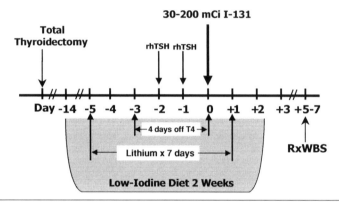

Figure 2. Protocol for using rhTSH prior to radioiodine therapy. We instruct the patient to discontinue thyroid hormone replacement three days prior to, and the day of, radioiodine administration. Unless there are contraindications to lithium use, we have the patient take lithium carbonate for 7 days, beginning 5 days prior to I-131 administration.

If radioiodine is given for therapeutic purposes, the next event in the protocol is to do a post-treatment whole body scan 5–7 days after the I-131 administration. These guidelines come from the large international multicenter trials that studied the efficacy of rhTSH in the management of differentiated thyroid carcinoma (Haugen 1999).

THE RATIONALE FOR STOPPING T4 FOR 4 DAYS WHEN USING rhTSH

We instruct the patient to discontinue thyroid hormone replacement three days prior to, and the day of, radioiodine administration (Fig. 2). We stop T4 for the same reason that we put the patient on a low-iodine diet. Standard doses of thyroid hormone contain enough iodine to interfere with the uptake of I-131. For example, the amount of iodine in a typical daily dose of L-thyroxine is about ten times the amount of iodine in 30 mCi of I-131 (approximately 50 μg versus 5 μg).

A recent study by Barbano et al. (2003) provides evidence that the iodine content in standard doses of L-thyroxin is likely to compromise I-131 therapy. These investigators compared the outcome of remnant ablation with 30 mCi I-131 in low-risk patients who were prepared with rhTSH compared with a control group that was prepared with 6 weeks of T4 deprivation. The only deviation from standard protocol was that T4 was stopped the day before the first injection of rhTSH and restarted the day after I-131 administration, amounting to 4 days of T4 withdrawal. All patients were instructed to consume a low-iodine diet for two weeks prior to receiving I-131. Urine iodine was measured in both treatment groups, as well as in an additional control group of patients who had no interruption in T4 replacement therapy prior to rhTSH stimulated diagnostic scans. The rate of successful ablation, defined as a negative diagnostic whole body scan and a serum thyroglobulin < 0.5 ng/mL, was higher when patients were prepared with rhTSH and 4 days off T4 (81%) than with six weeks of T4 deprivation (75%). In combination with the standard two-week low-iodine diet, patients taken off T4 for just four days had urine iodine levels (47μg/L) comparable to those observed following six weeks of T4 deprivation (39 μg/L), both of which were almost half those in the control group (76 μg/L) who were maintained on T4 continuously prior to diagnostic scanning with rhTSH preparation.

REFERENCES

Drug evaluation information related to rhTSH can be found on the web at http://cpip.gsm.com and then enter "Thyrotropin" or "Thyrogen" in the search window.

Haugen, BR, F Pacini, C Reiners, M Schlumberger, PW Ladenson, SI Sherman, DS Cooper, KE Graham, LE Braverman, MC Skarulis, TF Davies, LJ DeGroot, EL Mazzaferri, GH Daniels, DS Ross, M Luster, MH Samuels, DV Becker, HR Maxon III, RR Cavalieri, CA Spencer, K McEllin, BD Weintraub, and EC Ridgway. 1999. A comparison of recombinant human thyrotropin and thyroid hormone withdrawal for the detection of thyroid remnant or cancer. J Clin Endocrinol Metab **84**:3877–3885.

Vitale, G, GA Lupoli, A Ciccarelli, A Lucariello, MR Fittipaldi, F Fonderico, A Panico, and G Lupoli. 2003. Influence of body surface area on serum peak thyrotropin (TSH) levels after recombinant human TSH administration. J Clin Endocrinol Metab **88**:1319–1322.

5B.7. USING rhTSH PRIOR TO I-131 THERAPY

ROBERT J. AMDUR, MD AND ERNEST L. MAZZAFERRI, MD, MACP

The previous chapter explained the dose schedule and pharmacokinetics of using recombinant human thyroid stimulating hormone (rhTSH) prior to therapy or diagnostic testing. The purpose of this chapter is to explain the issues that effect the decision to use rhTSH to prepare patients for treatment with I-131.

POTENTIAL REASONS TO USE rhTSH

This section lists the potential indications or advantages of using rhTSH instead of thyroid hormone deprivation, to prepare a patient for diagnostic testing or radioiodine therapy:

Quality of life: The main rationale for using rhTSH is to avoid the symptoms of hypothyroidism that occur in virtually all patients who are deprived of thyroid hormone. With the typical thyroid hormone withdrawal protocol, most patients experience fatigue, difficulty with concentration, neuromuscular symptoms, constipation and other symptoms that compromise quality of life for at least four weeks. There are modifications of this protocol using shorter periods of withdraw, but they either fail to completely eradicate symptoms (Golger 2003) or have not quantitatively assessed symptoms (Serhal 2004). Symptoms of hypothyroidism do not occur with rhTSH. In a large U.S. and European multicenter trial (Haugen 1999) of the efficacy of rhTSH in which patients underwent both rhTSH and thyroid hormone withdrawal studies, patients had essentially no symptoms or signs of hypothyroidism after rhTSH administration compared with thyroid hormone withdrawal. There were statistically significant differences between rhTSH administration and thyroid hormone withdrawal for all 14 symptoms and signs of hypothyroidism on the Billewicz scale (a questionnaire for evaluating hypothyroidism symptoms). Patients reported significantly better quality of life scores (SF-36 instrument, a validated health survey developed for outcomes study) after rhTSH administration in areas including performance of physical activities, problems with daily activities as a result of physical health, bodily pain, and emotional problems compared with those after thyroid hormone withdrawal.

Cardiac disease: Hypothyroidism may exacerbate or precipitate serious problems in patients with ischemic heart disease, particularly when levothyroxine therapy is restarted.

Renal disease: Hypothyroidism normally causes a measurable but transient decline in renal function, which can be serious in patients with preexisting renal disease.

Psychiatric problems: Hypothyroidism may precipitate or exacerbate depression or psychosis in patients who are predisposed to these problems.

Conditions that impair endogenous TSH response to hypothyroidism: Old age, pituitary disease, concomitant high dose corticosteroid therapy, and patient noncompliance may make the TSH elevation suboptimal in response to the standard six-week period of hypothyroidism.

Gross tumor in critical areas: Complications from swelling or growth of metastatic disease in the brain or near the spinal cord, or adjacent to the airway or other vital structures might be more severe when a patient is deprived of thyroid hormone over an extended period than if they are prepared with rhTSH.

THE POTENTIAL DISADVANTAGE OF rhTSH

Gross tumor in critical areas: Tumor in critical areas such as the brain or near the spinal cord may rapidly enlarge in response to rhTSH injection, causing symptoms much as those occurring with thyroid hormone withdrawal, albeit with serum TSH elevations are of shorter duration. Also, bone metastases may become acutely painful with rhTSH administration.

Diagnostic studies (radioiodine DxWBS) may be less sensitive when the patient is prepared with rhTSH compared to thyroid hormone deprivation, although the multicenter study by Haugen et al. (1999) found no significant difference in uptake of I-131 between the methods of preparation. The rhTSH-stimulated serum thyroglobulin levels rise less than they do with thyroid hormone withdrawal, but adjusting the serum thyroglobulin cutoff levels circumvents this problem, making the rhTSH test at least as sensitive as thyroid hormone withdrawal in detecting tumor. Also FDG PET scans are more sensitive following rhTSH stimulation (see PET chapter).

Radioiodine therapy may be less effective in ablating the thyroid remnant and eliminating cancer if the patient is prepared with rhTSH. Differences in renal clearance and duration of TSH elevation are factors to consider:

Renal Clearance of radioiodine: Hypothyroidism decreases renal clearance of iodine, which recirculates back into normal or malignant follicular cells, thus increasing the time that radioiodine is concentrated in target cells (i.e., increased biologic half life). Several studies suggest thyroid hormone deprivation decreases renal clearance of radioiodine by approximately 50%.

Duration of TSH elevation: The length of time that target cells are stimulated to produce thyroglobulin or to concentrate I-131 is much longer when a patient is hypothyroid than following two injections of rhTSH. As explained in the previous chapter, serum TSH levels produced by rhTSH injections peak about 24 hours after the first injection and return to normal within about 4 days. Thyroid hormone withdrawal produces high serum TSH concentrations for 4 to 6 weeks or more, depending upon the withdrawal protocol. Moreover, renal clearance of I-131 remains normal after rhTSH administration, which reduces the effective half-life of I-131 in tumor.

In the final analysis, the choice of withdrawal over rhTSH is usually a matter of patient preference and remains a balance of competing factors. As a practical matter, most patients with serious metastatic disease who require multiple I-131 treatments over time rapidly become weary of undergoing thyroid hormone withdrawal and its attendant hypothyroidism, and many simply will not undergo repeated episodes of withdrawal.

STUDIES OF rhTSH FOR DIAGNOSTIC SCANNING

Reports like those shown in Figure 1 raise concern about the use of rhTSH to prepare patients for I-131 scans or therapy (Shlumberger 2000). However, two major phase III

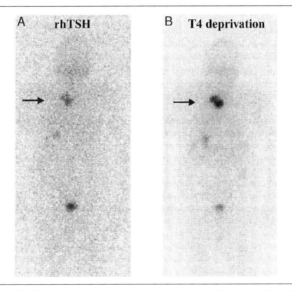

Figure 1. Sequential I-131 whole body scans in a patient with a vertebral metastasis (arrow). The scans were performed 48 hours after administration of 4 mCi I-131: first with stimulation with rhTSH (A) and subsequently with six weeks of thyroid hormone deprivation (B). Hormone deprivation was associated with more intense uptake on the scan and doubling of the time of retention of radioiodine. [From Fig. 1 in: Martin Schlumberger, Marcel Ricard and Furio Pacini. Clinical use of recombinant human TSH in thyroid cancer patients. European Journal of Endocrinology 2000, 143:557–563. Reproduced with permission from the Society of the European Journal of Endocrinology].

trials have compared the sensitivity of diagnostic whole body iodine scans and thyroglobulin measurements following preparation with rhTSH versus thyroid hormone withdrawal (Ladenson 1997; Haugen 1999). The study by Ladenson and colleagues (1997) showed a small increase in scan sensitivity with thyroid hormone withdrawal. The study published in 1999 by Haugen et al. was more meticulously controlled than the Ladenson study and showed no significant difference between rhTSH and thyroid hormone deprivation in both DxWBS and thyroglobulin sensitivity in detecting thyroid tumor and bed uptake. The Haugen study also compared two versus three 0.9 mg injections of rhTSH and found no difference in any of the study endpoints.

Based on these trials we believe that two injections of 0.9 mg rhTSH is a safe and effective alternative to thyroid hormone withdrawal for the preparation of patients for diagnostic scanning or thyroglobulin measurement. In our program all diagnostic testing is performed with rhTSH stimulation, unless the patient is unable to take the drug.

STUDIES OF rhTSH FOR THERAPEUTIC ADMINISTRATIONS

There are four important studies that compare the rate of successful remnant ablation following preparation with rhTSH versus thyroid hormone withdrawal. The studies by Ladenson et al. (2004), Robbins et al. (2001) and Barbaro et al. (2003) show no significant difference in ablation rates with rhTSH compared with thyroid hormone deprivation. The study by Pacini et al. (2002) reports a much higher failure rate of rhTSH than that after thyroid hormone withdrawal. In view of the controversy that exists about this issue a brief review of these studies is in order:

Robbins et al. (Memorial Sloan-Kettering, New York, 2002): This is the only published study that compares rhTSH and hormone deprivation in patients who receive standard therapeutic doses of I-131 (100–130 mCi) following total thyroidectomy. Approximately 10 months post ablation there was no significant difference in the chance of obtaining a negative total body scan (84% and 81%) or a TSH-stimulated thyroglobulin level <2 ng/mL (78% and 64%) following the two modalities of preparation (Fig. 2). The weak point of this study is that it is retrospective and thus selection criteria for receiving rhTSH and other aspects of the study were not standardized.

Pacini et al. (U. Pisa, Italy, 2002): This is a prospective study in which patients were sequentially assigned to treatment with either rhTSH or thyroid hormone deprivation prior to attempting remnant ablation with 30 mCi of I-131. The chance of a negative total body scan approximately 8 months post ablation was only 54% in patients treated with rhTSH compared to 84% following thyroid hormone deprivation (p <0.0001) (Fig. 3). Issues with this study are: 1) I-131 was given 48 hours, rather than the usual 24 hours, after the last rhTSH injection, 2) These results do not apply to patients who receive larger doses of I-131 (100–150 mCi,), and, 3) when using low dose therapy (30 mCi) the amount of iodine in thyroid hormone may have a major effect on the efficacy of a rhTSH-stimulated treatment. This final point is the subject of the Barbaro study.

Barbaro et al. (Spedali Riuniti, Italy 2003): This is similar to the Pacini et al. study in that patients were sequentially assigned to treatment with either rhTSH or thyroid hormone deprivation prior to the administration of 30 mCi I-131 in an attempt to ablate the thyroid remnant. In this study I-131 was administered at the usual time, 24 hours after

Remnant Ablation: Hypothyroid vs rhTSH

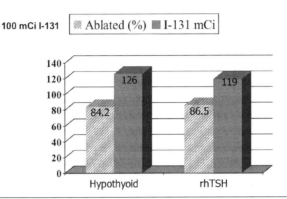

Figure 2. Retrospective study by Robbins et al. (2002) showing successful thyroid remnant ablation with 100 mCi I-131 following preparation with thyroid hormone withdrawal or rhTSH stimulation. Stripped bars represent the percent of patients achieving ablation and solid bars the average mCi I-131 necessary to achieve ablation. Drawn from the data of Robbins et al. J. Nucl. Med 2002 43:1482–1488.

Remnant Ablation: Hypothyroid vs rhTSH

30 mCi I-131 given <u>48 hrs</u> after last rhTSH dose

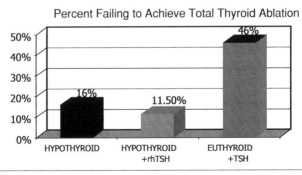

Figure 3. Prospective study of the remnant ablation results with 30 mCi I-131, shown as the percent failure rate in three groups of patients following preparation with rhTSH alone, rhTSH plus thyroid hormone withdrawal, and thyroid hormone withdrawal alone. I-131 was administered 48 hrs after the last dose of rhTSH. Drawn from the data of Pacini et al. J Clin Endocrinol Metab 2002; 87(9):4063–4068.

Remnant Ablation: Hypothyroid vs rhTSH

30 mCi I-131 given 24 hours after last rhTSH dose

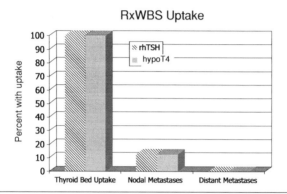

Figure 4. Prospective study of remnant ablation rates with 30 mCi I-131 in the protocol of Barbaro et al. that prepared patients with rhTSH with brief cessation of thyroid hormone. I-131 was administered 24 hours after the last injection of rhTSH. The ablation rate was similar following rhTSH preparation and thyroid hormone withdrawal. Drawn from the data of Barbaro et al. J Clin Endocrinol Metab 2003; 88(9):4110–4115.

the second injection of rhTSH. The unique factor in this study was that thyroid hormone was discontinued for three days prior to, and one day following, I-131 administration in the patients treated with rhTSH (Fig. 4). The rationale for this modification was that thyroid hormone replacement constitutes a significant source of dietary iodine. In contrast to the Pacini data, this study found no evidence of a worse outcome with rhTSH. Successful ablation (undetectable thyroglobulin and negative total body scan) was actually higher in patients prepared with rhTSH (81% versus 75%, p not significant).

Ladenson et al. Baltimore, 2004. This is a prospective study in which patients were randomized to receive rhTSH injections (n = 32) or to undergo thyroid hormone withdrawal (n = 28) in preparation for thyroid remnant ablation with 100 mCi I-131. Successful ablation was defined as 1) a negative DxWBS 2) if visible uptake, then RAIU <0.1%, 3) Tg< 2 ng/mL 72 hr. after the last injection of rhTSH. The results of this study, which are shown in Fig. 5, indicate that thyroid hormone withdrawal and rhTSH preparation are comparable in preparing patients for remnant ablation with 100 mCi I-131.

OUR VIEW OF THE ISSUE

Our position is that it is possible to use rhTSH in a way that does not compromise the results of treatment, and thus the outcome of patients with thyroid cancer. Elevating TSH is one of several important components of the preparatory regimen. Meticulous attention

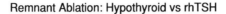

Remnant Ablation: Hypothyroid vs rhTSH

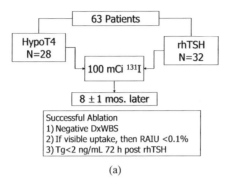

(a)

Remnant Ablation: Hypothyroid vs rhTSH

100 mCi I-131

	Thyroid Bed Uptake <0.1%	Serum Tg < 2 ng/mL	No Visible Thyroid Bed Uptake
HypoT4	100% 28/28	87% 20/32	86% 24/28
rhTSH	100% 32/32	96% 23/24	75% 24/32

(b)

Figure 5. Results of a prospective randomized study of remnant ablation with 100 mCi I-131 after preparation with either thyroid hormone withdrawl or rhTSH. (A) Criteria for ablation. (B) Results drawn from the data of Ladenson et al. (Ladenson PW, Pacini F, Schlumberger M et al. Endocrine Society ABSTRACT S35-1 New Orleans June 16–19 2004).

to depleting iodine stores prior to radioiodine administration will produce better results at any given level of TSH stimulation. In suitable patients, lithium therapy will increase the potency of a given dose of radioiodine to a significant degree by increasing the biologic half-life of I-131. These issues are the subjects of separate chapters in this part of the book.

In our opinion, the morbidity of the hypothyroidism that results from a 4–6 week period of thyroid hormone deprivation is such that the overall risk/benefit profile of using rhTSH to prepare patients for diagnostic studies or radioiodine therapy is favorable, assuming that other aspects of the preparatory regimen are optimized. We use rhTSH in all patients prior to diagnostic testing and in most patients prior to radioiodine therapy. The only setting in which we are undecided about the use of rhTSH in adults is the high-risk patient with distant metastases who tolerates hypothyroidism well. We do not use rhTSH in children.

REFERENCES

Barbaro, D, G Boni, G Meucci, U Simi, P Lapi, P Orsini, C Pasquini, F Piazza, M Caciagli, and G Mariani. 2003. Radioiodine treatment with 30 mCi after recombinant human thyrotropin stimulation in thyroid cancer: effectiveness for postsurgical remnants ablation and possible role of iodine content in ʟ-thyroxine in the outcome of ablation. J Clin Endocrinol Metab **88:**4110–4115.

Golger, A, TR Fridman, S Eski, IJ Witterick, JL Freeman, and PG Walfish. 2003. Three-week thyroxine withdrawal thyroglobulin stimulation screening test to detect low-risk residual/recurrent well-differentiated thyroid carcinoma. J Endocrinol Invest **26:**1023–1031.

Haugen, BR, F Pacini, C Reiners, M Schlumberger, PW Ladenson, SI Sherman, DS Cooper, KE Graham, LE Braverman, MC Skarulis, TF Davies, LJ DeGroot, EL Mazzaferri, GH Daniels, DS Ross, M Luster, MH Samuels, DV Becker, HR Maxon III, RR Cavalieri, CA Spencer, K McEllin, BD Weintraub, and EC Ridgway. 1999. A comparison of recombinant human thyrotropin and thyroid hormone withdrawal for the detection of thyroid remnant or cancer. J Clin Endocrinol Metab **84:**3877–3885.

Ladenson, PW, LE Braverman, EL Mazzaferri, F Brucker-Davis, DS Cooper, JR Garber, FE Wondisford, TF Davies, LJ DeGroot, GH Daniels, DS Ross, and BD Weintraub. 1997. Comparison of administration of recombinant human thyrotropin with withdrawal of thyroid hormone for radioactive iodine scanning in patients with thyroid carcinoma. N Engl J Med **337:**888–896.

Ladenson, PW, F Pacini, M Schlumberger, et al. 2004. Randomized study of remnant ablation using recombinant human TSH versus thyroid hormone withdrawal. The Endocrine Society Abstract S35-1, New Orleans, 16–19 June.

Mazzaferri, EL, and RT Kloos. 2005. Carcinoma of follicular epithelium: radioiodine and other treatment outcomes. In: Werner's & Ingbar's The Thyroid: A Fundamental and Clinical Text, 9th edn. Philadelphia: Lippincott Willams & Wilkins (Braverman LE, Utiger RD, eds) 934–966.

Pacini, F, E Molinaro, MG Castagna, F Lippi, C Ceccarelli, L Agate, R Elisei, and A Pinchera. 2002. Ablation of thyroid residues with 30 mCi (131)I: a comparison in thyroid cancer patients prepared with recombinant human TSH or thyroid hormone withdrawal. J Clin Endocrinol Metab **87:**4063–4068.

Robbins, RJ, and AK Robbins. 2003. Recombinant human thyrotropin and thyroid cancer management. J Clin Endocrinol Metab **88(5):**1933–1938.

Robbins, RJ, RM Tuttle, RN Sharaf, SM Larson, HK Robbins, RA Ghossein, A Smith, and WD Drucker. 2001. Preparation by recombinant human thyrotropin or thyroid hormone withdrawal are comparable for the detection of residual differentiated thyroid carcinoma. J Clin Endocrinol Metab **86:**619–625.

Schlumberger, M, M Ricard, and F Pacini. 2000. Clinical use of recombinant human TSH in thyroid cancer patients. Eur J Endocrinol **143:**557–563.

Serhal, DI, MP Nasrallah, and BM Arafah. 2004. Rapid rise in serum thyrotropin concentrations after thyroidectomy or withdrawal of suppressive thyroxine therapy in preparation for radioactive iodine administration to patients with differentiated thyroid cancer. J Clin Endocrinol Metab **89:**3285–3289.

PART 5C. THYROID REMNANT ABLATION

5C.1. I-131 THERAPY IN A PATIENT WITH A SMALL THYROID REMNANT

ROBERT J. AMDUR, MD AND ERNEST L. MAZZAFERRI, MD, MACP

The term thyroid remnant ablation is commonly used when the primary goal of I-131 therapy is to destroy normal residual thyroid tissue. It is important to understand that ablation of the normal thyroid remnant is not the only reason for giving I-131. When the risk of residual cancer is significant following thyroid surgery, then the goals of I-131 therapy are to destroy both residual cancer and the thyroid remnant.

SMALL VERSUS LARGE THYROID REMNANTS

The problems associated with a large thyroid remnant are described in the next chapter and in the chapter on hemithyroidectomy. The potential problems with a large thyroid remnant become important enough to change management recommendations when the size of the remnant reaches 2 grams (or cubic centimeters). We evaluate the size of the thyroid remnant by ultrasound. Thyroid remnants that are <2 grams are considered to be "small" and remnants ≥2 grams are considered "large". This information comes from a meta-analysis by Doi and Woodhouse (2000), that found that the size of the thyroid remnant is an important determinant predicting total thyroid ablation with I-131. Another study by Maxon et al. (1992), found that, 94% of patients had successful ablation when the surgeon left less than 2 grams of thyroid tissue as compared with a 68% success rate when the remnant was larger. Others have reported similar findings.

In general, patients with small thyroid remnants are those in whom the surgeon attempted to perform a total thyroidectomy. The purpose of this chapter is to present guidelines for treating patients with I-131 therapy following near total thyroidectomy.

Table 1. Summary of Main Points About Ablation of a Small Thyroid Remnant.

Small versus large thyroid remnant:
Small: <2 grams, large: ≥2 grams

Routine remnant ablation is controversial:
The argument against routine ablation of the thyroid remnant is that it has not been consistently shown to increase survival in patients with low-risk tumors.
The main arguments in favor of routine ablation of the thyroid remnant are:
* It is not possible to use the serum level of thyroglobulin as a sensitive measure of tumor status unless all normal thyroid tissue has been destroyed
* Remnant ablation may destroy residual cancer cells in the thyroid bed or elsewhere
* Ablating the thyroid remnant destroys residual follicular cells which are at risk for undergoing malignant transformation in the future
* The presence of a thyroid remnant may decrease the sensitivity of an iodine scan for the detection of nodal or distant metastasis by two mechanisms: tumor tissue produces a star burst effect that obscures neck and lung metastases, and a large remnant makes it difficult to raise TSH to a level that optimizes the uptake of radioiodine in residual tumor
* There are consistent data that remnant ablation decreases the risk of locoregional recurrence and distant metastases in both adults and children

Our policy regarding remnant ablation following (near) total thyroidectomy:
Our preference is to ablate the thyroid remnant in all patients who have undergone near total thyroidectomy
I-131 dose guidelines are shown in table 2
Ablation of the thyroid remnant is probably not necessary in patients with a solitary tumor of maximum dimension <1 cm that is confined to the thyroid with no areas of unfavorable differentiation, no vascular space invasion, and no nodal or distant metastasis

---

Radioiodine therapy in patients with a large thyroid remnant is the subject of the next chapter. Table 1 summarizes the major points from this chapter.

ROUTINE REMNANT ABLATION IS CONTROVERSIAL

Routine ablation of the thyroid remnant is controversial, especially in young patients with early stage disease. The article by Mazzaferri (1997) and the meta-analysis by Sawka et al. (2004) summarize the pertinent literature.

In the Sawka study (2004), pooled analyses showed a statistically significant treatment effect of ablation for the following 10-yr outcomes: locoregional recurrence (relative risk of 0.31, 95% CI, 0.2, 0.49) and distant metastases (absolute decrease in risk 3%, 95% CI, risk 1–4%). However, results have been inconsistent among centers for some outcomes, especially cancer specific mortality, mainly because of insufficient follow-up time. Thus, the incremental benefit of remnant ablation in low-risk patients treated with bilateral thyroidectomy and thyroid hormone suppressive therapy is unclear when measured in terms of enhanced survival.

Remnant ablation has not been consistently shown to improve cancer-specific survival except in the 1997 Mazzaferri study, which had the longest follow-up in the meta-analysis reported by Sawka et al., and in two other studies. Taylor et al. (1998) found that in patients with papillary cancer, radioiodine therapy was associated with improvement in cancer-specific mortality (RR 0.30) and disease progression (RR, 0.3), although when tall-cell variants were excluded, the effect on outcome was not significant.

After radioiodine therapy, patients with follicular thyroid cancer had improvement in overall mortality (RR, 0.17), cancer-specific mortality (RR, 0.12), disease progression (RR, 0.21), and disease-free survival (RR, 0.29). In the study by Lopez-Penabad et al. (2003) radioiodine conferred a survival benefit when used for adjuvant ablation therapy.

There are other important and practical arguments in favor of routine thyroid remnant ablation:

1. It is not possible to use the serum thyroglobulin level as a sensitive measure of tumor status in patients with residual normal thyroid tissue.
2. Remnant ablation may destroy residual cancer cells in the thyroid bed or thyroid remnant.
3. Ablating the thyroid remnant destroys residual follicular cells that are at risk for undergoing malignant transformation in the future. Sugg et al. (1998) found that multifocal intrathyroidal papillary thyroid carcinomas are not simply the result of lymphatic spread within the thyroid gland, but also have different RET/PTC oncogenes that give rise to *de novo* tumors in follicular cells that appear have an inherent predisposition to malignancy.
4. The presence of a large thyroid remnant may decrease the sensitivity of a radioiodine whole body scan for the detection of nodal or distant metastasis by two mechanisms. Normal thyroid tissue concentrates iodine more avidly than tumor tissue and a large thyroid remnant often shows a star burst effect that obscures metastases and makes it difficult to elevate TSH to a level that optimizes the uptake of radioiodine in residual tumor.

The ability to use thyroglobulin levels to detect recurrent disease long before it becomes visible on imaging studies is reason enough to ablate the thyroid remnant. The presence of a thyroid remnant makes it impossible to interpret serum thyroglobulin levels, unless they are clearly rising over time. This does not allow for early diagnosis of tumor. In order to signal the presence of persistent tumor, serum thyroglobulin levels must rise well above the already high serum thyroglobulin levels caused by a thyroid remnant; moreover, there is no clear cutoff for TSH-stimulated serum Tg levels to distinguish residual tumor. In contrast, after total thyroidectomy and remnant ablation, a TSH-stimulated serum thyroglobulin value >2 ng/mL >6 months after remnant ablation usually.

Thus there are a variety of reasons to believe that ablating the thyroid remnant will decrease cancer recurrence. Several large data sets support this claim. Figure 1 presents data from Ohio State University. The article by Mazzaferri and Kloos (2001) from which this figure is taken presents an in-depth analysis of the effect of remnant ablation on tumor outcome. The bottom line is that Cox regression demonstrated a statistically significant decrease in cancer recurrence, distant metastasis recurrence, and cancer mortality after a median follow-up of about 18 years in patients who underwent thyroid remnant ablation. A more recent study by Chow et al. (2002) found on Cox multivariate analysis that

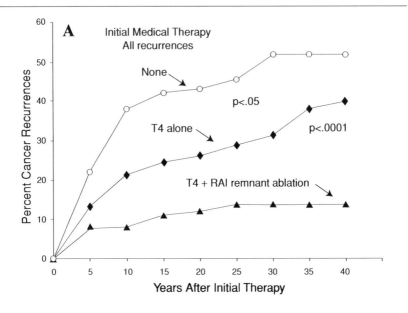

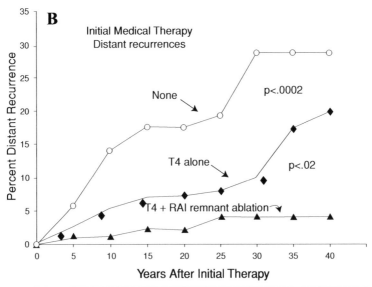

Figure 1. Effect of I-131 therapy to ablate the thyroid remnant on (A) the rate of cancer recurrence and (B) development of distant metastasis in 1,439 patients with differentiated thyroid carcinoma. Cancer recurrence is lowest in patients who had the thyroid remnant ablated soon after thyroidectomy. Modified from Fig. 3 in Mazzaferri EL and Kloos R.T. Current approaches to primary therapy for papillary and follicular thyroid cancer. J. Clin. Endocrinol. Metab 86(4), 1447–1463. 2001. Reproduced with permission of the Endocrine Society.

remnant ablation in patients with T1 N0 M0 tumor decreased the rate of locoregional recurrence by 70% and reduced the rate of distant metastases by 80%.

OUR POLICY REGARDING REMNANT ABLATION FOLLOWING (NEAR) TOTAL THYROIDECTOMY

Our preference is to ablate the thyroid remnant in all patients with differentiated thyroid cancer, including those with T1 N0 M0 tumors who have undergone a total thyroidectomy documented by ultrasonography and/or thyroid uptake measurement. Studies by Jarzab (2000) and Chow et al. (2004) show that this approach benefits children with thyroid cancer.

Perhaps the most cogent arguments against remnant ablation are that some low risk patients do not benefit from this treatment and are exposed to potentially harmful doses of radiation and painfully long periods of hypothyroidism. These are important arguments. They are clearly good reason to keep the activity of I-131 as low as possible for patients undergoing remnant ablation. Two recent studies help with this dilemma. The prospective randomized clinical trial by Bal et al. (1996) that was done to evaluate the optimal dose of I-131 for remnant ablation, found that increasing the empirical I-131 initial dose to more than 50 mCi results in a plateau of the dose-response curve, beyond which no further benefit is gained by increasing the amount of I-131. A second study by Bal et al. (2004) showed that patients receiving at least 25 mCi of I-131 had a three-fold better chance of achieving remnant ablation than did patients receiving less I-131, and any activity of I-131 between 25 and 50 mCi was adequate for remnant ablation.

The second concern about prolonged periods of hypothyroidism is also an important argument that has been addressed by several recent studies which show that rhTSH can prepare euthyroid patients (taking thyroid hormone) for remnant ablation with a success rate similar to that following thyroid hormone withdrawal. However, all but one of these rhTSH studies employed 100 mCi I-131 to achieve successful ablation. The prospective study by Barbaro et al. (2003) showed that the percentage of ablation (defined as an undetectable Tg and a negative WBS) was higher, although not reaching statistical significance, in patients treated with rhTSH (81.2%) compared with 75% for those undergoing thyroid hormone withdrawal.

Taken together, these data indicate that thyroid remnant ablation can be done with relatively low amounts of I-131, in the range of 25 to 50 mCi, following preparation with rhTSH, and that such therapy has substantial impact on locoregional recurrence and the appearance of new distant metastases, and can prolong survival. The protocol that we use is shown in Fig. 2.

Management decisions based only on overall survival data ignore the morbidity that an episode of cancer recurrence has on patients and their families. The specter of uncontrolled cancer is enormously distressing and subsequent therapy is often morbid and associated with a risk of permanent sequelae. There is no question that ablation of the thyroid remnant improves our ability to follow patients for tumor recurrence and decreases the chance of tumor relapse in most situations.

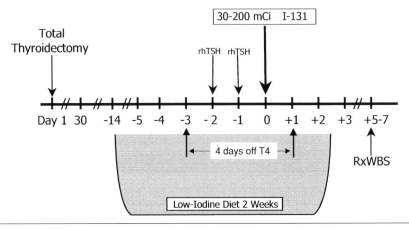

Figure 2. Protocol used in the authors' clinic for thyroid remnant ablation. In adults, we prefer to prepare patients for I-131 therapy with Recombinant Human TSH and four days of thyroid hormone withdrawl. Not shown in this figure is the administration of lithium for a total of 7 days, beginning 5 days prior to I-131 administration.

We discuss the rationale for, and arguments against, thyroid remnant ablation in all patients as part of the consent process. We recommend remnant ablation in all patients regardless of age and disease extent. Table 2 presents the guidelines that we use for prescribing I-131 when a goal of therapy is to ablate a small thyroid remnant.

The intensity with which we make the recommendation for thyroid remnant ablation depends on the likelihood of tumor recurrence. Clearly there are situations where the potential benefit of remnant ablation is extremely low. For example, ablation of the thyroid remnant is probably not necessary in patients with a solitary tumor of maximum dimension <1 cm that is confined to the thyroid with no areas of unfavorable differentiation (e.g., Tall cell features), no vascular space invasion, and no nodal or distant metastasis, especially if the basal serum Tg level is undetectable.

EXTERNAL BEAM RADIOTHERAPY

We mention external beam radiotherapy here to remind the reader that there are situations where we recommend treatment with both I-131 and external beam radiotherapy following thyroidectomy. Guidelines for external beam radiotherapy are the subject of separate chapters. Basically, in patients with no evidence of gross residual disease, we recommend both I-131 and external beam radiotherapy in patients older than 45 years if the thyroidectomy specimen demonstrates a positive margin, invasion of normal tissues that

Table 2. Guidelines for Ablation of the Thyroid Remnant Following (near) Total Thyroidectomy.

I-131 dose is based on risk catagory:		
Low risk	Stage[1] T1N0M0	50 mCi
Standard risk	All situations that do not qualify as low or high-risk	150 mCi
High risk	Stage[1] T4 or M1 or any situation where there is known to be residual disease	200 mCi

Lithium carbonate[2]:
Lithium is used in all patients unless there is a specific contraindication

Preparation with rhTSH instead of T4 deprivation[2]:
We use rhTSH in all situations except when the patient is a child, the cost of rhTSH is prohibitive, or the patient prefers T4 deprivation

Thyroid remnant ablation in children[2]:
Dose prescriptions are not standardized to the degree that they are in adults. In children who are well below adult size and stage of development we usually prescribe an amount of I-131 adjusted by the child's total body surface area that makes it comparable to that given to an adult (see chapter on lung metastases)

As with adults, we use lithium in all cases unless there are specific contraindications to its use

We do not use rhTSH in children unless there are contraindications to making the patient hypothyroid. The optimal safe dose of rhTSH in children has not yet been established

---

[1] 6th edition of the AJCC staging system.
[2] Seperate chapters are devoted to these topics.

define a stage T4 primary tumor, or nodal metastasis with extensive extracapsular tumor extension. Our preference is to deliver I-131 therapy before external beam treatments.

REFERENCES

Bal, CS, A Kumar, and GS Pant. 2004. Radioiodine dose for remnant ablation in differentiated thyroid carcinoma: a randomized clinical trial in 509 patients. J Clin Endocrinol Metab **89(4):**1666–1673.

Bal, C, AK Padhy, S Jana, GS Pant, and AK Basu. 1996. Prospective randomized clinical trial to evaluate the optimal dose of ^{131}I for remnant ablation in patients with differentiated thyroid carcinoma. Cancer **77:**2574–2580.

Barbaro, D, G Boni, G Meucci, U Simi, P Lapi, P Orsini, C Pasquini, F Piazza, M Caciagli, and G Mariani. 2003. Radioiodine treatment with 30 mCi after recombinant human thyrotropin stimulation in thyroid cancer: effectiveness for postsurgical remnants ablation and possible role of iodine content in L-thyroxine in the outcome of ablation. J Clin Endocrinol Metab **88(9):**4110–4115.

Chow, SM, SC Law, WM Mendenhall, SK Au, PT Chan, TW Leung, CC Tong, IS Wong, and WH Lau. 2002. Papillary thyroid carcinoma: prognostic factors and the role of radioiodine and external radiotherapy. Int J Radiat Oncol Biol Phys **52(3):**784–795.

Chow, SM, SC Law, WM Mendenhall, SK Au, S Yau, O Mang, and WH Lau. 2004. Differentiated thyroid carcinoma in childhood and adolescence-clinical course and role of radioiodine. Pediatr Blood Cancer **42(2):**176–183.

Doi, SA, and NJ Woodhouse. 2000. Ablation of the thyroid remnant and ^{131}I dose in differentiated thyroid cancer. Clin Endocrinol (Oxford) **52(6):**765–773.

Jarzab, B, JD Handkiewicz, J Wloch, B Kalemba, J Roskosz, A Kukulska, and Z Puch. 2000. Multivariate analysis of prognostic factors for differentiated thyroid carcinoma in children. Eur J Nucl Med **27(7):**833–841.

Lopez-Penabad, L, AC Chiu, AO Hoff, P Schultz, S Gaztambide, NG Ordonez, and SI Sherman. 2003. Prognostic factors in patients with Hurthle cell neoplasms of the thyroid. Cancer **97:**1186–1194.

Maxon, HR, EE Englaro, SR Thomas, VS Hertzberg, JD Hinnefeld, LS Chen, H Smith, D Cummings, and MD Aden. 1992. Radioiodine-131 therapy for well-differentiated thyroid cancer—a quantitative radiation dosimetric approach: outcome and validation in 85 patients. J Nucl Med **33:**1132–1136.

Mazzaferri, EL. 1997. Thyroid remnant ^{131}I ablation for papillary and follicular thyroid carcinoma. Thyroid **7(2):**265–271.

Mazzaferri, EL, and RT Kloos. 2001. Current approaches to primary therapy for papillary and follicular thyroid cancer. J Clin Endocrinol Metab **86(4):**1447–1463.

Sawka, AM, K Thephamongkhol, M Brouwers, L Thabane, G Browman, and HC Gerstein. 2004. Clinical review 170: a systematic review and metaanalysis of the effectiveness of radioactive iodine remnant ablation for well-differentiated thyroid cancer. J Clin Endocrinol Metab **89(8):**3668–3676.

Sugg, SL, S Ezzat, IB Rosen, JL Freeman, and SL Asa. 1998. Distinct multiple RET/PTC gene rearrangements in multifocal papillary thyroid neoplasia. J Clin Endocrinol Metab **83:**4116–4122.

5C.2. I-131 THERAPY IN A PATIENT WITH A LARGE THYROID REMNANT

ROBERT J. AMDUR, MD AND ERNEST L. MAZZAFERRI, MD, MACP

A thyroid remnant is considered to be "large" when it is ≥ 2 grams (or cubic centimeters). We measure the size of a thyroid remnant with ultrasound. The purpose of this chapter is to explain the issues that are important to consider when using I-131 therapy in a patient with a large thyroid remnant. Table 1 summarizes the main points from this chapter.

THE PROBLEM WITH A LARGE THYROID REMNANT

The problem with a large thyroid remnant is explained in the chapters in this book that discuss hemithyroidectomy and I-131 therapy in patients with a small thyroid remnant. The main argument for leaving a large thyroid remnant is that it decreases the chance of complications from thyroid cancer surgery, most notably recurrent laryngeal nerve injury and hypoparathyroidism. In contrast, the main rationale for total thyroidectomy is to decrease the chance of tumor recurrence and to improve the probability of achieving complete remnant ablation with low doses of I-131. Leaving a large thyroid remnant makes it difficult to achieve these goals. For example, in the study by Ozata et al. (1995) 75% of the patients who underwent partial thyroidectomy without I-131 remnant ablation had, during thyroid hormone suppression of TSH, serum Tg concentrations of TSH >3 ng/mL and 20% had levels >10 ng/mL, well in the range suggesting persistent tumor.

Table 1. Summary of the Major Points About Ablation of a Large Thyroid Remnant.

Definition of a "large" thyroid remnant:
A "large" thyroid remnant is ≥ 2 grams (cubic centimeters)

Reasons to ablate a thyroid remnant of any size:
It is not possible to use the serum level of thyroglobulin as a sensitive measure of tumor status unless all normal thyroid tissue has been destroyed
Remnant ablation may destroy residual cancer cells in the thyroid remnant
Ablating the thyroid remnant destroys residual follicular cells which are at risk for undergoing malignant transformation in the future

Problems specific to a large thyroid remnant:
Decreased effectiveness of radioiodine therapy and decreased sensitivity of iodine imaging by two mechanisms:
Normal thyroid tissue concentrates iodine more avidly than tumor tissue and a large thyroid remnant may produce a star burst effect obscuring cervical and lung metastases, and it may cause difficulties in elevating the TSH in response to thyroid hormone withdrawal to a level that optimizes the uptake of radioiodine in residual tumor
Complete ablation of a large thyroid remnant often requires multiple radioiodine treatments. This may require multiple I-131 treatments if the goal of therapy is to have no uptake on the thyroid DxWBS and undetectable TSH-stimulated Tg levels
Radioiodine therapy in a patient with a large thyroid remnant occasionally causes severe neck edema or dysphagia or thyroid storm

We prefer to never be in the position of delivering I-131 to a patient with a large thyroid remnant, and usually advise completion thyroidectomy
We advocate completion thyroidectomy for a large thyroid remnant unless there are factors that make the risk of the procedure high- such as underlying medical problems or a recurrent laryngeal nerve paralysis from the initial thyroidectomy procedure

I-131 dose when we do treat a patient with a large thyroid remnant:
30 mCi I-131
We usually prepare adults with rhTSH rather than T4 deprivation
We usually use lithium to increase I-131 potency

OUR FIRST CHOICE IS COMPLETION THYROIDECTOMY

Our preference is to never be in a situation where we are treating a patient with a large thyroid remnant with radioiodine. We advocate completion thyroidectomy in all patients with thyroid cancer who are referred to our clinic with a large thyroid remnant unless there are factors that make the risk of the procedure high, such as serious underlying medical problems or a recurrent laryngeal nerve paralysis from the initial thyroidectomy procedure. The intensity of our recommendation for additional surgery is low when the prognosis is so favorable that there is no need for additional treatment. This usually occurs in a patient with a unifocal tumor < 1 cm in diameter, with a negative surgical margin, no extrathyroid extension, no unfavorable histologic features, no vascular space invasion, and no nodal or distant metastasis.

ABLATION OF A LARGE THYROID REMNANT WITH I-131

Some disagree with the recommendation for completion thyroidectomy in patients with a large thyroid remnant when the primary tumor is larger than 1 cm. The study by Randolph and Daniels (2002) supports the view that radioiodine ablation of a large thyroid remnant is effective in destroying enough thyroid tissue to raise the TSH and reduce the uptake in the DxWBS and might be associated with less morbidity than completion thyroidectomy. However, stringent criteria for complete remnant ablation comprising absent uptake of radioiodine on DxWBS and an undetectable serum TSH-stimulated Tg level were not met in this study. It has been our experience that multiple I-131 treatments are required following hemithyroidectomy to achieve a negative iodine scan, and that thyroglobulin levels frequently remain elevated. Moreover, there are acute side effects when radioiodine is given to treat large remnants—especially neck edema, dysphagia, or severe neck pain and rarely even thyroid storm.

The study by Bal et al. (2003) documents the need for multiple radioiodine treatments to achieve a negative DxWBS in patients with a large thyroid remnant. The major criterion for ablation in this study was a negative DxWBS, and the minor criteria were a 48 h uptake of I-131 (RAIU) of <0.2% and a thyroglobulin value of $\leq$10 ng/mL. Only 57% of patients achieved a negative DxWBS after a single radioiodine treatment averaging 30 mCi, and 8% required three treatments to achieve ablation goals. The results would have been considerably worse if a negative DxWBS and TSH-stimulated thyroglobulin level of <2 ng/ml had been used as the criteria for successful ablation.

There is a large body of data demonstrating that ablating the thyroid remnant following total thyroidectomy decreases the likelihood of cancer recurrence, including those at distant sites such as the lung. This implies that any compromise in the thoroughness of remnant ablation is likely to reduce the chance of cancer cure. In our opinion, the acute morbidity and long term risks of multiple radioiodine treatments are not insignificant. For these reasons we prefer to surgically remove all gross thyroid tissue (i.e., completion thyroidectomy) prior to using radioiodine to ablate the thyroid remnant in patients where the risks of a completion thyroidectomy are likely to be acceptable.

OUR GUIDELINES FOR ABLATION OF A LARGE THYROID REMNANT

Table 2 summarizes the guidelines that we use for managing patients with a large thyroid remnant. Our standard policy is to give 30 mCi I-131 when the goal is to ablate a large thyroid remnant in patients who cannot or will not undergo completion thyroidectomy.

Table 2. Our Guidelines for Ablation of a Large Thyroid Remnant.

When there are no unusual risks to completion thyroidectomy[1]:
We recommend completion thyroidectomy in all patients

When the risk of completion thyroidectomy is high[1]:
Thyroid remnant ablation with 30 mCi I-131

Lithium carbonate[2]:
Lithium is used in all patients unless there is a specific contraindication

Preparation with rhTSH instead of T4 deprivation[2]:
We use rhTSH in all situations except when the patient is a child, the cost of rhTSH is prohibitive, or the patient prefers T4 deprivation
When using rhTSH in patients with a large thyroid remnant, we prescribe Propranolol XL 60 mg per day for approximately 4 weeks to decrease the chance of cardiac problems from excessive T4 production

---

[1] Relative contraindications to completion thyroidectomy include underlying medical problems that make the procedure high-risk or unilateral recurrent laryngeal nerve paralysis from the initial thyroidectomy procedure.
[2] Seperate chapters are devoted to these topics.

An approach that uses the results of a radioiodine uptake study to prescribe the dose for remnant ablation is described by Zidan et al. (2004) and is summarized in the chapter on choosing the dose of I-131 for therapy.

REFERENCES

Bal, CS, A Kumar, and GS Pant. 2003. Radioiodine lobar ablation as an alternative to completion thyroidectomy in patients with differentiated thyroid cancer. Nucl Med Commun **24(2):**203–208.

Ozata, M, H Bayhan, N Bingöl, S Dündar, Z Beyhan, A Corakci, and MA Gundogan. 1995. Sequential changes in serum thyroid peroxidase following radioiodine therapy of patients with differentiated thyroid carcinoma. J Clin Endocrinol Metab **80:3**634–3638.

Randolph, GW, and GH Daniels. 2002. Radioactive iodine lobe ablation as an alternative to completion thyroidectomy for follicular carcinoma of the thyroid. Thyroid **12(11):**989–996.

Zidan, J, E Hefer, G Iosilevski, K Drumea, M Stein, A Kuten, and O Israel. 2004. Efficacy of I-131 ablation therapy using different doses as determined by postoperative thyroid scan uptake in patients with differentiated thyroid cancer. IJROPB **59(5):**1330–1336.

PART 5D. SUPPRESSION OF THYROTROPIN AND THE POTENTIAL TOXICITY OF I-131 THERAPY

5D.1. EFFECTS OF SUPPRESSING THYROTROPIN ON TUMOR GROWTH AND RECURRENCE

ERNEST L. MAZZAFERRI, MD, MACP

It is common practice to prescribe levothyroxine (L–T4) to patients with differentiated thyroid carcinoma following initial therapy. This chapter will summarize the rationale for this treatment and the prevailing opinion concerning its use and the degree of suppression of Thyrotropin (Thyroid Stimulating Hormone, TSH) that is optimal in this setting.

TSH stimulates both the growth and functional activity of thyroid follicular cells, including activity of the sodium iodine symporter that transports iodine into the cell. There is now direct evidence that *in vitro* stimulation of the TSH receptor is sufficient to initiate thyroid tumorigenesis (Ludgate 1999). TSH also stimulates the growth and activity of malignant follicular cells in man, which forms the basis for the use of L–T4 in the treatment of this disease. Like normal thyroid tissue, most papillary and follicular carcinomas contain functional TSH receptors and sodium iodine symporters (Shen 2001), but whether postoperative L–T4 alone improves survival is less certain. There have been no prospective randomized trials of this question, but there is evidence that TSH stimulates tumor growth.

Tumors in patients with Graves' disease may be more aggressive, which is thought to be the result of stimulatory effects of circulating TSH receptor antibodies (Belfiore 2001). Rapid tumor growth sometimes follows L–T4 withdrawal in preparation for I-131 therapy. Moreover, L–T4 given as an adjunct following surgical and I-131 therapy is effective. Tumor recurrence rates are higher if L–T4 is not given after surgery. We found that there were significantly fewer recurrences after 30 years' follow-up of patients treated with L-T4 as compared with no adjunctive therapy and that there were fewer cancer deaths in the L-T4 group (6% vs. 12% P<0.001) (Mazzaferri 1994). As a result of these findings it has been common practice to use L-T4 in the management of patients with differentiated thyroid carcinoma, usually in doses sufficient to lower the serum TSH to less than 0.1 mIU/L.

POTENTIAL ADVERSE EFFECTS OF L-T4 THERAPY

Patients with thyroid carcinoma are usually treated with L-T4 to lower TSH secretion below normal, thereby deliberately causing subclinical if not overt thyrotoxicosis. There are several potentially serious negative consequences of this practice. One is bone mineral loss that can even occur in children (Hung 2002). TSH suppression contributes to osteoporosis in postmenopausal women with thyroid carcinoma (Faber 1994; Dulgeroff 1994; Uzzan 1996), which may be prevented by estrogen or antiresorptive therapy. Still, using the smallest L-T4 dose necessary to suppress TSH has no significant effects on bone metabolism and bone mass in men or women with thyroid carcinoma (Marcocci 1997).

Cardiovascular abnormalities are well recognized in endogenous subclinical thyrotoxicosis, and also occur in patients taking suppressive doses of L-T4 and may be ameliorated by beta–adrenergic blockade. Subclinical thyrotoxicosis causes an increased risk of atrial fibrillation, (Sawin 1994) a higher 24-hour heart rate, more atrial premature contractions than normal, increased cardiac contractility and ventricular hypertrophy, systolic and diastolic dysfunction and increased cardiovascular mortality (Biondi 1993; Fazio 1995; Shapiro 1997; Parle 2001).

THE OPTIMAL L-T4 DOSE

Patients with thyroid carcinoma who have undergone total thyroid ablation require more L-T4 than those with spontaneously occurring primary hypothyroidism. In one study, the average dose of L-T4 that resulted in an undetectable basal serum TSH concentration and no increase in serum TSH after thyrotropin-releasing hormone (TRH) was 2.7 ± 0.4 (SD) μg/kg/day (Bartalena 1987). Younger patients needed larger doses than older patients and TSH suppression was more likely when the therapy had been prolonged. In a comparative study of patients with thyroid carcinoma and patients with non–carcinoma related hypothyroidism, the dose of L-T4 required to reduce serum TSH concentrations to normal was 2.11 and 1.62 μg/Kg/day, respectively (Burmeister 1992). These results suggest that some L-T4 is secreted from residual thyroid tissue in patients who have spontaneously occurring hypothyroidism. In this same study, the maximal suppression of serum thyroglobulin was produced by doses of L-T4 which reduced circulating TSH to 0.4 mU/L.

A study by Pujol et al. (1996) found that a constantly suppressed TSH (≤0.05 μU/mL) was associated with a longer relapse-free survival than when serum TSH levels were always 1 μU/mL or greater, and that the degree of TSH suppression was an independent predictor of recurrence. Another large study by (Cooper 1999) found that disease stage, patient age and I-131 therapy independently predicted disease progression, but that the degree of TSH suppression did not.

The most appropriate dose of L–T4 for most patients with thyroid carcinoma reduces the serum TSH concentration to just below the lower limit of the normal range. Some prefer greater suppression, for example serum TSH concentrations between 0.05 to 0.1 μU/mL in low risk patients and less than 0.01 μU/mL in high risk patients, (Dulgeroff 1994) and a few advocate the latter target for all patients. However, there is no published evidence that maintaining serum TSH concentrations less than 0.01 μU/mL has benefits, and it does have some risks.

A recent meta-analysis by McGriff et al. (2002) evaluated the effect of thyroid hormone suppressive therapy on the likelihood of major adverse clinical events, including disease progression, recurrence and death. Among 4,174 patients with thyroid cancer 69% (2,880) were reported as being on thyroid hormone suppression therapy. Meta-analysis showed that the group of patients who received thyroid hormone suppression therapy had a decreased risk of major adverse clinical events. Furthermore, by applying a Likert scale, 88% (15/17) of interpretable studies showed either a 'likely' or 'questionable' beneficial effect of thyroid hormone suppression of TSH, and assessment of causality between this practice and reduction of major adverse clinical events suggested a probable association. The authors of this study concluded that thyroid hormone suppression of TSH appears justified in patients with thyroid cancer following initial therapy.

In conclusion, we recommend TSH suppression to just below 0.1 mU/L for high-risk thyroid cancer patients, while maintaining the TSH at or slightly below the lower limit of normal (0.1–0.5 mU/L) in patients at low risk of having recurrence.

REFERENCES

Bartalena, L, E Martino, A Pacchiarotti, L Grasso, F Aghini Lombardi, L Buratti, G Bambini, M Breccia, and A Pinchera. 1987. Factors affecting suppression of endogenous thyrotropin secretion by thyroxine treatment: retrospective analysis in athyreotic and goitrous patients. J Clin Endocrinol Metab **64**:849–855.

Belfiore, A, D Russo, R Vigneri, and S Filetti. 2001. Graves' disease, thyroid nodules and thyroid cancer. Clin Endocrinol (Oxford) **55**:711–718.

Biondi, B, S Fazio, C Carella, G Amato, A Cittadini, G Lupoli, L Saccà, A Bellastella, and G Lombardi. 1993. Cardiac effects of long term thyrotropin-suppressive therapy with levothyroxine. J Clin Endocrinol Metab **77**:334–338.

Burmeister, LA, MO Goumaz, CN Mariash, and JH Oppenheimer. 1992. Levothyroxine dose requirements for thyrotropin suppression in the treatment of differentiated thyroid cancer. J Clin Endocrinol Metab **75**:344–350.

Cooper, DS, B Specker, M Ho, M Sperling, PW Ladenson, D Ross, KB Ain, ST Bigos, JD Brierley, BR Haugen, I Klein, J Robbins, SI Sherman, T Taylor, and HR Maxon III. 1999. Thyrotropin suppression and disease progression in patients with differentiated thyroid cancer: results from the National Thyroid Cancer Treatment Cooperative Registry. Thyroid **8**:737–744.

Dulgeroff, AJ, and JM Hershman. 1994. Medical therapy for differentiated thyroid carcinoma. Endocrinol Rev **15**:500–515.

Faber, J, and AM Galloe. 1994. Changes in bone mass during prolonged subclinical hyperthyroidism due to ʟ-thyroxine treatment: a meta-analysis. Acta Endocriol (Copenhagen) **130**:350–356.

Fazio, S, B Biondi, C Carella, D Sabatini, A Cittadini, N Panza, G Lombardi, and L Saccà. 1995. Diastolic dysfunction in patients on thyroid-stimulating hormone suppressive therapy with levothyroxine: beneficial effect of β-blockade. J Clin Endocrinol Metab **80**:2222–2226.

Hung, W, and NJ Sarlis. 2002. Current controversies in the management of pediatric patients with well-differentiated non-medullary thyroid cancer: a review. Thyroid **12**:683–702.

Ludgate, M, V Gire, M Crisp, R Ajjan, A Weetman, M Ivan, and D Wynford-Thomas. 1999. Contrasting effects of activating mutations of GαS and the thyrotropin receptor on proliferation and differentiation of thyroid follicular cells. Oncogene **18**:4798–4807.

Marcocci, C, F Golia, E Vignali, and A Pinchera. 1997. Skeletal integrity in men chronically treated with suppressive doses of L-thyroxine. J Bone Miner Res **12**:72–77.

Mazzaferri, EL, and SM Jhiang. 1994. Long-term impact of initial surgical and medical therapy on papillary and follicular thyroid cancer. Am J Med **97**:418–428.

McGriff, NJ, G Csako, L Gourgiotis, CG Lori, F Pucino, and NJ Sarlis. 2002. Effects of thyroid hormone suppression therapy on adverse clinical outcomes in thyroid cancer. Ann Med **34**:554–564.

Parle, JV, P Maisonneuve, MC Sheppard, P Boyle, and JA Franklyn. 2001. Prediction of all-cause and cardio-vascular mortality in elderly people from one low serum thyrotropin result: a 10-year cohort study. Lancet **358**:861–865.

Pujol, P, JP Daures, N Nsakala, L Baldet, J Bringer, and C Jaffiol. 1996. Degree of thyrotropin suppression as a prognostic determinant in differentiated thyroid cancer. J Clin Endocrinol Metab **81**:4318–4323.

Sawin, CT, A Geller, PA Wolf, AJ Belanger, E Baker, P Bacharach, PWF Wilson, EJ Benjamin, and RB D'Agostino. 1994. Low serum thyrotropin concentrations as a risk factor for atrial fibrillation in older persons. N Engl J Med **331**:1249–1252.

Shapiro, LE, R Sievert, L Ong, EL Ocampo, RA Chance, M Lee, M Nanna, K Ferrick, and MI Surks. 1997. Minimal cardiac effects in asymptomatic athyreotic patients chronically treated with thyrotropin-suppressive doses of L-thyroxine. J Clin Endocrinol Metab **82**:2592–2595.

Shen, DH, RT Kloos, EL Mazzaferri, and SM Jhiang. 2001. Sodium iodide symporter in health and disease. Thyroid **11**:415–425.

Uzzan, B, J Campos, M Cucherat, P Nony, JP Boissel, and GY Perret. 1996. Effects on bone mass of long term treatment with thyroid hormones: a meta-analysis. J Clin Endocrinol Metab **81**:4278–4289.

5D.2. POTENTIAL SIDE EFFECTS AND COMPLICATIONS OF I-131 THERAPY

ROBERT J. AMDUR, MD AND ERNEST L. MAZZAFERRI, MD, MACP

The purpose of this chapter is to explain the potential side-effects and complications that may result from I-131 therapy. From the standpoint of patient management, we find it useful to classify potential effects into two main categories: the potential side-effects and complications that we discuss with the "typical" patient (Table 1) versus toxicities that are rare in the absence of specific risk factors (Table 2).

TOXICITIES THAT WE DISCUSS WITH THE "TYPICAL" PATIENT

Table 1 lists the potential side-effects and complications that we discuss with the typical patient prior to I-131 therapy. In this setting a typical patient is a person with a thyroid remnant that is < 2 grams, no evidence of gross tumor, cumulative I-131 dose thus far < 250 mCi, current prescribed I-131 dose < 200 mCi, and no factors that would clearly increase the chance of a complication from I-131 (e.g., low peripheral blood counts, renal insufficiency, xerostomia from prior head and neck radiotherapy or collagen vascular disease).

Nausea

Nausea is the most common side effect of I-131 therapy with at least 50% of patients experiencing nausea to some degree. Nausea usually begins within a few hours of taking I-131 and usually resolves 24–36 hours later. The mechanism of nausea from I-131 therapy may be radiation-induced gastritis from the concentration of radioiodine in the parietal cells of the stomach. Nausea is more likely and more severe with increasing I-131 dose, and is most common when > 200 mCi is administered or if the patient is

Table 1. The Potential Side-Effects and Complications that we Discuss with the "Typical" Patient Prior to I-131 Therapy*.

Temporary side-effects	Permanent complications
Nausea	Second malignancy
Taste disturbance	Dry mouth +/− dental problems
Salivary gland swelling	Early menopause
Menstrual cycle disturbance	Female reproductive problems
	Male reproductive problems

* The "typical" patient is a person with a thyroid remnant that is < 2 grams, no evidence of gross tumor, cumulative I-131 dose thus far < 250 mCi, current prescribed I-131 dose < 200 mCi, and no factors that would clearly increase the chance of a complication from I-131 (e.g., low peripheral blood counts, renal insufficiency, xerostomia from prior head and neck radiotherapy or collagen vascular disease).

Table 2. Side-Effects and Complications that are Rare in the Absence of High-Risk Factors.

The major risk factor is probably a large thyroid remnant
Thyroiditis
Thyrotoxicosis
Recurrent Laryngeal nerve weakness

The major risk factor is probably a dose per administration > 200 mCi
Bone marrow suppression: temporary
Facial nerve weakness
Stomatitis

The major risk factor is probably a high total cumulative dose (> 500 mCi)
Bone Marrow Suppression: Permanent
Salivary duct obstruction
Nasolacrimal duct obstruction
Conjunctivitis/Ocular dryness
Alopecia
Epistaxis

The major risk factor is widespread lung metastases
Pneumonitis with or without lung fibrosis

The major risk factor is brain or vertebral metastases
Mass effect problems in the brain or spinal cord

taking lithium. We give all of our patients a prescription for Promethazine (25 mg PO q 6hr PRN nausea, #6) in preparation for I-131 therapy. In our experience nausea to the point of vomiting occurs in about 10% of patients who receive 150 mCi. It is desirable to prevent vomiting both from the standpoint of patient comfort and therapeutic efficacy. In our experience, when vomiting occurs it usually begins 7–12 hours after I-131 administration and can last as long as 2 or 3 days.

Taste Disturbance

Both major and minor salivary glands concentrate iodine (Fig. 1). Transient but unpleasant changes in taste occur in the majority of patients who receive I-131 for thyroid cancer. Most patients say that they first become aware of this affect the day following I-131

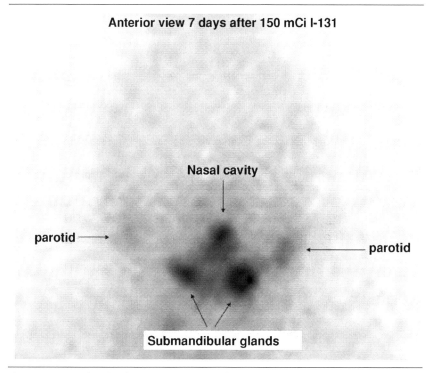

Figure 1. Pattern of uptake of I-131 in salivary tissue. The rate of iodine clearance from the parotid glands is such that little radioiodine remains in the parotids 7 days after administration. Concentration of radioiodine in salivary tissue may cause taste disturbance, xerostomia, stomatitis, salivary duct obstruction, or facial nerve weakness. Similar concentration in the lacrimal glands and serous glands in the nasal cavity may result in dry eye symptoms, nasolacrimal duct obstruction or epistaxis.

administration and taste usually returns to normal over the next weeks. On examination the patient's tongue is often smooth and shiny with diminished papillae. I-131 disturbs taste in two ways. Radiation damage to von Ebner's glands decreases the transport of food particles to the taste buds in the circumvallate papilla of the tongue. Radiation damage to the major salivary glands decreases salivary flow and changes salivary composition.

Salivary Gland Swelling

In our experience approximately 30% of patients experience symptomatic swelling and tenderness of the major salivary glands within 24 hours of receiving 100–150 mCi I-131. The parenchymal cells of serous glands concentrate iodine and thus suffer radiation damage similar to the follicular cells of the thyroid. Radiation injury in the major salivary glands activates the inflammatory cascade and leads to the problems related to taste, xerostomia, and obstruction that are discussed in other sections of this chapter.

Parotid Duct Stricture Following I-131 Therapy

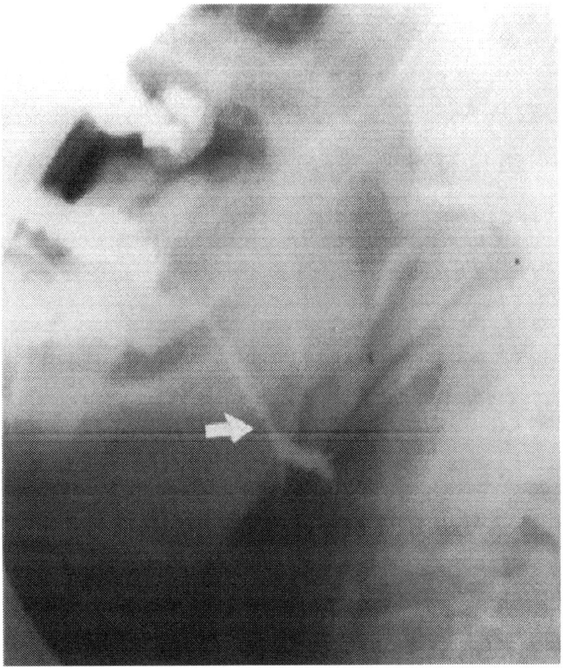

Figure 2. Parotid duct stenosis (arrow) 17 months following I-131 therapy in a patient with symptoms of obstruction of the parotid duct. (From Mandel SJ and Mandel L. Radioactive Iodine and the Salivary Glands. Thyroid 13(3): 265–271, 2003. Reproduced with permission from Mary Ann Liebert, Inc.)

In the usual patient acute salivary gland swelling resolves spontaneously within 7 days. Staying well hydrated, non-narcotic analgesics, and sucking on sour candy will decrease the duration and severity of this reaction. If symptoms are severe, a short course of steroids (Prednisone 30 mg per day tapered over two weeks) may be helpful.

During the year following I-131 treatment patients may experience painless swelling of the parotid glands that generally lasts less than a day. This is due to a plug of damaged epithelial cells that temporarily blocks Stensen's duct (Fig. 2). Mild massage of the parotid area (Fig. 3) usually alleviates the swelling and the patient typically experiences a salty taste when the duct becomes unblocked. We warn patients about this complication because they otherwise may seek medical attention in Emergency rooms or may be seen by other health care providers who mistake this scenario for a parotid duct stone and begin treatment with antibiotics or even perform imaging studies of the parotid glands.

Parotid Massage To Relieve Obstruction

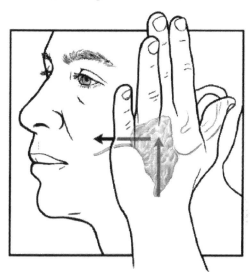

Figure 3. Technique of parotid massage to relieve symptoms of parotid duct obstruction. (From Mandel SJ and Mandel L. Radioactive Iodine and the Salivary Glands. Thyroid 13(3): 265–271, 2003. Reproduced with permission from Mary Ann Liebert, Inc.)

Neck Edema

Generalized, painless edema of the subcutaneous tissues of the neck occurs in about 10% of our patients and is a separate reaction from that described in the section on salivary gland swelling and thyroiditis. Neck edema generally begins 1–2 days after I-131 administration and resolves spontaneously by day 7 after treatment. The pathophysiology of edema from I-131 treatment is not clear. The degree of neck swelling is usually mild but may be significant if there is a large thyroid remnant in which case the patient may develop acute painful radiation thyroiditis. There are reports of severe neck edema causing airway compromise. Corticosteroids, such as prednisone 30 mg per day, are useful if treatment is needed.

Second Malignancy

Ionizing radiation is a carcinogen such that there is no question in our mind that there are patients who will get leukemia or a solid tumor as a result of I-131 therapy. However, there are several well-done studies that do not demonstrate an increase in the risk of leukemia or any particular solid tumor as a result of I-131 therapy. At this point in time we are not comfortable quantifying the risk of a second malignancy as a result of I-131 therapy. Similarly, some studies suggest that the risk of leukemia increases when total cumulative I-131 activity exceeds 500–1000 mCi, the interval between I-131 administrations is less than 12 months, or when the total blood dose per administration exceeds 2 Gy. We assume that increasing the intensity of I-131 therapy will increase the likelihood of cancer induction in some organ systems but think that the details of this relationship are not known at this time.

The two articles on second malignancies after I-131 that we include in the reference list at the end of this chapter summarize the most recent and reliable data on this subject. The Rubino article is the most comprehensive analysis in the literature and presents data that supports the conclusion that higher doses of I-131 increase the incidence of second malignancies. These authors suggest that the excess absolute risk of second cancers from I-131 therapy is 14.4 for solid cancers and 0.8 for leukemias per 27 mCi per 100,000 person–years of follow–up. This means that if we give 100 mCi of I-131 to 10,000 patients and then follow those patients for 10 years we will observe 53 solid cancers and 3 leukemias that were caused by radiation exposure.

It is a challenge to find a way to explain risk statistics in a way that is meaningful to the average clinician and patient. We find it most useful to explain risk in this setting as the percentage of patients who will develop a radiation–induced malignancy over the next 40 years from a given dose of I-131 (total cumulative dose). We choose 40 years for the calculation because it is a rough estimate of the life expectancy of a 30–50 year old person. If we ignore the possibility of multiple malignancies in a single person, the 40-year risk of a radiation-induced malignancy from a 150 mCi dose of I-131 is given by the equation:

$$\% \text{ risk} = (14.4 + 0.8)\,(4000)(150) \div (100{,}000)(27) = 3.4$$

In this equation 14.4 and 0.8 are the number of radiation-induced solid tumors and leukemia from 27 mCi I-131 per 100,000 person-years follow-up from the Rubino study, 4000 is the number of person-years follow-up that results from following 100 patients for 40 years, and 150 is the dose of I-131 in this example. We explain the risk of a radiation-induced malignancy by saying: "A patient has a 3% chance of developing cancer over the next 40 years from a cumulative dose of I-131 of 150 mCi". Using this approach, the 40-year risk of a radiation-induced malignancy based on cumulative I-131 dose is: 2% after 100 mCi, 3% after 150 mCi, 6% after 300 mCi, and 10% after 450 mCi.

We present the predictions from the Rubino paper because this is the most comprehensive study of this issue. The major criticism of this study is that the control group (no I-131 therapy) that was used for the relative risk calculations is the general population rather than patients with cancer who did not receive I-131. It is known that having one kind of cancer increases the risk of developing a second malignancy, independent of radiation exposure. Therefore, the estimates presented in the Rubino paper may overestimate the risk of second cancer induction as a result of I-131. Again, our opinion is that I-131 therapy increases the risk of a second malignancy in a dose dependent fashion but the details of this relationship are not known to a degree that permits us to quantify this risk for a given patient in any setting.

Dry Mouth and Dental Problems

Serous salivary glands concentrate iodine (Fig. 1). The cumulative dose of I-131 is likely the most important factor in the development of permanent salivary gland damage. One frequently referenced study demonstrated decreased salivary gland function in 80% of patients who receive a total of 500 mCi. A more recent study demonstrated decreased salivary clearance rates of approximately 40% in 75% of patients with an average cumulative I-131 dose of 375 mCi. Many patients with objective decreases in salivary gland function are not symptomatic.

We inform all patients who are to be treated with I-131 that they are likely to have less, or thicker, saliva forever following therapy. If the total cumulative dose of I-131 is going to be less than 200 mCi we tell them that they are unlikely to notice this change but that they should assume that they are at increased risk for cavity formation. We instruct all patients to meet with their dentist a few months after I-131 therapy to inform them of the need to monitor their teeth carefully and to institute a more aggressive cleaning schedule as needed. To decrease the chance of problems from xerostomia we instruct patients to remain well hydrated and suck on sour candy for three days after taking I-131 and we prescribe pilocarpine 5 mg PO TID beginning two days prior, the day of, and for two days after I-131 administration. We prescribe a high-fluoride toothpaste called Prevident 5000 for all patients who receive a cumulative I-131 dose of >200 mCi.

Menstrual Cycle Disturbance and Early Menopause

It is well documented that I-131 therapy may cause transient amenorrhea and hot flashes during the first year after therapy. A frequently referenced study on this subject found that these symptoms occurred in approximately 30% of patients with a cumulative I-131 dose of 270 mCi (Raymond 1989). The frequency of amenorrhea did not correlate with I-131 dose but did correlate with patient age. Similarly, there are data showing that standard dose I-131 decreases the age of menopause. In the main study on this subject approximately 60% of women were menopausal at age 50 with an average cumulative I-131 dose of approximately 100 mCi compared to 40% for a control group that did not receive I-131 (Ceccarelli 2001).

Female Infertility, Miscarriage, Prematurity, and Birth Defects

There is no question that ionizing radiation can cause ovarian damage to a degree that will affect fertility and the ability to give birth to a normal, full-term baby. As we increase the dose and intensity of I-131 therapy, or the proximity of therapy to conception, the risk of reproductive problems is going to increase. Having said this, it is comforting to note that the available data suggests that the risk of reproductive problems from standard-dose I-131 therapy for cancer is extremely low. The major studies on this subject demonstrate no association between I-131 therapy and fertility, birth weight, and birth defects. The data on preterm delivery are conflicting. A recent study from Hong Kong shows an increase in pre term births in patients who were treated with I-131 for cancer (9% versus 5%) but several other studies do not support this finding. The data on spontaneous miscarriage is also conflicting. Several studies show no increase in miscarriage rate with I-131 therapy but a major study from France found that the miscarriage rate increased from 18% to 40% if I-131 was administered within one year of conception (Chow 2004).

Our interpretation of the literature is that it is unlikely that < 200 mCi of I-131 will increase the chance of infertility, an abnormal birth, or a defective baby. The literature supports the concept that the interval between I-131 administration and conception influences the chance of problems. We instruct our patients not to get pregnant for at least 6 months following I-131 therapy.

Testicular Damage Causing Infertility or Birth Defects

Testicular germinal epithelium is extremely sensitive to ionizing radiation. Multiple studies demonstrate that standard doses of I-131 (100–150 mCi) decrease FSH levels and increase sperm abnormalities. In patients with normal sperm production prior to treatment, the effects of I-131 are transient with the duration and severity of the effect being proportional to the administered dose. Prolonged or permanent oligospermia has been reported after high (> 500 mCi) cumulative doses but even with cumulative doses of 500–1000 mCi the majority of patients remain fertile. In the majority of cases FSH levels normalize within 9 months of treatment. There are no data to suggest that birth defects are more likely in children whose fathers where treated with I-131. Testosterone levels remain normal in the great majority of patients even with cumulative I-131 doses above 500 mCi.

In summary, for patients treated with a single < 200 mCi dose of I-131 testicular function recovers within 6 months and the risk of long-term infertility from this therapy is minimal. The risk of fertility problems increases rapidly with cumulative dose. Prior to I-131 therapy we discuss sperm banking with all male patients who are interested in maintaining fertility but recommend it only in patients who have been previously treated with I-131 or in whom multiple administrations are likely (e.g., patients who are known to have lung metastases at presentation). To decrease the chance of testicular damage from I-131 therapy we stress the importance of hydration and cathartics during our pretreatment education sessions.

TOXICITIES FOR WHICH THE MAJOR RISK FACTOR IS PROBABLY A LARGE THYROID REMNANT

Thyroiditis

Inflammation of a large thyroid remnant causes dysphagia, thyroid tenderness, and ear pain. The major risk factor is the size of the thyroid remnant but I-131 dose is clearly important as moderate to severe symptoms are unusual with doses below 30 mCi. Thyroiditis usually presents a few days after I-131 administration. Symptoms usually resolve within 7–10 days but severe cases with airway compromise have been reported. Mild discomfort is usually managed with nonnarcotic analgesics and for more severe cases we prescribe prednisone 30 mg per day.

Thyrotoxicosis

Thyrotoxicosis is a well recognized side-effect of I-131 therapy in patients with large thyroid remnants or functioning metastatic tumor. Elevations in T4 are usually found in patients with symptoms of thyroiditis but thyrotoxicosis may occur in the absence of inflammatory symptoms. Hyperthyroid symptoms usually begin a few days after I-131 administration. The severity of symptoms is usually mild to moderate but severe problems can occur and deaths have been reported. Severe problems are more likely with larger thyroid remnants, large volume functional metastases, and high I-131 dose. Management is as described for thyroiditis with the addition of beta blockers to reduce the heart rate and control the symptoms of thyrotoxicosis.

Recurrent Laryngeal Nerve Weakness

There are reports of vocal cord dysfunction soon after I-131 therapy. We have never seen this complication but it is reasonable to predict that it will occur given that residual thyroid tissue or tumor frequently surrounds the recurrent laryngeal nerve as it enters the larynx. Risk factors likely include a large thyroid remnant and high dose per administration.

TOXICITIES FOR WHICH THE MAJOR RISK FACTOR IS PROBABLY A LARGE I-131 DOSE ADMINISTRATION

Acute Radiation Sickness

A syndrome of headache, fatigue, malaise, and nausea occurs in about two thirds of patients who receive an administered dose of ≥ 200 mCi I-131. Symptoms usually begin about 4 hours after administration and resolve 36 hours later. The severity of these symptoms is directly related to the dose per administration.

Bone Marrow Suppression: Temporary but Serious

Peripheral blood red cell, white cell, and platelet counts drop after standard dose I-131 therapy with nadir values 4–6 weeks after administration and usually return to the normal range by week 12 after the date of administration. In patients with normal peripheral blood counts and renal function prior to therapy, the degree of bone marrow suppression rarely causes symptoms following < 200 mCi administrations. Severe or prolonged depressions in the peripheral counts have been reported and are more likely with increasing whole blood dose above 2 Gy. We check blood counts and renal function prior the I-131 therapy but do not check blood counts following treatment unless the counts were low before therapy, the total cumulative dose is > 500 mCi, or the patient has symptoms that could be due to bone marrow suppression.

Facial Nerve Weakness

There are reports of transient facial nerve weakness after I-131 therapy. This appears to be an extremely rare complication but one that is not unreasonable to expect with high-dose administrations (> 200 mCi) given the course of the facial nerve through the parotid gland.

Stomatitis

There is one brief report of what appears to be a case of generalized stomatitis causing pain and difficultly with oral function a few days after I-131 therapy with 200 mCi. It is reasonable to expect that some patients will get generalized irritation of the oral mucosa in response to high I-131 concentration in the saliva and minor salivary glands of the oral mucosa. Treatment depends on the severity of the problem and the presence of secondary bacterial or fungal infection.

TOXICITIES FOR WHICH THE MAJOR RISK FACTOR IS PROBABLY A LARGE CUMULATIVE I-131 DOSE

Bone Marrow Suppression: Permanent

In the absence of leukemia, permanent suppression of the bone marrow to a clinically important degree is rare with cumulative activities < 1000 mCi. Factors that increase the chance of this complication are very large (>500) single admistrations of I-131 without calculated dosimetry, advanced age, impaired renal function, short interval (<6 month) between I-131 administrations, or marginal blood counts before therapy.

Salivary Duct Obstruction

Permanent damage to the parotid or submandibular glands results in decreased salivary flow, increased saliva viscosity, decreased salt resorption, and Stensen's duct narrowing (Figs. 2 and 3). These changes result in intermittent swelling and tenderness of the gland that may present a few months after I-131 therapy and recur throughout the patients life. The underlying problem is a jelly-like plug of debris that blocks major ducts. Time, hydration, sour tastes, and massage usually cause the plug to be broken down or expelled. When this happens the patient often experiences a salty taste in the mouth followed by decreased swelling over the next few hours. To decrease the chance of salivary gland damage at the time of I-131 therapy we instruct patients to remain well hydrated and suck on sour candy for three days after taking I-131 and we prescribe pilocarpine 5 mg PO TID beginning two days prior, the day of, and for two days after I-131 administration.

Nasolacrimal Duct Obstruction

The nasolacrimal glands and duct contains sodium–iodide symporters, and thus concentrate I-131. There are now multiple reports of both temporary and permanent obstruction of the nasolacrimal duct as a result of I-131 therapy. In almost all cases the cumulative dose has been > 200 mCi. Symptoms of epiphora begin anywhere from 3–16 months following I-131 administration and often go undiagnosed for long periods of time. As permanent duct obstruction may be prevented by early intervention, it is important to question the patient about this symptom and to refer patients with this problem promptly to an ophthalmologist. Some respond to dilatation of the duct, but the most serious cases require surgical repair of the nasolacrimal duct.

Conjunctivitis and Ocular Dryness

I-131 is taken up by both major and minor lacrimal glands. One study reports that about 25% of patients report symptoms of dry eye and conjunctivitis three months after I-131 therapy. In some cases these are chronic problems that do not completely resolve over time. The relationship of dry eye symptoms to the therapeutic dose of I-131 is unclear but it is reasonable to suggest that the factors affecting the lacrimal glands will be similar to those that cause symptomatic problems with the salivary glands.

Alopecia

Transient, mild, generalized scalp alopecia is not unusual in patients who receive multiple I-131 treatments. It begins a few weeks after I-131 administration and usually normalizes over the next three months. While this might result from radiation damage to follicle cells, it is nearly always due to transient periods of hypothyroidism that patients undergo during thyroid hormone withdrawal to prepare for I-131 treatment. This same phenomenon of hair loss occurs when thyrotoxic patients are treated with I-131 and become hypothyroid; hair loss becomes evident during the transition of thyroid function but spontaneously subsides after about three months of euthyroidism. The best explanation for this is that normal hair follicles spontaneously lose hair at regular intervals, but the timing of these cycles is different among the follicles. This cycling hair loss stops during hypothyroidism; however, when the patient becomes euthyroidism the hair follicles all begin loosing hair at the same time, which is very evident to patients. This process stops in about three months when the hair follicles resume their usual random cycles.

Epistaxis

There are reports of transient epistaxis and extreme nasal dryness 1–2 weeks after high-dose I-131 therapy. The nasal mucosa has sodium–iodide symporters, which is why nasal I-131 uptake is often seen on post-treatment whole body scans. It is reasonable to assume that I-131 therapy may compromise the nasal mucosa by direct radiation effects from I-131 in the nasal secretions or by destruction of the minor salivary glands that line the nasal cavity. Dehydration, smoking, a history of radiotherapy to the nasal cavity, and dose of I-131 are likely to be important risk factors for nasal problems.

THE MAJOR RISK FACTOR FOR PNEUMONITIS IS WIDESPREAD LUNG METASTASES AND A HIGH DOSE OF I-131 PER ADMINISTRATION

Pneumonitis is the term for a symptom complex that usually includes dyspnea, cough, and pulmonary infiltrates. The risk of pneumonitis probably increases with disease burden but this is not a clinically useful indicator of the likelihood of pneumonitis in patients who are known to have lung metastases because both lungs are diffusely involved with tumor deposits in most patients and because moderate to severe pneumonitis is unusual even when there is diffuse uptake of I-131, or when metastases are visible on a chest radiograph.

The most important factor in the development of symptomatic pneumonitis in patients with lung metastases is the administered amount of I-131 per treatment and the biologic half-time of I-131 in the lung metastases. Specifically, there are reports of pneumonitis soon after the administration of > 250 mCi I-131 and over a wide range of total cumulative doses. More precise data are scarce. Some studies suggest that it is possible to identify patients who are at high risk for developing pneumonitis by measuring the whole body retention of I-131 at 48 hours. The dogma that is replicated throughout the literature is that pneumonitis is rare if the whole body retention of I-131 at 48 hours is < 80 mCi.

In our program we do not measure 48 hour I-131 retention or other dosimetric parameters to make the decision to treat a patient with lung metastases with I-131 therapy. In patients without pulmonary symptoms, we do not perform additional testing related to predicting the risk of pneumonitis as long as each individual treatment is 200 mCi or less and the cumulative I-131 dose following the planned administration will be ≤ 500 mCi. In patients who we retreat multiple times for lung metastases we use the standard pulmonary function tests to make the decision about additional I-131 therapy. The most important parameter to measure is the oxygen diffusion capacity (DLCO). We consider patients with an abnormal DLCO to be at high risk for problems from pneumonitis to the point that we rarely deliver additional I-131 therapy in patients with a major decrease in this parameter.

Patients who develop pneumonitis must be watched closely as pulmonary collapse can occur quickly. When symptoms are progressive, or severe, steroid therapy is usually indicated. We do not advocate using steroids prophylactically prior to I-131 therapy as the withdrawal of steroids may precipitate radiation pneumonitis in a patient who would otherwise not develop this problem.

THE MAJOR RISK FACTOR FOR A NEUROLOGIC EVENT IS BRAIN OR VERTEBRAL METASTASES

Enlargement of brain or vertebral metastasis may occur in response to TSH stimulation, either from thyroid hormone withdrawal or administration of rhTSH or hemorrhage or edema may occur from the cytotoxic effects of I-131. Volume changes in metastatic deposits may cause acute neurologic deficits that require emergent care. It is therefore important to image the brain and spine prior to I-131 therapy if there is any question that metastatic disease may be present in these areas. Pretreatment with steroids (Dexamethasone 4 mg PO QID) decreases the chance of edema but surgical resection or external beam radiotherapy to metastatic sites prior to I-131 may be the best option.

REFERENCES

Ceccarelli, C, W Bencivelli, D Morciano, A Pinchera, and F Pacini. 2001. [131]I therapy for differentiated thyroid cancer leads to an earlier onset of menopause: results of a retrospective study. J Clin Endocrinol Metab **86(8):**3512–3515.

Chow, S, S Yau, S Lee, W Leung, and SC Law. 2004. Pregnancy outcome after diagnosis of differentiated thyroid carcinoma: no deleterious effect after radioactive iodine treatment. Int J Radiat Oncol Biol Phys **59(4):**992–1000.

Mandel, SJ, and L Mandel. 2003. Radioactive iodine and the salivary glands. Thyroid **13(3):**265–271.

Raymond, JP, M Izembart, V Marliac, F Dagousset, RE Merceron, M Vulpillat, et al. 1989. Temporary ovarian failure in thyroid cancer patients after thyroid remnant ablation with radioactive iodine. J Clin Endocrinol Metab **69:**186–190.

Rubino, C, F de Vathaire, ME Dottorini, P Hall, C Schvartz, JE Couette, MG Dondon, MT Abbas, C Langlois, and M Schlumberger. 2003. Second primary malignancies in thyroid cancer patients. Br J Cancer **89(9):**1638–1644.

5D.3. MANAGEMENT OF XEROSTOMIA, TASTE IMPAIRMENT AND DENTAL PROPHLAXIS

ROBERT J. AMDUR, MD, PAMELA L. SANDOW, DMD, WILLIAM M. MENDENHALL, MD, AND ERNEST L. MAZZAFERRI, MD, MACP

Radioiodine therapy has the potential to damage salivary glands and taste buds in a dose-dependent fashion. Some clinicians assume that the effects of standard-dose radioiodine therapy on oral function are insignificant because it is often difficult to correlate problems with dry mouth, tooth decay, or decreased taste with previous radioiodine therapy. In our opinion, the long-term effects of radioiodine therapy on oral health are underestimated. Specific studies are discussed in the review article by Mandel (2003) and in the chapter on radioiodine toxicity that is presented in a previous section of this book. The purpose of this chapter is to explain the instructions that we give patients, and products that we have found most useful, for managing the effects of radioiodine on the mouth. Table 1 summerizes the recommendations.

XEROSTOMIA

Many commercial products are available without prescription for xerostomia and all work well in some patients. We have had the most reliable results with the Biotene products (mouthwash, toothpaste, chewing gum, and Oralbalance gel) (Fig. 1). When xerostomia is not relieved by hydration and over-the-counter products, we prescribe one of the two cholinergic agonists that have demonstrated efficacy in relieving xerostomia. Pilocarpine hydrochloride (trade name Salagen) is the only product that is approved by the Food and Drug Administration (FDA) for relief of xerostomia from radiation therapy. The usual adult dose of pilocarpine is 5 mg three times a day. The second drug for xerostomia is cevimeline hydrochloride (trade name Evoxac), with the usual adult

Table 1. Medications for Xerostomia, Taste Loss, and Dental Prophylaxis.

Treatment of Xerostomia:
- Stay well hydrated
- Avoid caffeine and alcohol (in beverages and mouthwashes)
- Biotene products: mouthwash, toothpaste, chewing gum, Oralbalance gel
- Pilocarpine (Salagen) 5 mg TID or Cevimeline (Evoxac) 30 mg TID

Treatment of decreased taste sensation:
- Zinc Sulfate 220 mg BID

Prevention of tooth decay and periodontal disease:
Single I-131 treatment:
- Professional cleaning every 3–6 months
More than one I-131 treatment and no current dental problems:
- Professional cleaning every 3–6 months
- Brush daily with Prevident 5000 toothpaste
More than one I-131 treatment and current dental problems:
- Professional cleaning every 3 months
- Daily treatment with 1.1% sodium fluoride in custom trays

dose of 30 mg three times per day. Cevimeline is currently only FDA approved to treat xerostomia in patients with Sjogren's disease. The potential advantage of cevimeline over pilocarpine is a longer duration of action.

DECREASED TASTE

Persistent taste alteration following radioiodine therapy is mainly the result of decreased saliva or changes in salivary composition. For this reason, the first line treatment for taste disturbance is to relieve xerostomia as much as possible. However, a treatment that is aimed specifically at improving taste perception is zinc sulfate. Zinc is considered a dietary supplement and therefore available without prescription. Multiple studies suggest that zinc supplements improve taste in some situations. Side effects are almost nonexistent. Many supermarkets and drug stores in our area stock 220 mg tablets of zinc sulfate that we recommend to be taken twice daily with meals.

TOOTH DECAY

Even minor decreases in salivary volume, or changes in salivary composition, increase the susceptibility to tooth decay. Data are scarce on the long-term effects of radioiodine therapy on dental health but in our experience, it is an area that should be addressed. Our consent document recommends that patients inform their dentists that the therapy they have received may increase tooth decay. In patients who have received radioiodine therapy, we recommend a professional dental cleaning and dental examination at least every 6 months throughout their lifetime.

In patients who receive only one radioiodine treatment, we do not recommend more frequent cleanings, or special fluoride treatments. However, for patients who receive more than one radioiodine treatment, we recommend brushing at least once-a-day with a prescription toothpaste that contains a high fluoride concentration. Specifically, at

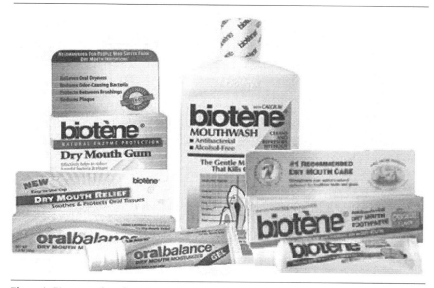

Figure 1. Biotene products for xerostomia: mouthwash, toothpaste, chewing gum, and oral gel (Reproduced with permission from Laclede, Inc). For more information see website: http://www.biotene.net/

the time of the second radioiodine treatment we give the patient a prescription that reads: "Prevident 5000 toothpaste. Use to brush teeth for several minutes at bedtime. Do not rinse mouth, eat or drink for at least 30 minutes after brushing. Dispense one tube. Refill as needed". This product contains 1.1% sodium fluoride and costs about $15–20 per 1.8 oz. tube. A high-fluoride toothpaste is more effective in reducing tooth decay than a liquid fluoride rinse because the fluoride paste stays in contact with the teeth for a longer period of time.

In any patient that demonstrates progressive problems with periodontal disease or tooth decay following radioiodine therapy, we recommend the daily use of a con-centrated fluoride gel in a custom-made tray and professional dental cleaning every 3 months.

REFERENCE

Mandel, SJ, and L Mandel. 2003. Radioactive iodine and the salivary glands. Thyroid **13(3)**:265–271.

PART 6. FOLLOW-UP PROTOCOL AND TREATMENT OF RECURRENT OR METASTATIC DIFFERENTIATED THYROID CANCER

6.1. AN OVERVIEW OF FOLLOW-UP OF DIFFERENTIATED THYROID CANCER

ERNEST L. MAZZAFERRI, MD, MACP

Follow-up paradigms for patients with differentiated thyroid carcinoma (DTC) have changed considerably in the last five years. Before then, patients underwent periodic testing with serum thyroglobulin (Tg) measurements made during thyroid hormone suppression of TSH, and with diagnostic whole-body scans (DxWBS). Over the past 5 years, however, the shortcomings of DxWBS and serum Tg measurements made during thyroid hormone suppression of TSH have been widely recognized, particularly in patients who are at low risk of having recurrent or persistent disease. There is good agreement between investigators in the US (Mazzaferri 2003) and Europe (Schlumberger 2004) that follow-up for low risk patients (about 85% of postoperative patients) who have undergone total or near-total thyroidectomy and I-131 remnant ablation should be based mainly on TSH-stimulated serum Tg measurements and neck ultrasonography.

Follow-up is somewhat different in patients at low and high risk of having persistent or recurrent disease. Thus, before discussing the follow-up paradigms, it is necessary to define risk of persistent or recurrent disease in the context of follow-up.

ESTIMATION OF RISK AFTER INITIAL THERAPY

Low risk patients have ALL of the following characteristics after initial surgery and remnant ablation:

[1] No known distant metastases
[2] All macroscopic tumor has been resected

[3] There is no tumor invasion of locoregional tissues or structures

[4] The tumor is not of aggressive histology (tall cell, columnar cell, diffuse sclerosing, Hürthle cell variants) and does not invade vascular spaces or beyond the thyroid capsule

[5] There is no I-131 uptake outside the thyroid bed on the first DxWBS (Schlumberger 2004; Toubeau 2004; Rouxel 2004)

High risk patients have ANY of the following characteristics after initial surgery and I-131 remnant ablation therapy:

[1] Macroscopic invasive tumor at the time of surgery to extra thyroid structures

[2] Distant metastases

[3] I-131 uptake outside the thyroid bed on the post thyroid remnant ablation whole body scan (RxWBS) (Cailleux 2000; Bachelot 2002)

Intermediate Risk patients have ANY of the following characteristics after initial surgery and I-131 remnant ablation:

[1] Microscopic invasion of tumor into the perithyroidal soft tissues at initial surgery

[2] Tumor with aggressive histology (e.g., tall cell, insular, columnar cell carcinoma)

[3] Tumor with vascular invasion (Wenig 1998; Prendiville 2000; Akslen 2000; Gardner 2000)

CRITERIA FOR ABSENCE OF PERSISTENT TUMOR (NO EVIDENCE OF DISEASE)

Current criteria for substantiating disease-free status in patients with differentiated thyroid carcinoma who have undergone total or near total thyroidectomy and thyroid remnant ablation comprise ALL of the following:

[1] No clinical evidence of tumor

[2] No imaging evidence of tumor (no uptake outside the thyroid bed on the RxWBS after remnant ablation or the last I-131 treatment, and negative cervical ultrasonography)

[3] Undetectable serum thyroglobulin during TSH suppression and stimulation

[4] No serum anti-thyroglobulin antibodies

The follow-up of patients with differentiated thyroid carcinoma is divided into three phases, during which certain tasks are performed:

Phase 1 Follow-up (1 to 2 Months After Surgery) (Figure 1)

This is the evaluation that occurs immediately after surgery, which comprises a complete review of the surgical procedure and the tumor pathology, a physical examination and neck ultrasonography- although neck edema often compromises exam quality. The

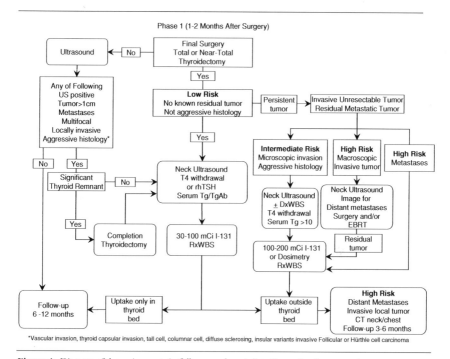

Figure 1. Diagram of the main events in follow-up phase 1 (1 to 2 months after surgery).

patient's calcium should be checked if the serum calcium was low postoperatively or the patient has symptoms of hypocalcemia: circumoral paresthesias, tingling of the fingers, or a positive Chvostek's sign (gently tapping over the facial nerve near the parotid causes twitching of the face or lips). The serum TSH should be determined to assess the need to change the dose of levothyroxine.

The main issues during this phase are to determine the extent of residual gross tumor and thyroid tissue, and to have a meaningful discussion with the patient concerning the thyroid remnant ablation and its potential complications. The issues of conception should be discussed with men and women of childbearing age. A flow sheet should be started for the patient's chart that contains all the pertinent details concerning the surgery and follow-up (APPENDIX).

Phase 2 (6–12 Months) (Figure 2)

During this evaluation the main issues are determining the extent of tumor shown on the thyroid ablation RxWBS. The follow-up from this point depends heavily on whether

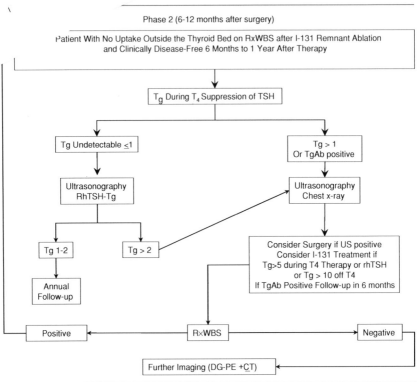

Figure 2. Diagram of the main events in follow-up phase 2 (6–12 months after surgery).

the patient has uptake only in the thyroid bed. The serum Tg and TSH are measured and neck ultrasonography is performed.

Figure 2 shows the questions posed during this phase. Most patients (~85%) appear to be free of tumor and have low or undetectable serum Tg levels with a suppressed TSH. Patients should be warned at this point about the potential complications of I-131 therapy, including dry mouth, parotid swelling, and nasolacrimal duct obstruction.

Phase 3 (6–12 Months) (Figure 3)

Patients reach this stage when there is every indication that they are free of disease. The main thing to do at this point is to emphasize the need for long term follow-up on an annual basis, measure serum Tg and TSH levels, adjust the dose of levothyroxine as necessary, and assess the patient for any complications of surgery or I-131 therapy.

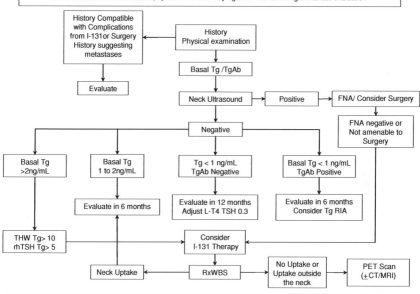

Figure 3. Diagram of the main events in follow-up phase 3 (> 12 months after surgery).

Thyroid Cancer Flow Sheet — E. Mazzaferri, MD										
Patient Name										
Hospital Number										
Birth date										
Diagnosis Information	**Initial Therapy**			**Treatment**			**Treatment**			
Date of Surgery										
Age at time of Surgery										
Time (months since initial treatment)										
City										
Head & Neck Irradiation										
Pathology – histology										
Thyroid Tumor size (cm)										
Number of tumors										
Location (left, right ,etc)										
Local Invasion (yes/no)										
Lymph nodes (number)										
Lymph node location										
Distant metastases (site)										
Thyroid surgery (type)										
Lymph node surgery										
External Radiation (dose)										
Other therapy										
Follow-up	**Date**	**Time**	**L-T4**	**TSH**	**Tg**	**Tg Ab**	**Dx WBS**	**PET**	**CT**	**Other**
Visit 1										
Visit 2										
Visit 3										
Visit 4										
Visit 5										
Visit 6										

Thyroid Cancer Flow Sheet — E. Mazzaferri, MD										
Patient Name										
Hospital Number										
Follow-up	**Date**	**Time**	**L-T4**	**TSH**	**Tg**	**Tg Ab**	**Dx WBS**	**PET**	**CT**	**Other**
Visit 7										
Visit 8										
Visit 9										
Visit 10										
Visit 11										
Visit 12										
Visit 13										
Visit 14										
Visit 15										
Visit 16										
Visit 17										
Visit 18										
Visit 19										
Visit 20										
Visit 21										
Visit 22										
Visit 23										
Visit 24										
Visit 25										
Visit 26										
Visit 27										
Visit 28										
Visit 29										
Visit 30										

REFERENCES

Akslen, LA, and VA LiVolsi. 2000. Prognostic significance of histologic grading compared with subclassification of papillary thyroid carcinoma. Cancer **88:**1902–1908.

Bachelot, A, AF Cailleux, M Klain, E Baudin, M Ricard, N Bellon, B Caillou, JP Travagli, and M Schlumberger. 2002. Relationship between tumor burden and serum thyroglobulin level in patients with papillary and follicular thyroid carcinoma. Thyroid **12:**707–711.

Cailleux, AF, E Baudin, JP Travagli, M Ricard, and M Schlumberger. 2000. Is diagnostic iodine-131 scanning useful after total thyroid ablation for differentiated thyroid cancer? J Clin Endocrinol Metab **85:**175–178.

Gardner, RE, RM Tuttle, KD Burman, S Haddady, C Truman, YH Sparling, L Wartofsky, RB Sessions, and MD Ringel. 2000. Prognostic importance of vascular invasion in papillary thyroid carcinoma. Arch Otolaryngol Head Neck Surg **126:**309–312.

Mazzaferri, EL, RJ Robbins, CA Spencer, LE Braverman, F Pacini, L Wartofsky, BR Haugen, SI Sherman, DS Cooper, GD Braunstein, S Lee, TF Davies, BM Arafah, PW Ladenson, and A Pinchera. 2003. A consensus report of the role of serum thyroglobulin as a monitoring method for low-risk patients with papillary thyroid carcinoma. J Clin Endocrinol Metab **88:**1433–1441.

Prendiville, S, KD Burman, MD Ringel, BM Shmookler, ZE Deeb, K Wolfe, N Azumi, L Wartofsky, and RB Sessions. 2000. Tall cell variant: an aggressive form of papillary thyroid carcinoma. Otolaryngol Head Neck Surg **122:**352–357.

Rouxel, A, G Hejblum, MO Bernier, PY Boelle, F Menegaux, G Mansour, C Hoang, A Aurengo, and L Leenhardt. 2004. Prognostic factors associated with the survival of patients developing loco-regional recurrences of differentiated thyroid carcinomas. J Clin Endocrinol Metab **89:**5362–5368.

Schlumberger, M, G Berg, O Cohen, L Duntas, F Jamar, B Jarzab, E Limbert, P Lind, F Pacini, C Reiners, FS Franco, A Toft, and WM Wiersinga. 2004. Follow-up of low-risk patients with differentiated thyroid carcinoma: a European perspective. Eur J Endocrinol **150:**105–112.

Toubeau, M, C Touzery, P Arveux, G Chaplain, G Vaillant, A Berriolo, JM Riedinger, C Boichot, A Cochet, and F Brunotte. 2004. Predictive value for disease progression of serum thyroglobulin levels measured in the postoperative period and after (131)I ablation therapy in patients with differentiated thyroid cancer. J Nucl Med **45:**988–994.

Wenig, BN, LDR Thompson, CF Adair, B Shmookler, and CS Heffess. 1998. Thyroid papillary carcinoma of columnar cell type—a clinicopathologic study of 16 cases. Cancer **82:**740–753.

6.2. FOLLOW-UP OF DIFFERENTIATED THYROID CANCER USING SERUM THYROGLOBULIN MEASUREMENTS

ERNEST L. MAZZAFERRI, MD, MACP

Serum thyroglobulin (Tg) measurements play a central role in the follow-up of patients with thyroid cancer. It is clearly the most sensitive means of detecting persistent tumor, but there are a number of things that the practitioner must know to use this test effectively. This chapter discusses the role of serum Tg measurements in the follow-up of patients with differentiated thyroid carcinoma.

BACKGROUND AND KEY POINTS

Serum Tg and tumor mass

- *Serum Tg levels reflect the mass of normal or malignant follicular cells*

Tg is secreted by normal and malignant follicular cells and is accordingly elevated by residual tumor, *which can only be identified after the patient has undergone total thyroidectomy and I-131 ablation*. Serum Tg levels rise in response to TSH, whether evoked by thyroid hormone withdrawal or rhTSH stimulation, and are suppressed by lowering the serum TSH levels with levothyroxine therapy. Still, Burmeister et al. (1992) found that maximal Tg suppression occurs when the TSH level reaches 0.4 mIU/L, which has major relevance during follow-up. The Tg response to an endogenous rise in TSH (levothyroxine withdrawal) is typically 2-fold that which occurs following rhTSH stimulation (Haugen 1999; Baloch 2003). According to the National Academy of Clinical Biochemistry (Baloch 2003), 1 gram of normal thyroid tissue produces a serum Tg level of 1 ng/mL when TSH levels are normal and produces a Tg level of 0.5ng/mL when the TSH is suppressed to 0.1 mIU/L, yet this is only a rule of thumb because tumors differ substantially in their ability to secrete Tg.

- *Tg cutoff levels to detect persistent tumor*

The serum Tg increases to > 2 ng/mL after two consecutive injections of 0.9 mg recombinant human TSH α (rhTSH or Thyrogen®) in about 20% of patients who are clinically free of disease and have serum Tg levels < 1 ng/mL during thyroid hormone suppression of TSH (Mazzaferri 2003). About one-third of this group have persistent tumor (Mazzaferri 2003). Similar observations have been made with thyroid hormone withdrawal (THW) (Cailleux 2000). Although there is good evidence that a Tg cutoff level above 2 ng/mL following rhTSH stimulation is highly sensitive in identifying patients with persistent tumor the cutoff differs among medical centers and laboratories and should be determined for each institution (Haugen 1999; David 2001; Mazzaferri & Kloos, 2002; Haugen 2002; Lima 2002; Wartofsky 2002; Mazzaferri 2003). Using serum Tg measurements in the follow-up of patients with differentiated thyroid cancer must be done in patients without interference from a variety of sources and using Tg assays that meet the requirements summarized below.

- *Accuracy of serum Tg testing*

Unfortunately, the positive predictive value (PPV) of the initial Tg level off thyroid hormone (Tg-off) is low, ranging from 42% to 53%, respectively, for Tg levels of 5 ng/mL and 10 ng/mL (Baudin 2003). The same is true for the PPV of a Tg above 2 ng/mL stimulated by rhTSH (Tg-rhTSH), which is only around 50% (Robbins 2001; Mazzaferri & Kloos 2002; Robbins 2002). However, all these data are from the first TSH-stimulated Tg test done during follow-up, and TSH-stimulated serum Tg levels measured just before I-131 remnant ablation have a high predictive value (Roelants 1997; Duren 1999; Toubeau 2004). Serial Tg measurements have a higher sensitivity for detecting tumor than does a single Tg measurement (Lima 2002; Baudin 2003). In the study by Baudin et al. (2003), the PPV was 83% if the slope of the Tg-off curve increased over time as determined by a 50% rise from the initial Tg-off levels to subsequent follow-up Tg-off values. However, serial Tg measurements must be done in the same laboratory using the same Tg method, because Tg serum specimens measured in different laboratories show large intra-laboratory differences, despite the standardization of Tg assays (Morris 2002; Ferrari 2003). *Thus, serial serum Tg measurements must be done by the same laboratory, using the same testing method.*

- *Combining serum Tg measurements with other tests*

There is good evidence that TSH-stimulated serum Tg measurements may fail to identify patients with residual tumor in cervical lymph nodes (Frasoldati 2003; Torlontano 2004). For this reason most centers now combine serum Tg measurements with neck ultrasonography, which changes the accuracy of the tests. An important study by Pacini et al. (2002) found that when other tests, especially neck ultrasonography, are added to TSH-stimulated Tg measurement, the PPV of the combined tests approaches 100%.

- *The negative predictive value (NPV) of an undetectable TSH-stimulated serum Tg*

It is important to emphasize that the NPV of a TSH-stimulated Tg that remains undetectable, even when done as the only test, is very high, ranging around 99% in most studies of both thyroid hormone withdrawal and rhTSH stimulation (Mazzaferri &

Kloos 2002; Pacini 2002; Mazzaferri 2003). A high NPV is of major importance because it assures both patients and physicians alike that the patient is free of disease. With this finding and a negative neck ultrasound examination, the likelihood of having a recurrence is so small that physicians can relax the requirements for TSH suppression and the follow-up testing.

- **Serum Tg measurements measured by different methods**
Tg is most commonly measured by immunometric assay (Tg-IMA) but also can be measured by radioimmunoassay (Tg-RIA). A meta-analysis done by Eustatia-Rutten et al. (2004) found that Tg-IMA was consistently more sensitive than Tg-RIA. If rhTSH stimulation was used as a substitute for THW, sensitivity remained high at ∼93%.

- **Tg can only be accurately measured after total thyroidectomy and remnant ablation**
Patients who have not undergone total or near-total thyroidectomy and I-131 remnant ablation have serum Tg levels in the range found in patients with persistent differentiated thyroid cancer (Ozata 1994; Van Wyngaarden 1997; Randolph 2002). To rectify this by administering 30 mCi of I-131 may destroy sufficient residual thyroid tissue to raise serum TSH levels, but does not render Tg undetectable (Randolph 2002). Administering 100 to 400 mCi of I-131 after hemi-thyroidectomy can achieve total ablation and may render Tg undetectable (Dietlein 2005), but this is not widely practiced and can cause severe radiation thyroiditis and thus should only be viewed as an alternative to completion thyroidectomy in patients who cannot or will not undergo this surgical procedure.

- **Spuriously high Tg measurements**
The usual half-life of Tg in the circulation is 3–4 days and rises for as long as 4 to 6 weeks after surgery and after I-131 therapy as the result of injured tissues leaking Tg into the blood (Feldt-Rasmussen 1982; Izumi 1986; Hocevar 1997; Baloch 2003). Serum heterophile antibodies (HAB) seriously interfere with Tg measurements (see below).

- **Spuriously low Tg measurements**
Undifferentiated thyroid cancers display a low basal Tg and a blunted or no increase in serum Tg levels in response to TSH stimulation (Baloch 2003). Also, the "hook" effect in Tg IMA methods can cause falsely low values (see below). In others, the serum Tg occasionally fails to rise during thyroid hormone withdrawal, but this can be avoided by simultaneously measuring serum TSH levels, which should always be done during Tg-off testing. In contrast, TSH measurements should *not* be routinely done after rhTSH stimulation because the TSH levels rise and fall so quickly that the TSH is usually in the normal range if it is measured 72 hours after the last rhTSH injection, which is when the serum Tg should be measured.

- **Tg can not be measured accurately in serum that contains anti–Tg antibodies (TgAb)**
This is a serious problem, since about 25% of patients with differentiated thyroid carcinoma have detectable serum TgAb as compared to only 10% of the general population. This usually renders Tg-IMA levels undetectable, regardless of the serum concentrations

of either Tg or TgAb. Although there is less TgAb interference with Tg measured by RIA (Spencer 2004), most commercial laboratories use Tg-IMA tests. Moreover, TgAb-positive patients typically show a blunted or absent Tg response to thyroid hormone withdrawal or rhTSH stimulation, regardless of the assay used to measure Tg, including Tg-RIA tests that normally undergo somewhat less TgAb interference than Tg-IMA (Baloch 2003; Spencer 2004). Serum TgAb should be screened by sensitive IMA testing, not with the older heterophile antibody tests fail to detect low levels of TgAb that seriously affect the Tg-IMA results.

So called "recovery" Tg assays, which estimate the affects of TgAb in sera by measuring the recovery of Tg added to the serum specimen, are used in several large centers in the U.S.A and Europe that report good results as measured against clinical findings (Cailleux 2000; Robbins 2002); still, the National Academy of Clinical Biochemistry strongly advises that recovery assays should not be used (Spencer 1996; Spencer 1998; Baloch 2003).

Tg mRNA measured in peripheral blood has been suggested to solve the problem of TgAb interference (Ringel 1998; Wingo 1999); however, clinical testing has resulted in inconsistent results and the test is not routinely used (Bojunga 2000; Biscolla 2000; Bellantone 2001; Takano 2001; Fugazzola 2002; Denizot 2003; Elisei 2004).

• *TgAb is a surrogate marker for serum Tg measurements*
TgAb is a tumor marker, rising when tumor is present and falling when it has been destroyed (Spencer 1998). An important study by Chiovato et al. (2003) of 116 patients followed for as long as 18 years found that the median time for TgAb to become undetectable in patients with thyroid cancer was 3 years and ranged from about 2 to 4 years. There was a statistically significant correlation between the complete disappearance of thyroid tissue and that of thyroid antibodies, thus supporting the concept that continued antibody production depends on the persistence of autoantigen. The coexistence of thyroid cancer with either Hashimoto thyroiditis or Graves' disease did not modify the pattern of thyroid antibody disappearance compared with that in patients with focal autoimmune thyroiditis, which is commonly found in papillary thyroid carcinoma thyroid specimens. As a practical matter in the follow-up of patients with TgAb, we usually measure Tg in a laboratory with a reliable RIA method, and if the initial Tg is not above about 2 ng/mL, we simply follow the patient with serial TgAb measurements and neck ultrasonography.

• *Tg immunometric assays (IMA) may be seriously altered by heterophile antibodies*
Unlike the situation with TgAb, interference with Tg-IMA methods by heterophile antibodies (HAB) have not been well recognized by laboratories or clinicians as causing problems with Tg assays. This is an extremely serious problem because HAB interference usually results in false positive Tg results. A large study by Preissner et al. (2003) found that the prevalence of HAB interference was about 3% in 1,106 consecutive specimens with Tg IMA values greater than 1 ng/ml. Some of the falsely elevated Tg levels were well into the range that empiric I-131 therapy is often advised. Tg HAB interference should be suspected when the Tg levels fail to change during TSH stimulation or suppression, and

when diluted Tg specimens fail to give a proportionately lower Tg levels in the assay, and when high Tg levels do not fit the clinical situation. The scope of this problem is uncertain, but may be larger than acknowledged. Only a few laboratories run specific tests for HAB, such as described in the Mayo Clinic Laboratories by Preissner et al. (2003).

- *Laboratory methodology of clinical importance to the clinician*
In addition to using the international Tg standard, Tg IMA methods should have the following features to assure reliability of the results:

(a) Sufficient sensitivity (at least 1 ng/mL) to detect small amounts of thyroid tissue when serum TSH is low
(b) Screens for the "hook effect," which occurs with very high levels of antigen, i.e., thyroglobulin, that interferes with the IMA assay at a certain point, giving spuriously low Tg results
(c) All sera should be screened for TgAb with a sensitive TgAb immunoassay (not hemagglutination)
(d) Serum TgAb concentration should be reported because it gives an indication of the amount of residual tumor that persists
(e) Serial serum Tg tests must be measured in the same laboratory

- *High-sensitivity Tg Assays*
Highly sensitive Tg Assays can accurately measure serum Tg levels as low as 0.03–0.8 ng/mL suggesting that they may supplant TSH-stimulated Tg measurements (Marquet 1996; Wunderlich 2001; Zophel 2003; Iervasi 2004). These tests are not yet widely available and have not been extensively tested on large cohorts of patients.

REFERENCES

Baloch, Z, P Carayon, B Conte-Devolx, LM Demers, U Feldt-Rasmussen, JF Henry, VA Livosli, P Niccoli-Sire, R John, J Ruf, PP Smyth, CA Spencer, and JR Stockigt. 2003. Laboratory medicine practice guidelines. Laboratory support for the diagnosis and monitoring of thyroid disease. Thyroid **13**:3–126.
Baudin, E, CD Cao, AF Cailleux, S Leboulleux, JP Travagli, and M Schlumberger. 2003. Positive predictive value of serum thyroglobulin levels, measured during the first year of follow-up after thyroid hormone withdrawal, in thyroid cancer patients. J Clin Endocrinol Metab **88**:1107–1111.
Bellantone, R, CP Lombardi, M Bossola, A Ferrante, P Princi, M Boscherini, L Maussier, M Salvatori, V Rufini, F Reale, L Romano, G Tallini, G Zelano, and A Pontecorvi. 2001. Validity of thyroglobulin mRNA assay in peripheral blood of postoperative thyroid carcinoma patients in predicting tumor recurrences varies according to the histologic type: results of a prospective study. Cancer **92**:2273–2279.
Biscolla, RP, JM Cerutti, and RM Maciel. 2000. Detection of recurrent thyroid cancer by sensitive nested reverse transcription-polymerase chain reaction of thyroglobulin and sodium/iodide symporter messenger ribonucleic acid transcripts in peripheral blood. J Clin Endocrinol Metab **85**:3623–3627.
Bojunga, J, S Roddiger, M Stanisch, K Kusterer, R Kurek, H Renneberg, S Adams, E Lindhorst, KH Usadel, and PM Schumm-Draeger. 2000. Molecular detection of thyroglobulin mrna transcripts in peripheral blood of patients with thyroid disease by RT-PCR. Br J Cancer **82**:1650–1655.
Burmeister, LA, MO Goumaz, CN Mariash, and JH Oppenheimer. 1992. Levothyroxine dose requirements for thyrotropin suppression in the treatment of differentiated thyroid cancer. J Clin Endocrinol Metab **75**:344–350.
Cailleux, AF, E Baudin, JP Travagli, M Ricard, and M Schlumberger. 2000. Is diagnostic iodine-131 scanning useful after total thyroid ablation for differentiated thyroid cancer? J Clin Endocrinol Metab **85**:175–178.

Chiovato, L, F Latrofa, LE Braverman, F Pacini, M Capezzone, L Masserini, L Grasso, and A Pinchera. 2003. Disappearance of humoral thyroid autoimmunity after complete removal of thyroid antigens. Ann Intern Med **139**:346–351.

David, A, A Blotta, M Bondanelli, R Rossi, E Roti, LE Braverman, L Busutti, and EC Degli Uberti. 2001. Serum thyroglobulin concentrations and (131)I whole-body scan results in patients with differentiated thyroid carcinoma after administration of recombinant human thyroid-stimulating hormone. J Nucl Med **42**:1470–1475.

Denizot, A, C Delfino, A Dutour-Meyer, F Fina, and L Ouafik. 2003. Evaluation of quantitative measurement of thyroglobulin mRNA in the follow-up of differentiated thyroid cancer. Thyroid **13**:867–872.

Dietlein, M, WA Luyken, H Schicha, and A Larena-Avellaneda. 2005. Incidental multifocal papillary microcarcinomas of the thyroid: is subtotal thyroidectomy combined with radioiodine ablation enough? Nucl Med Commun **26**:3–8.

Duren, M, AE Siperstein, W Shen, QY Duh, E Morita, and OH Clark. 1999. Value of stimulated serum thyroglobulin levels for detecting persistent or recurrent differentiated thyroid cancer in high- and low-risk patients. Surgery **126**:13–19.

Elisei, R, A Vivaldi, L Agate, E Molinaro, C Nencetti, L Grasso, A Pinchera, and F Pacini. 2004. Low specificity of blood thyroglobulin messenger ribonucleic acid assay prevents its use in the follow-up of differentiated thyroid cancer patients. J Clin Endocrinol Metab **89**:33–39.

Eustatia-Rutten, CF, JW Smit, JA Romijn, EP Van Der Kleij-Corssmit, AM Pereira, MP Stokkel, and J Kievit. 2004. Diagnostic value of serum thyroglobulin measurements in the follow-up of differentiated thyroid carcinoma, a structured meta-analysis. Clin Endocrinol (Oxford) **61**:61–74.

Feldt-Rasmussen, U, PH Petersen, J Date, and CM Madsen. 1982. Serum thyroglobulin in patients undergoing subtotal thyroidectomy for toxic and nontoxic goiter. J Endocrinol Invest **5**:161–164.

Ferrari, L, D Biancolini, E Seregni, G Aliberti, A Martinetti, C Villano, F Pallotti, C Chiesa, and E Bombardieri. 2003. Critical aspects of immunoradiometric thyroglobulin assays. Tumori **89**:537–539.

Frasoldati, A, M Pesenti, M Gallo, A Caroggio, D Salvo, and R Valcavi. 2003. Diagnosis of neck recurrences in patients with differentiated thyroid carcinoma. Cancer **97**:90–96.

Fugazzola, L, A Mihalich, L Persani, N Cerutti, M Reina, M Bonomi, E Ponti, D Mannavola, E Giammona, G Vannucchi, AM Di Blasio, and P Beck-Peccoz. 2002. Highly sensitive serum thyroglobulin and circulating thyroglobulin mRNA evaluations in the management of patients with differentiated thyroid cancer in apparent remission. J Clin Endocrinol Metab **87**:3201–3208.

Haugen, BR, F Pacini, C Reiners, M Schlumberger, PW Ladenson, SI Sherman, DS Cooper, KE Graham, LE Braverman, MC Skarulis, TF Davies, LJ Degroot, EL Mazzaferri, GH Daniels, DS Ross, M Luster, MH Samuels, DV Becker, HR Maxon III, RR Cavalieri, CA Spencer, K Mcellin, BD Weintraub, and EC Ridgway. 1999. A comparison of recombinant human thyrotropin and thyroid hormone withdrawal for the detection of thyroid remnant or cancer. J Clin Endocrinol Metab **84**:3877–3885.

Haugen, BR, EC Ridgway, BA Mclaughlin, and MT Mcdermott. 2002. Clinical comparison of whole-body radioiodine scan and serum thyroglobulin after stimulation with recombinant human thyrotropin. Thyroid **12**:37–43.

Hocevar, M, M Auersperg, and L Stanovnik. 1997. The dynamics of serum thyroglobulin elimination from the body after thyroid surgery. Eur J Surg Oncol **23**:208–210.

Iervasi, A, G Iervasi, A Bottoni, G Boni, C Annicchiarico, P Di Cecco, and GC Zucchelli. 2004. Diagnostic performance of a new highly sensitive thyroglobulin immunoassay. J Endocrinol **182**:287–294.

Izumi, M, I Kubo, M Taura, S Yamashita, I Morimoto, S Ohtakara, S Okamoto, LF Kumagai, and S Nagataki. 1986. Kinetic study of immunoreactive human thyroglobulin. J Clin Endocrinol Metab **62**:410–412.

Lima, N, H Cavaliere, E Tomimori, M Knobel, and G Medeiros-Neto. 2002. Prognostic value of serial serum thyroglobulin determinations after total thyroidectomy for differentiated thyroid cancer. J Endocrinol Invest **25**:110–115.

Marquet, PY, A Daver, R Sapin, B Bridgi, JP Muratet, DJ Hartmann, F Paolucci, and B Pau. 1996. Highly sensitive immunoradiometric assay for serum thyroglobulin with minimal interference from autoantibodies. Clin Chem **42**:258–262.

Mazzaferri, EL, and RT Kloos. 2002. Is diagnostic iodine-131 scanning with recombinant human TSH (rhTSH) useful in the follow-up of differentiated thyroid cancer after thyroid ablation? J Clin Endocrinol Metab **87**:1490–1498.

Mazzaferri, EL, RJ Robbins, CA Spencer, LE Braverman, F Pacini, L Wartofsky, BR Haugen, SI Sherman, DS Cooper, GD Braunstein, S Lee, TF Davies, BM Arafah, PW Ladenson, and A Pinchera. 2003. A consensus report of the role of serum thyroglobulin as a monitoring method for low-risk patients with papillary thyroid carcinoma. J Clin Endocrinol Metab **88**:1433–1441.

Morris, LF, AD Waxman, and GD Braunstein. 2002. Interlaboratory comparison of thyroglobulin measurements for patients with recurrent or metastatic differentiated thyroid cancer. Clin Chem **48**:1371–1372.

Ozata, M, S Suzuki, T Miyamoto, RT Liu, F Fierro-Renoy, and LJ Degroot. 1994. Serum thyroglobulin in the follow-up of patients with treated differentiated thyroid cancer. J Clin Endocrinol Metab **79**:98–105.

Pacini, F, M Capezzone, R Elisei, C Ceccarelli, D Taddei, and A Pinchera. 2002. Diagnostic 131-iodine whole-body scan may be avoided in thyroid cancer patients who have undetectable stimulated serum Tg levels after initial treatment. J Clin Endocrinol Metab **87**:1499–1501.

Preissner, CM, DJ O'kane, RJ Singh, JC Morris, and SK Grebe. 2003. Phantoms in the assay tube: heterophile antibody interferences in serum thyroglobulin assays. J Clin Endocrinol Metab **88**:3069–3074.

Randolph, GW, and GH Daniels. 2002. Radioactive iodine lobe ablation as an alternative to completion thyroidectomy for follicular carcinoma of the thyroid. Thyroid **12**:989–996.

Ringel, MD, PW Ladenson, and MA Levine. 1998. Molecular diagnosis of residual and recurrent thyroid cancer by amplification of thyroglobulin messenger ribonucleic acid in peripheral blood. J Clin Endocrinol Metab **83**:4435–4442.

Robbins, RJ, JT Chon, M Fleisher, S Larson, and RM Tuttle. 2002. Is the serum thyroglobulin response to recombinant human TSH sufficient, by itself, to monitor for residual thyroid carcinoma? J Clin Endocrinol Metab **87**:3242–3247.

Robbins, RJ, RM Tuttle, RN Sharaf, SM Larson, HK Robbins, RA Ghossein, A Smith, and WD Drucker. 2001. Preparation by recombinant human thyrotropin or thyroid hormone withdrawal are comparable for the detection of residual differentiated thyroid carcinoma. J Clin Endocrinol Metab **86**:619–625.

Roelants, V, P De Nayer, A Bouckaert, and C Beckers. 1997. The predictive value of serum thyroglobulin in the follow-up of differentiated thyroid cancer. Eur J Nucl Med **24**:722–727.

Spencer, CA. 1996. Recoveries cannot be used to authenticate thyroglobulin (Tg) measurements when sera contain Tg autoantibodies. Clin Chem **42**:661–663.

Spencer, CA. 2004. Challenges of serum thyroglobulin (Tg) measurement in the presence of Tg autoantibodies. J Clin Endocrinol Metab **89**:3702–3704.

Spencer, CA, M Takeuchi, M Kazarosyan, CC Wang, RB Guttler, PA Singer, S Fatemi, JS Lopresti, and JT Nicoloff. 1998. Serum thyroglobulin autoantibodies: prevalence, influence on serum thyroglobulin measurement, and prognostic significance in patients with differentiated thyroid carcinoma. J Clin Endocrinol Metab **83**:1121–1127.

Takano, T, A Miyauchi, H Yoshida, Y Hasegawa, K Kuma, and N Amino. 2001. Quantitative measurement of thyroglobulin mrna in peripheral blood of patients after total thyroidectomy. Br J Cancer **85**:102–106.

Torlontano, M, M Attard, U Crocetti, S Tumino, R Bruno, G Costante, G D'azzo, D Meringolo, E Ferretti, R Sacco, F Arturi, and S Filetti. 2004. Follow-up of low risk patients with papillary thyroid cancer: role of neck ultrasonography in detecting lymph node metastases. J Clin Endocrinol Metab **89**:3402–3407.

Toubeau, M, C Touzery, P Arveux, G Chaplain, G Vaillant, A Berriolo, JM Riedinger, C Boichot, A Cochet, and F Brunotte. 2004. Predictive value for disease progression of serum thyroglobulin levels measured in the postoperative period and after (131)I ablation therapy in patients with differentiated thyroid cancer. J Nucl Med **45**:988–994.

Van Wyngaarden, K, and IR Mcdougall. 1997. Is serum thyroglobulin a useful marker for thyroid cancer in patients who have not had ablation of residual thyroid tissue? Thyroid **7**:343–346.

Wartofsky, L. 2002. Management of low-risk well-differentiated thyroid cancer based only on thyroglobulin measurement after recombinant human thyrotropin. Thyroid **12**:583–590.

Wingo, ST, MD Ringel, JS Anderson, AD Patel, YD Lukes, YY Djuh, B Solomon, D Nicholson, PL Balducci-Silano, MA Levine, GL Francis, and RM Tuttle. 1999. Quantitative reverse transcription-PCR measurement of thyroglobulin mRNA in peripheral blood of healthy subjects. Clin Chem **45**:785–789.

Wunderlich, G, K Zophel, L Crook, S Smith, BR Smith, and WG Franke. 2001. A high-sensitivity enzyme-linked immunosorbent assay for serum thyroglobulin. Thyroid **11**:819–824.

Zophel, K, G Wunderlich, and BR Smith. 2003. Serum thyroglobulin measurements with a high sensitivity enzyme-linked immunosorbent assay: is there a clinical benefit in patients with differentiated thyroid carcinoma? Thyroid **13**:861–865.

6.3. OVERVIEW OF MANAGEMENT OF DIFFERENTIATED THYROID CARCINOMA IN PATIENTS WITH NEGATIVE WHOLE BODY RADIOIODINE SCANS AND ELEVATED SERUM THYROGLOBULIN LEVELS

ERNEST L. MAZZAFERRI, MD, MACP

Among patients with differentiated thyroid carcinoma (DTC), the main objective of follow-up is to identify tumor at the earliest possible stage while simultaneously identifying those who are free of disease. Although a thin diagnostic line lies between the two groups, it is important to differentiate them because treatment will have its greatest potential to extend survival in those with a minimal tumor burden, while the others are assured that they are free of disease thus avoiding further unnecessary treatment, especially TSH suppression with its potential for adverse cardiac events and bone loss. Tumor is generally in its earliest stages when the only evidence of its presence is a rise in serum thyroglobulin (Tg) in response to TSH. The criteria used to identify patients who have no evidence of disease are summarized in the 1st chapter in this section, and consist of a negative whole body scan after the last I-131 treatment, a negative neck ultrasound, and an undetectable serum Tg that does not rise in response to TSH.

THE PROBLEM OF DELAYED IDENTIFICATION OF TUMOR

Using older, less sensitive, follow-up techniques results in identifying persistent and often advanced stage tumor late in its course, often 10 or more years after initial therapy (Mazzaferri & Kloos 2000). This increases the likelihood that advanced tumor will be found when it is less responsive to therapy, which results in an increase of cancer mortality rates. This can happen by failing to recognize cancer in a thyroid nodule (Yeh 2004) or by performing contralateral lobectomy (completion thyroidectomy) more than 6 months after hemithyroidectomy (Scheumann 1996), or by failure to identify persistent tumor shortly after surgery (Mazzaferri & Kloos 2000).

CLINICAL EVALUATION

Serum Tg Levels

- ### *High Serum Tg Concentrations and Tumor Mass*

Any alteration in the serum Tg level usually reflects a change in tumor mass providing total thyroidectomy and I-131 remnant ablation have been done and the TSH level is stable (Bachelot 2002). Still, an undetectable basal Tg level during thyroid hormone suppression of TSH (Tg-on) is not a reliable criterion to exclude persistent tumor (Bachelot 2002; Mazzaferri 2003; Schlumberger 2004). The incremental serum Tg level in response to TSH stimulation provides a much better estimate of tumor mass, and patients with the highest serum Tg levels generally have the most extensive disease (Mazzaferri & Kloos 2002; Mazzaferri 2003; Schlumberger 2004). Thus, accurate measurement and interpretation of Tg levels is a major prerequisite for distinguishing patients who are free of disease from those with tumor.

The Differential Diagnosis of High Serum Tg Levels

Several things should be considered when the serum Tg level is elevated and imaging studies are negative, especially considering the trend of empirically treating high serum Tg levels with I-131.

- ### *High serum Tg and negative diagnostic whole body scan (DxWBS)*

We do few DxWBS studies because they are often falsely negative. Instead we usually treat patients with I-131 if we believe there is persistent tumor, providing neck ultrasonography is negative. There are five situations in which the basal serum Tg is high (>1 ng/mL) or rises above 2 ng/mL during TSH stimulation and the whole body radioiodine scan is negative (Mazzaferri 1995):

1. TSH is too low (< 30 mIU/L) to maximally stimulate I-131 uptake
2. Iodine contamination, usually from radiographic contrast material or drugs
3. Metastases too small to see on the I-131 whole body scan
4. Heterophile antibody interference with Tg assays
5. Insufficient I-131 administered
6. Tumor undifferentiation with reduced/absent sodium–iodine symporter function

- ### *High Tg and Negative post therapy whole body scan (RxWBS)*

This is a considerably more serious problem than a high Tg and negative DxWBS. When the RxWBS fails to show uptake after ≥100 mCi of I-131, the usual presumption is that the tumor does not concentrate the isotope. Yet before this idea can be accepted, one must be absolutely certain that there were no technical problems in the preparation of the patient and administration of the isotope, and that "stunning" from a prior DxWBS did not occur. These technical problems are common, particularly when physicians are unfamiliar with the optimal routines for preparing patients for I-131 treatment.

• *Insufficient TSH Stimulation of I-131 Uptake*

To maximize the therapeutic effect of I-131, one must adhere closely to a protocol that ensures serum TSH levels reach at least 30 mIU/L. This may be done by discontinuing levothyroxine, and administering oral T_3 (liothyronine, Cytomel®) alone for 4 weeks then withdrawing it for 2 weeks. The serum TSH usually rises to about 70 mIU/L, but typically ranges from just barely over 30 to 300 mIU/L or more, depending upon the size of the thyroid remnant, which is why a serum TSH should always be measured after thyroid hormone withdrawal before I-131 is administered. High serum TSH levels can also be achieved with 0.9 mg of rhTSH IM on two successive days, after which serum rhTSH levels peak to ~180 mIU/L and rapidly return to baseline within 5 days. In this situation, however, TSH is ordinarily not measured because the Tg is obtained 72 hours after the last injection, well after the serum TSH has returned to baseline. In the past 5 years rhTSH has been used both for diagnostic and therapeutic purposes (Robbins 2002; Barbaro 2003; Jarzab 2003). The latter is an off-label use of the drug but is associated with greater compliance and improved patient comfort as compared with thyroid hormone withdrawal (Berg 2002). Of major importance, the half-life of I-131 in thyroid remnants and metastases may be shorter than usual after preparation with rhTSH for I-131 therapy.

• *Lithium Augmentation of I-131 Therapy*

This is the subject of another chapter, but to briefly summarize, studies by Koong et al. (1997) from the NIH show that lithium is a useful adjuvant for I-131 therapy of thyroid cancer, augmenting the retention of I-131 in both tumor and thyroid remnants. It may result in a 50% increase in the biological half-life (cell retention) in tumors and 90% in remnants and is proportionally greater in lesions with poor I-131 retention. The increase in accumulated I-131 and the lengthening of the biologic half-life (retention time + I-131 half-life) combines to increase the estimated I-131 radiation dose in metastases nearly threefold, without increasing the total body radiation levels. Its use is particularly helpful to enhance uptake in tumors of small volume with short retention times that may be causing a negative RxWBS.

• *Iodine Contamination*

Before I-131 treatment is administered; the total body iodine pool should be low with urine iodine levels ~ 50 μg/24 hours. This requires at least two full weeks of a low-iodine diet and absolute avoidance of iodine-containing medicines or iodinated radiographic contrast materials, which may expand the iodine pool for 3 to 6 months or even longer, depending upon the contrast material and the patient's age and renal function.

• *Metastases Too Small to See on RxWBS*

Most commonly this is due to lymph node metastases that usually can be detected by ultrasonography. If the ultrasound examination is negative, the patient may have lung metastases or tumor at other distant sites. When this is the case, serum Tg levels usually rise gradually over time.

- ***Tumor Dedifferentiation with Impaired Sodium–Iodine Symporter Function***
Tumor without functional sodium–iodine symporters fails to concentrate I-131 after the patient has been carefully prepared for treatment, including high TSH levels, lithium pretreatment and low urine iodine excretion and a 4 day suspension of thyroid hormone therapy just before I-131 therapy is given to patients prepared with rhTSH stimulation. No further I-131 treatment is given to these patients, especially when an FDG–PET reveals tumor.

- ***Serum Heterophile Antibody***
One of the main concerns in a patient with a high Tg and negative imaging studies is the presence of heterophile antibodies (HAB) that interfere with Tg measurements made by immunometric assays, falsely raising the Tg result. When the Tg results do not fit the clinical picture or fail to rise and fall with changes in the serum TSH levels, HAB should be suspected.

- ***Measuring Serum Tg Levels Over Time***
Serum Tg levels sometimes decline spontaneously over several years to undetectable levels without further treatment (Pacini 2001; Baudin 2003). The trend of serial serum Tg levels over time is more useful than an isolated value (Baudin 2003), providing the Tg is measured in the same laboratory using the same assay method (Baloch 2003). This can avoid unnecessary I-131 therapy in patients without viable tumor.

Testing Sequence

The testing sequence varies among clinicians, but the one we use is shown in Figure 1. The exact Tg level at which one should consider empiric I-131 therapy is a matter of debate, but the higher the Tg level at the time of treatment, the more likely I-131 uptake will be seen on the RxWBS, providing the patient is properly prepared and the tumor has functional sodium–iodine symporters. The serum Tg levels we use to consider I-131 therapy are 5 ng/mL following rhTSH stimulation and 10 ng/mL after thyroid hormone withdrawal. Giving empiric I-131 therapy to patients with lower TSH-stimulated serum Tg levels on this basis alone results in unnecessary treatment of a substantial number of patients.

TREATMENT

Choice of Therapy

- ***Contraindications to I-131 Therapy***
Patients with high serum Tg levels should not be treated with I-131 if they have any of the following six conditions:

1) HAB Tg interference
2) No uptake on prior RxWBS after adequate preparation
3) Rapidly rising Tg after I-131 therapy with minimal I-131 uptake on RxWBS
4) FDG PET with intense uptake of large tumor deposits

5) Anatomical imaging such as ultrasonography or CT showing tumor deposits amenable to surgery

6) Macroscopic tumor previously not responsive to I-131 therapy

- *The Arguments Concerning Efficacy of I-131 Therapy*

When the DxWBS and neck ultrasonography are both negative, patients are often empirically treated with ≥100 mCi I-131, both to locate and treat persistent tumor (Cailleux 2000). Whether this benefits patients has sparked much controversy (Schlumberger 1997; McDougall 1997; Mazzaferri & Kloos 2001; Fatourechi 2002). One consistent observation, however, is that Tg levels decline when I-131 uptake is seen on the RxWBS after empiric treatment with 100 to 150 mCi, particularly in patients with lung metastases (Pineda 1995; Pacini 2001).

- *Summary of efficacy of therapy*

Empiric I-131 treatment must be considered in light of studies that show a spontaneous fall in serum Tg levels months to years after I-131 ablation without further treatment (Pacini 2001; Baudin 2003). Survival benefit from I-131 therapy is inversely related to tumor mass. Schlumberger and Pacini (1999), for example, reported complete remission and 10-year survival rates, respectively, of 96% and 100% in 19 patients with tumor found only on a positive RxWBS, compared with 83% and 91% among 55 patients with metastases seen on both the DxWBS and RxWBS, and 53% and 63% among 64 patients with micronodules seen on chest x-ray, and with 14% and 11% among 77 patients with macronodules seen on chest x-ray.

In a study by Van Tol et al. (2003), 56 patients with differentiated thyroid carcinoma were treated with 150 mCi of I-131 because of an elevated serum Tg level after thyroid hormone withdrawal and a negative 10 mCi I-131 DxWBS. After empiric therapy, half had I-131 uptake on the RxWBS and half did not. After a median of 4.2 years (0.5 to13.5 yr.) and a median cumulative I-131 activity of 150 mCi, 64% of the 28 patients with positive RxWBS achieved complete remission defined as a negative RxWBS and a serum Tg <1.5 µg/L on thyroid hormone suppressive therapy, compared with only 36% of the 28 patients who had negative RxWBS. None of those with a positive RxWBS died of thyroid cancer, whereas 9 without I-131 uptake died of cancer, producing a 5-year survival rate of 100% in the former and 76% in the latter (P < 0.001). Still, ascertainment bias may have shaded this study, because the patients who did not concentrate I-131 in their metastases likely had tumors that were less differentiated and did not concentrate I-131 for that purpose.

Eleven studies of empiric I-131 therapy are summarized in Table 1. About one-third of the patients with persistent tumor had locoregional disease and another third had metastases, usually in the lungs. We found that 13% of 89 consecutive paired DxWBS and RxWBS studies in 79 patients (15%) with serum THW-Tg levels usually above 15 ng/mL and a negative DxWBS had I-131 uptake in the lung on the RxWBS (Mazzaferri & Kloos 2001). Two to 4 years later, three of them (25%) all under age 45 years, had no uptake on RxWBS and a serum Tg levels < 5 µg/L during THW. In another study of 23 patients treated with I-131 for diffuse pulmonary metastases

Table 1. Studies of I-131 Therapy in Patients with Elevated Serum Thyroglobulin and Negative Diagnostic Scan.

| Authors | Number of Patients | | | Follow-up duration | Results |
	Total in Study	Negative DxWBS and empirically treated	Positive RxWBS after empiric treatment		
Pachucki & Burmeister (1997)	21	7 (33%)	4(57%)	1.5–34 months	No data
Mazzaferri & Kloos (2001)	10	10 (100%)	8(80%)	2–4 years	3 no uptake on RxWBS and Tg-off <5 µg/L
Ronga (1990)	61	11 (18%)	8(73%)	Not given	No follow-up data in pos. RxWBS group. One of 3 patients with neg. RxWBS had progressive disease within 5 months
de Keizer (2001)	22	16 (73%)	11(69%)	1 year	Decrease in Tg-off in 9 patients RxWBS-pos. and in 3 with RxWBS- neg. Tg-off 8–608 µg/L
Pacini (1987)	17	17 (100%)	16(16%)	12 patients; 30 months to 5 years	At last follow-up decrease in serum Tg (-off?) in 7 and an increase in 1 patient
Pineda et al. (1995)	17	17 (100%)	16(94%)	6 months to 5 years	Decrease in Tg-off in 81% after 1st empiric treatment and in 5 patients after 3rd empiric I-131 treatment. 50% of patients had Tg-on< 5 µg/L. RxWBS neg. in 50%; Tg-off never <5 µg/L
Fatourechi (2002)	24	24 (100%)	6(25%)	6–33 months	Tg-on increased after I-131 in 75% of patients; 5 died, 4 with negative RxWBS, 1 with partial neg. RxWBS (no uptake in bone metastases)
Schaap (2002)	39	39 (100%)	22(60%)	Up to 15 months	Tg-on after in RxWBS—pos. decreased and increased in RxWBS—neg. group (P = 0.006.)
Pacini (2001)	70	42 (60%)	30(71%)	Mean 6.7 years ± 3.8 years	Decrease in Tg-off in 19 patients with RxWBS— pos. Complete remission in 33% of patients with RxWBS—pos., in 17% with RxWBS—neg. and in 68% of untreated group
Van Tol (2003)	56	56 (100%)	28 (50%)	Mean 4.5 ± 2.9 years	No change in Tg-off before and after empiric I-131 therapy in both groups. Complete remission in 64% of patients with RxWBS—pos. and in 36% with RxWBS—neg. 5-year cancer survival 100% in RxWBS—pos. and 76% in RxWBS—neg. group
Koh (2003)	60	28 (47%)	12 (43%)	23.8 ± 19.6 months	Tg-on and Tg-off decreased, respectively 41% and 37% in treated group vs. a Tg rise of 44% and 67%, respectively in untreated group.
Bal (2004)	28	9 (32%)	9 (100%)	102.8 ± 70.5 months	Negative RxWBS and undetectable serum Tg 5/9 (56%) Negative RxWBS and high Tg2/9(22%) Not ablated 1 (11%) Lost to follow-up 1 (11%)

Updated and Modified from van Tol et al. (2003). DxWBS is diagnostic I-131 whole body scan; RxWBS is posttreatment whole body scan; Tg-on is Serum Tg measured during thyroid hormone therapy and Tg-off is Tg measured off thyroid hormone or under rhTSH stimulation; pos. Is positive and neg. is negative.

detected only by I-131 imaging, 87% had no lung uptake on subsequent scans (Schlumberger 1988). After I-131 therapy, serum Tg became undetectable and lung CT scans showed disappearance of the micronodules in almost half the patients, while lung biopsy showed no evidence of disease in two. Others also report a substantial fall in serum Tg levels after I-131 treatment with little or no progression of disease compared to a rise in serum Tg over time and progression of disease in patients who have been treated (Pineda 1995). Others report a reduction of metastatic disease in most patients whose lung metastases concentrate I-131, but find that a complete remission is uncommon (Sisson 1996; Samuel 1998). Still, a partial response with reduction of metastatic disease is usually possible and patients generally have a good quality of life with no further disease progression.

The best responses occur in children and young adults with diffuse pulmonary metastases not seen on any imaging studies except on the RxWBS (Casara 1993; Schlumberger 1997). This is not uncommon. The study by Bal et al. (2004) is an important study in children with pulmonary metastases. In this study, 9 of 28 children (32%) had pulmonary metastases seen only on the RxWBS. In 2 of these children the RxWBS was positive only after two I-131 treatments. After a follow-up of 102.8 ± 70.5 months, 56 % (5/9) of the group were considered to be free of disease, defined by a negative RxWBS and undetectable serum Tg off levothyroxine, 22% had a partial remission, defined as no uptake on the last RxWBS but a high Tg ranging from 18.4 to 29.6 ng/mL, and one patient each did not achieve remission or was lost to follow-up.

REFERENCES

Bachelot, A, AF Cailleux, M Klain, E Baudin, M Ricard, N Bellon, B Caillou, JP Travagli, and M Schlumberger. 2002. Relationship between tumor burden and serum thyroglobulin level in patients with papillary and follicular thyroid carcinoma. Thyroid. **12:**707–711.

Bal, CS, A Kumar, P Chandra, SN Dwivedi, and S Mukhopadhyaya. 2004. Is chest x-ray or high-resolution computed tomography scan of the chest sufficient investigation to detect pulmonary metastasis in pediatric differentiated thyroid cancer? Thyroid. **14:**217–225.

Bal, CS, AK Padhy, and A Kumar. 2001. Clinical features of differentiated thyroid carcinoma in children and adolescents from a sub-Himalayan iodine-deficient endemic zone. Nucl Med Commun **22:**881–887.

Baloch, Z, P Carayon, B Conte-Devolx, LM Demers, U Feldt-Rasmussen, JF Henry, VA LiVosli, P Niccoli-Sire, R John, J Ruf, PP Smyth, CA Spencer, and JR Stockigt. 2003. Laboratory medicine practice guidelines. Laboratory support for the diagnosis and monitoring of thyroid disease. Thyroid **13:**3–126.

Barbaro, D, G Boni, G Meucci, U Simi, P Lapi, P Orsini, C Pasquini, F Piazza, M Caciagli, and G Mariani. 2003. Radioiodine treatment with 30 mCi after recombinant human thyrotropin stimulation in thyroid cancer: effectiveness for postsurgical remnants ablation and possible role of iodine content in L-thyroxine in the outcome of ablation. J Clin Endocrinol Metab **88:**4110–4115.

Baudin, E, CD Cao, AF Cailleux, S Leboulleux, JP Travagli, and M Schlumberger. 2003. Positive predictive value of serum thyroglobulin levels, measured during the first year of follow-up after thyroid hormone withdrawal, in thyroid cancer patients. J Clin Endocrinol Metab **88:**1107–1111.

Berg, G, G Lindstedt, M Suurkula, and S Jansson. 2002. Radioiodine ablation and therapy in differentiated thyroid cancer under stimulation with recombinant human thyroid-stimulating hormone. J Endocrinol Invest **25:**44–52.

Cailleux, AF, E Baudin, JP Travagli, M Ricard, and M Schlumberger. 2000. Is diagnostic iodine-131 scanning useful after total thyroid ablation for differentiated thyroid cancer? J Clin Endocrinol Metab **85:**175–178.

Casara, D, D Rubello, G Saladini, G Masarotto, A Favero, ME Girelli, and B Busnardo. 1993. Different features of pulmonary metastases in differentiated thyroid cancer: natural history and multivariate statistical analysis of prognostic variables. J Nucl Med **34:**1626–1631.

de Keizer, B, HP Koppeschaar, PM Zelissen, CJ Lips, PP Van Rijk, A van Dijk, and JM de Klerk. 2001. Efficacy of high therapeutic doses of iodine-131 in patients with differentiated thyroid cancer and detectable serum thyroglobulin. Eur J Nucl Med **28**:198–202.

Fatourechi, V, ID Hay, H Javedan, GA Wiseman, BP Mullan, and CA Gorman. 2002. Lack of impact of radioiodine therapy in Tg-positive, diagnostic whole-body scan-negative patients with follicular cell-derived thyroid cancer. J Clin Endocrinol Metab **87**:1521–1526.

Jarzab, B, D Handkiewicz-Junak, J Roskosz, Z Puch, Z Wygoda, A Kukulska, B Jurecka-Lubieniecka, K Hasse-Lazar, M Turska, and A Zajusz. 2003. Recombinant human TSH-aided radioiodine treatment of advanced differentiated thyroid carcinoma: a single-centre study of 54 patients. Eur J Nucl Med Mol Imaging **30**:1077–1086.

Koh, JM, ES Kim, JS Ryu, SJ Hong, WB Kim, and YK Shong. 2003. Effects of therapeutic doses of ^{131}I in thyroid papillary carcinoma patients with elevated thyroglobulin level and negative ^{131}I whole-body scan: comparative study. Clin Endocrinol (Oxford) **58**:421–427.

Koong, SS, JC Reynolds, EG Movius, AM Keenan, KB Ain, MC Lakshmanan, and J Robbins. 1999. Lithium as a potential adjuvant to ^{131}I therapy of metastatic, well differentiated thyroid carcinoma. J Clin Endocrinol Metab **84**:912–916.

Mazzaferri, EL. 1995. Treating high thyroglobulins with radioiodine. A magic bullet or a shot in the dark? J Clin Endocrinol Metab **80**:1485–1487.

Mazzaferri, EL, and RT Kloos. 2000. Using recombinant human TSH in the management of well-differentiated thyroid cancer: current strategies and future directions. Thyroid **10**:767–778.

Mazzaferri, EL, and RT Kloos. 2001. Current approaches to primary therapy for papillary and follicular thyroid cancer. J Clin Endocrinol Metab **86**:1447–1463.

Mazzaferri, EL, and RT Kloos. 2002. Is diagnostic iodine-131 scanning with recombinant human TSH (rhTSH) useful in the follow-up of differentiated thyroid cancer after thyroid ablation? J Clin Endocrinol Metab **87**:1490–1498.

Mazzaferri, EL, RJ Robbins, CA Spencer, LE Braverman, F Pacini, L Wartofsky, BR Haugen, SI Sherman, DS Cooper, GD Braunstein, S Lee, TF Davies, BM Arafah, PW Ladenson, and A Pinchera. 2003. A consensus report of the role of serum thyroglobulin as a monitoring method for low-risk patients with papillary thyroid carcinoma. J Clin Endocrinol Metab **88**:1433–1441.

McDougall, IR. 1997. [131]I treatment of ^{131}I negative whole body scan, and positive thyroglobulin in differentiated thyroid carcinoma: what is being treated? Thyroid **7**:669–672.

Pachucki, J, and LA Burmeister. 1997. Evaluation and treatment of persistent thyroglobulinemia in patients with well-differentiated thyroid cancer. Eur J Endocrinol **137**:254–261.

Pacini, F, L Agate, R Elisei, M Capezzone, C Ceccarelli, F Lippi, E Molinaro, and A Pinchera. 2001. Outcome of differentiated thyroid cancer with detectable serum Tg and negative diagnostic 131-I whole body scan: comparison of patients treated with high 131-I activities versus untreated patients. J Clin Endocrinol Metab **86**:4092–4097.

Pacini, F, F Lippi, N Formica, R Elisei, S Anelli, and C Ceccarelli. 1987. Therapeutic doses of iodine-131 reveal undiagnosed metastases in thyroid cancer patients with detectable serum thyroglobulin levels. J Nucl Med **28**:1888–1891.

Pineda, JD, T Lee, K Ain, J Reynolds, and J Robbins. 1995. Iodine-131 therapy for thyroid cancer patients with elevated thyroglobulin and negative diagnostic scan. J. Clin. Endocrinol. Metab. **80**:1488–1492.

Robbins, RJ, SM Larson, N Sinha, A Shaha, C Divgi, KS Pentlow, R Ghossein, and RM Tuttle. 2002. A retrospective review of the effectiveness of recombinant human TSH as a preparation for radioiodine thyroid remnant ablation. J Nucl Med **43**:1482–1488.

Ronga, G, A Fiorentino, E Paserio, A Signore, V Todino, MA Tummarello, M Filesi, and I Baschieri. 1990. Can iodine-131 whole-body scan be replaced by thyroglobulin measurement in the post-surgical follow-up of differentiated thyroid carcinoma? J Nucl Med **31**:1766–1771.

Samuel, AM, B Rajashekharrao, and DH Shah. 1998. Pulmonary metastases in children and adolescents with well-differentiated thyroid cancer. J Nucl Med **39**:1531–1536.

Schaap, J, CF Eustatia-Rutten, M Stokkel, TP Links, M Diamant, EA van der Velde, JA Romijn, and JW Smit. 2002. Does radioiodine therapy have disadvantageous effects in non-iodine accumulating differentiated thyroid carcinoma? Clin Endocrinol (Oxford) **57**:117–124.

Scheumann, GFW, H Seeliger, TJ Musholt, O Gimm, G Wegener, H Dralle, H Hundeshagen, and R Pichlmayr. 1996. Completion thyroidectomy in 131 patients with differentiated thyroid carcinoma. Acta Chir Eur J Surg **162**:677–684.

Schlumberger, MJ. 1999. Diagnostic follow-up of well-differentiated thyroid carcinoma: historical perspective and current status. J Endocrinol Invest **22(Suppl. 11)**:3–7.

Schlumberger, M, O Arcangioli, JD Piekarski, M Tubiana, and C Parmentier. 1988. Detection and treatment of lung metastases of differentiated thyroid carcinoma in patients with normal chest X-rays. J Nucl Med **29:**1790–1794.

Schlumberger, M, G Berg, O Cohen, L Duntas, F Jamar, B Jarzab, E Limbert, P Lind, F Pacini, C Reiners, FS Franco, A Toft, and WM Wiersinga. 2004. Follow-up of low-risk patients with differentiated thyroid carcinoma: a European perspective. Eur J Endocrinol **150:**105–112.

Schlumberger, M, F Mancusi, E Baudin, and F Pacini. 1997. 131-I therapy for elevated thyroglobulin levels. Thyroid **7:**273–276.

Sisson, JC, TJ Giordano, DA Jamadar, EA Kazerooni, B Shapiro, MD Gross, SA Zempel, and SA Spaulding. 1996. 131-I treatment of micronodular pulmonary metastases from papillary thyroid carcinoma. Cancer **78:**2184–2192.

Van Tol, KM, PL Jager, EG De Vries, DA Piers, HM Boezen, WJ Sluiter, RP Dullaart, and TP Links. 2003. Outcome in patients with differentiated thyroid cancer with negative diagnostic whole-body scanning and detectable stimulated thyroglobulin. Eur J Endocrinol **148:**589–596.

Yeh, MW, O Demircan, P Ituarte, and OH Clark. 2004. False-negative fine-needle aspiration cytology results delay treatment and adversely affect outcome in patients with thyroid carcinoma. Thyroid **14:**207–215.

6.4. TREATMENT GUIDELINES WHEN THE ONLY EVIDENCE OF DISEASE IS AN ELEVATED SERUM THYROGLOBULIN LEVEL

ROBERT J. AMDUR, MD AND ERNEST L. MAZZAFERRI, MD, MACP

The previous chapter discusses the issues and controversies about treating patients when the only evidence of residual disease is an elevated serum thyroglobulin (Tg) level. The purpose of this chapter is to summarize our treatment guidelines in this situation. Table 1 lists the main points from this chapter.

These guidelines do not apply to patients with known metastases that do not concentrate I-131. It is not necessary to measure serial serum Tg levels in patients with bulky metastases that do not concentrate I-131, since the test serves no useful purpose. Patients with metastases that are unresponsive to I-131 therapy should be considered for surgery or external beam radiotherapy (EBRT) or should be enrolled in protocols studying new forms of therapy, or under hospice care.

THE LENGTH OF TIME THAT Tg PRODUCTION MAY CONTINUE FOLLOWING I-131 THERAPY

An issue that is related to the empiric treatment of elevated serum Tg levels is the time that it takes for serum Tg to spontaneously become undetectable after all residual cancer has been eliminated by I-131 therapy, EBRT or surgery. In all these cases, the serum Tg level may remain detectable for a year or more before becoming undetectable. It is for this reason that we recommend measuring the serum Tg level every 6 months for the first few years after treatment. The same is true when anti-thyroglobulin antibodies are present. The guidelines in this chapter apply only to patients without any detectable tumor on physical examination and neck ultrasonography or on the last posttreatment whole body scan (RxWBS).

Table 1. Guidelines for Treatment when the only Evidence of Disease is an Elevated Serum Tg Level.

Serum Tg evaluation:
A serum Tg level of 5 ng/mL after rhTSH or 10 ng/mL after thyroid hormone withdrawal indicates residual cancer
Anti-Tg antibodies (TgAb) produce falsely low Tg results with an immunometric assay
When TgAb are present, Tg measured by RIA may be helpful
Falling TgAb levels are an indication of improving tumor status and vice versa

Usually, the only studies we obtain prior to retreating with I-131 or surgery are:
Chest radiograph
Cervical ultrasound, ultrasound guided FNA
MR of the mediastinum if surgery is planned (positive FNA)

FDG PET:
FDG PET is a first choice test to rule out metastases that do not concentrate radioiodine
Perform FDG PET with TSH stimulation

Chest CT and Tc-99 bone scan:
Our second choice to rule out metastases that do not concentrate radioiodine

Diagnostic Whole Body Scan with radioiodine (DxWBS):
We almost never perform a DxWBS prior to I-131 therapy

Brain MR scan:
We perform a MR of the brain if there is any question of a brain metastasis

We retreat with I-131 for elevated serum Tg level unless:
The patient has previously been shown to have metastases that do not concentrate I-131
The last RxWBS was negative for tumor uptake and was done following at least 100 mCi I-131 with adequate preparaton
The patient prefers to be observed without additional treatment
The risks of additional I-131 therapy are high: low blood counts or renal insufficiency

Dose of I-131:
Adults: 150 mCi
Children: Dose adjusted for body surface area (see the chapter on Lung metastases)
We usually use rhTSH injections for adults and T4 deprivation in children
We prescribe lithium unless there are contraindications to this drug

External Beam Radiotherapy (EBRT):
We do not recommend EBRT when the only evidence of disease is an elevated serum Tg level

THE Tg LEVEL THAT INDICATES RESIDUAL CANCER FOLLOWING REMNANT ABLATION

Most experts agree that a serum Tg level > 2 ng/mL after rhTSH stimulation, or > 5 ng/mL after thyroid hormone withdrawal, are the cutoffs above which the patient should be investigated—but not empirically treated. At these levels, the elevated serum Tg is not likely to spontaneously fall to an undetectable level. There is an even greater likelihood of persistent tumor when the serum Tg level is > 5 ng/mL after rhTSH stimulation and >10 ng/mL after thyroid hormone withdrawal.

There is disagreement about the threshold serum Tg level that should prompt empiric therapy when the tumor site is not apparent. We usually recommend I-131 therapy with the higher Tg levels (> 5 ng/mL with rhTSH and > 10 ng/mL with thyroid hormone withdrawal) mentioned above providing the levels have been increasing over time. This is a critical point because the highest probability of persistent tumor occurs when the serum Tg is rising as compared with employing rigid cutoffs.

We set the rhTSH-stimulated Tg threshold at 2 ng/mL because there is an abundant literature that this is the most sensitive threshold for detecting thyroid cancer linked with the highest negative predictive value. With these issues in mind, we currently use the following guidelines based on three main scenarios:

1. *The basal serum Tg level is <1 ng/mL on thyroid hormone suppression of TSH*
   With this scenario, the patient undergoes rhTSH stimulation and if the level remains at 2 ng/mL or lower, then we follow the patient with neck ultrasonography and repeat the basal and rhTSH-stimulated serum Tg measurement at yearly intervals until both are undetectable.
2. *The basal serum Tg level is > 1 ng/mL but less 2 ng/mL on thyroid hormone*
   With this scenario, the patient undergoes annual rhTSH stimulation until both the basal and rhTSH-stimulated levels are undetectable. This usually is not an indication of residual disease and we follow the patient until we have clearly established that the Tg is rising or falling (usually a change of 50% over time). If the Tg is rising and the rhTSH-stimulated level is above 5 ng/mL and tumor cannot be found on ultrasonography, we consider empiric I-131 therapy.
3. *Anti-Tg antibodies (TgAb) are positive and serum Tg is undetectable*
   With this scenario, ultrasonography is the most informative test. It is impossible to conclude that the patient is free of disease based upon serum Tg measurements. The presence of TgAb renders TSH stimulation of serum Tg unreliable, done either by rhTSH or thyroid hormone withdrawal. We obtain a serum Tg in a laboratory that reliably measures Tg by radioimmunoassay (RIA), which undergoes less interference with anti-Tg than does Tg measured by immunometric assays. If the baseline RIA Tg level is < 2 ng/mL on thyroid hormone suppression of TSH, we simply follow TgAb levels over time. If TgAb levels are consistently lower with each 6-month measurement, we do no further testing other than ultrasonography. If TgAb levels plateau or rise, which is a signal of residual cancer, or if the Tg measured by RIA is rising and reaches 5–10 ng/mL, we consider empiric I-131 therapy.

REQUIRED IMAGING STUDIES

Chest radiograph: Lung metastases are the most common site of distant metastasis from thyroid cancer. We perform the standard two-view radiograph of the chest in all patients because the morbidity of this study is extremely low.

Neck ultrasound: In all patients, we image the neck for gross disease because this finding usually indicates a need for surgery if we can prove by ultrasound guided FNA that the tissue is malignant, or I-131 therapy if the nodes are very small (<5 mm) and cannot be proven by ultrasound-guided FNA to be malignant. When we are uncertain, we simply evaluate the neck with ultrasound every 6 months until the situation becomes clear. MR and CT imaging are rarely done in this setting since both are far less sensitive for cervical disease. If there is a suspicion of mediastinal disease, MR imaging is a good choice.

18 Flourodeoxyglucose Positron Emission Tomography (FDG PET): The main indication for this test in the follow-up of patients with thyroid cancer is when the serum Tg is > 10 ng/mL and the RxWBS is negative after a therapeutic dose of at least 100 mCi.

The FDG PET gives therapeutic information, sometimes leading to successful surgical intervention, and it gives prognostic information that is helpful in making decisions about further studies. Insurance carries frequently will not pay for FDG PET unless a recent whole body iodine scan is negative, which is not a problem in these patients because, by definition, the RxWBS is negative and the Tg is > 10 ng/mL. When there are obstacles to performing FDG PET, we evaluate distant metastases with the combination of a CT scan of the chest and a Tc-99 bone scan (without TSH stimulation). We perform the CT with contrast because we do not consider additional I-131 therapy in this group of patients.

Chest Compound Tomography (CT) and Technesium-99m bone scan to rule out metastases that do not concentrate radioiodine: In most patients, we find these studies are not necessary, although some investigators find them useful in the setting of a high serum Tg with a negative DxWBS. Usually the only imaging studies that we obtain prior to treating a patient with I-131 for an elevated serum Tg level are a chest radiograph and a neck ultrasound. We perform a more thorough evaluation when the patient has symptoms of distant metastasis or when we think that the patient may have distant metastases that do not concentrate radioiodine. Our usual indication for imaging for distant metastasis prior to retreating with I-131 is a high baseline serum Tg level (> 50 ng/mL on thyroid hormone) in a patient with a previously negative RxWBS.

Diagnostic whole body scans with radioiodine (DxWBS): The previous chapter explains why we rarely perform a DxWBS.

Brain MR scan: We obtain a brain MR scan if there is any question of a brain metastasis. A markedly elevated serum Tg level (> 50) in a patient with no other evidence of disease may be a sign of a disease in the brain.

I-131 THERAPY FOR ELEVATED SERUM Tg LEVEL

When the only evidence of disease is an elevate serum Tg level that is rising, we retreat the patient with I-131 when the risk of retreatment with I-131 is acceptable and: 1) the patient has had uptake on the RxWBS following the last empiric I-131 treatment, or 2) the patient has not previously received an I-131 treatment with proper preparation as described in other chapters, or 3) the only evidence of a negative whole body scan is from a negative DxWBS. We do not retreat patients if we know that their disease is resistant to I-131 therapy.

EXTERNAL BEAM RADIOTHERAPY (EBRT)

We do not use EBRT when the only evidence of disease is an elevated serum Tg level.

6.5. TREATMENT OF RESIDUAL DIFFERENTIATED THYROID CANCER IN THE NECK AND MEDIASTINUM

ROBERT J. AMDUR, MD AND ERNEST L. MAZZAFERRI, MD, MACP

The previous chapter explains the treatment of patients who are Tg-positive and scan-negative. The following chapters explain the management of patients with distant metastases. The purpose of this chapter is to discuss the management of patients in whom a comprehensive imaging workup is positive only in the neck and/or superior mediastinum. We use the term "residual" to refer to either residual or recurrent disease. Table 1 summarizes the main points from this chapter.

SURGICALLY REMOVE RESIDUAL TUMOR WHENEVER POSSIBLE

Optimal therapy of recurrent tumor in the neck or upper mediastinum begins with a surgical procedure when it is likely that the surgeon will be able to remove all gross disease with acceptable morbidity. Following surgery, we retreat with I-131 and/or external beam radiotherapy depending on the likely tumor burden and prior history of I-131 therapy.

RETREAT WITH I-131 WHEN IT MAY BE BENEFICIAL

Following resection of recurrent tumor, we retreat the patient with I-131 when the risk of retreatment with I-131 is acceptable (adequate blood counts and renal function) and additional I-131 therapy will increase the chance of cure. We do not retreat patients with a history of tumor recurrence following multiple high-quality I-131 treatments.

Table 1. Management of Recurrent Tumor in the Neck or Superior Mediastinum.

The first step is repeat surgery if:
Resection of all gross tumor is likely based on an estimate of the extent of disease
The predicted morbidity and risk of gross total resection is acceptable

Following salvage surgery the second step is retreatment with I-131 if:
The risk of retreatment with I-131 is acceptable based on hematologic status
The patient has not previously received multiple high-quality I-131 treatments[1]

Following repeat surgery the second step is external beam radiotherapy if:
Age > 45 years
Retreatment with I-131 is a poor option due to low blood counts or a history of multiple prior I-131 treatments under high-quality conditions
The surgical specimen demonstrates a positive margin, invasion of subcutaneous soft tissues, larynx, trachea, esophagus, recurrent laryngeal nerve, or prevertebral fascia, or tumor encasement of the carotid artery or mediastinal vessels, or nodal metastasis with extracapsular tumor extension

Following repeat surgery and retreatment with I-131, the third step is external beam radiotherapy if:
Age > 45 years
The surgical specimen demonstrates a positive margin, or there is gross tumor invasion of subcutaneous soft tissues, larynx, trachea, esophagus, recurrent laryngeal nerve, or prevertebral fascia, or tumor encasement of the carotid artery or mediastinal vessels, or nodal metastasis with gross extracapsular tumor extension

Details of I-131 retreatment:
Adults: 150 mCi with a negative surgical margin, 200 mCi otherwise
Children: Dose based on body surface area (see the chapter on Lung metastases)
We usually use rhTSH injections for adults and T4 deprivation in children
Lithium is given in all cases in which there are no contraindications to using the drug

Details of External beam radiotherapy:
Usual program: 63 or 72 Gy depending on risk factors with Intensity Modulated Radiation Therapy

---

[1] It is not reasonable to expect the chance of cure to be increased by additional I-131 therapy when tumor has recurred following multiple high-quality I-131 treatments.

USE EXTERNAL BEAM RADIOTHERAPY (EBRT) IN OLDER ADULTS WITH HIGH-RISK FINDINGS

In patients > 45 years old, we recommend EBRT to the neck and upper mediastinum for recurrent disease that is unresectable or when the surgical specimen demonstrates a positive margin, invasion of subcutaneous soft tissues, larynx, trachea, esophagus, recurrent laryngeal nerve, or prevertebral fascia, or tumor encasement of the carotid artery or mediastinal vessels, or nodal metastasis with extracapsular tumor extension. The role of EBRT in younger patients with these high-risk findings is unclear. We rarely use EBRT in younger patients unless there is unresectable disease that is likely to cause serious problems in the near future.

6.6. TREATMENT OF LUNG METASTASES FROM DIFFERENTIATED THYROID CANCER

ROBERT J. AMDUR, MD AND ERNEST L. MAZZAFERRI, MD, MACP

Approximately 10% of adults and 20% of younger children with differentiated thyroid cancer develop lung metastases sometime in the course of their disease. In approximately half of the cases, lung metastases are found at the time of initial diagnosis and approximately 25% do not present until 20 to 30 years after initial therapy, an observation that is likely to change dramatically with newer surveillance techniques (Fig. 1).

The purpose of this chapter is to summarize the management of lung metastases in patients without metastatic disease elsewhere. Table 1 summarizes the guidelines discussed in this chapter. Radiographic images of patients with lung metastases are presented in part 2 of this book.

PROGNOSIS

Lung metastases from differentiated thyroid cancer are potentially curable, particularly in children and young adults, who often live for decades with diffuse pulmonary metastases that have been appropriately treated. Still, the prognosis depends upon the burden of disease, details of treatment and the intensity of radioiodine uptake by the tumor, and the inherent growth characteristics of the tumor. Tables 2 and 3 summarize data from two series with long-term follow-up of relatively large groups of patients with lung metastases as the only site of distant tumor. These studies show that long-term survival is especially high when lung metastases are too small to see on the standard chest radiograph or CT. Ten-year survival rates are 100% when the metastases are only evident on the posttreatment whole body scan. The 10-year survival rates steadily decline as the metastases become larger, falling to about 40% when there are micronodules (<1cm)

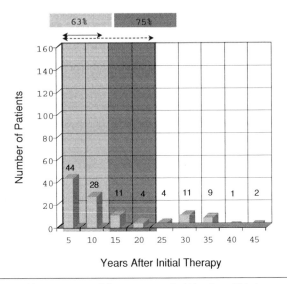

Figure 1. Time of first recognition of distant metastases in 114 patients. This shows graphically the problem of late recognition of distant metastases in patients with differentiated thyroid cancer. Drawn from the data of Mazzaferri and Kloos (2001).

on the chest x-ray, and about 15% when the nodules are larger than 1 cm. Powerful prognosticators are age over 45 years at the time of diagnosis and the tumor's ability to trap I-131.

In short, the prognostic features are quite different depending upon the nature and stage of the tumor and the patient's age at the time of diagnosis. Bilateral diffuse pumonary uptake in children and young adults with no other metastases has a reasonably good prognosis because the tumor usually takes up I-131 and not infrequently can be completely ablated. At the other end of the spectrum, large lung metastases in patients over age 45 years that concentrate I-131 have a less favorable prognosis, and the prognosis of bulky metastases that do not concentrate I-131 is poor.

MANAGEMENT WHEN METASTASES ARE DETECTED PRIOR TO ABLATION OF THE THYROID REMNANT

The usual scenario is to find lung metastases on the routine preoperative chest radiograph, which almost never happens in young patients but increases in frequency with advancing age. Occasionally metastases are found on chest CT or an FDG PET scan done prior to referral to our group. We ordinarily do not perform imaging studies other than ultrasonography and chest radiography prior to surgery, and do not perform a diagnostic

Table 1. Management of Patients with Lung Metastases from Differentiated Thyroid Cancer.

Factors that apply to all situations:
These guidelines assume normal peripheral blood counts and normal renal function
In these guidelines "I-131 therapy for lung metastases" means:
Adults: 200 mCi I-131
Children: usually estimated from body surface area and decreased to an amount of I-131 comparable to
    treating an adult with 200 mCi (see figures and tables)
TSH elevation is usually via rhTSH in adults and T4 deprivation in children
We use lithium in all situations unless there are contraindications to its use

When lung metastases are detected prior to ablation of a large thyroid remnant:
First use completion thyroidectomy or 30 mCi I-131 to destroy the thyroid remnant
Deliver I-131 therapy for lung metastases after ablation of the thyroid remnant

When lung metastases are detected prior to ablation of a small thyroid remnant:
Deliver I-131 therapy for lung metastases (and to ablate the thyroid remnant)

When lung metastases are detected on a RxWBS:
This finding does not change the follow-up or treatment plan unless I-131 therapy consisted of 30 mCi to
    ablate a large thyroid remnant

When lung metastases are detected > 3 months following I-131 therapy:
Deliver I-131 therapy for lung metastases
I-131 therapy for lung metastases is repeated multiple times for persistent disease as long as lung metastases
    continue to concentrate I-131 and the risk of additional I-131 therapy is acceptable

Symptomatic lung metastases:
Symptomatic lung disease indicates advanced and usually incurable disease
I-131 therapy is rarely useful as first line therapy, especially in older patients
External beam radiotherapy is usually first line therapy to relieve symptoms
Consider adding I-131 therapy following local therapy

Pulmonary complications of I-131 therapy for lung metastases:
Pneumonitis or pulmonary fibrosis is rare if the single dose per administration is < 250 mCi
We use oxygen diffusing capacity to identify patients who are at high risk for pulmonary complications from
    I-131 therapy for lung metastases

whole body scan with radioiodine (DxWBS) before I-131 remnant ablation. The post treatment whole body scan (RxWBS) is about four times more likely to be positive when lung metastases are present than the DxWBS.

Thyroid tissue usually concentrates radioiodine much more avidly than metastatic cancer to the point that it is usually not possible to effectively treat lung metastases with I-131 in a patient with a large thyroid remnant. Thus when lung metastases are discovered prior to remnant ablation, the therapeutic paradigm depends on the size of the thyroid remnant.

Large (> 2 gram) thyroid remnant: Management of patients with a large thyroid remnant is the subject of a previous chapter. We recommend completion thyroidectomy in patients with a large remnant when the risk of additional surgery is acceptable. In the few cases in which completion thyroidectomy is not an option, we first ablate the thyroid remnant with 30 mCi of I-131 before attempting to treat the lung metastases. Six months later we image the neck with ultrasound, and if the remnant is small (< 2 grams) we treat the lung metastases. If not, we administer an additional 30 mCi of I-131 and again reassess the situation with an ultrasound examination in six months. This is generally not

Table 2. Outcome of Patients with Lung as the Only Site of Distant Metastases: Schlumberger Series[1].

	Complete remission	10-year survival
Elevated serum Tg and positive RxWBS[2]	96%	100%
Normal chest x-ray and positive DxWBS[3]	83%	91%
Micronodules on chest radiograph	53%	63%
Macronodules on chest radiograph	11%	14%

[1] Schlumberger. J. Endocrinol. Invest 22, Suppl 11, 3–7. 1999.
[2] RxWBS = post-treatment I-131 whole body scan.
[3] DxWBS = Diagnostic radioiodine total body scan.

a favorable situation, because considerable time may be lost before the lung metastases can be effectively treated with large amounts of I-131.

Small (< 2 gram) thyroid remnant: A wide range of I-131 activities have been used to treat lung metastases. We use a fixed-dose approach to I-131 therapy and prescribe 200 mCi of I-131 for adults regardless of the extent or size of the lung metastases. When diffuse pulmonary metastases are found, limiting single treatments to 200 mCi is almost always sufficient to avoid serious lung injury, but higher cumulative amounts of I-131 given over an extended period increase the risk of causing lung fibrosis. Treatment of children with lung metastases is done in the same way, except the amount of I-131 administered is adjusted to the child's size (body surface area).

Treatment of lung metastases in children: An elegant study by Reynolds (1994) can be used to estimate the fraction of an adult fixed dose of I-131 that can be given to a child. This study showed that the increased radiation dose to children is due to the activity being distributed in smaller organ volumes as well as the shorter distance between organs, thus increasing the likelihood of cross radiation. He calculated a relative exposure and relative dose for 18 target organs other than the thyroid. The relative dose for children is defined as the administered mCi that gives the same exposure as 1 mCi administered to an adult.

Table 3. Outcome of Patients with Lung as the Only Site of Distant Metastases: Ronga Series[1].

	10-year survival	20-year survival	Log–rank test
Age at diagnosis ≤ 45 versus > 45 years	83% vs 37%	68% vs 14%	p < 0.001
Histology Follicular versus Papillary	48% vs 64%	38% vs 46%	p NS
Metastases visible on chest radiograph or CT scan No versus Yes	75% vs 47%	61% vs 26%	p < 0.001
Metastases concentrate I-131 Yes versus No	76% vs 25%	59% vs 0%	p < 0.001

[1] Ronga et al., Q J Nucl Med Mol Imaging. 2004 Mar;48(1):12–19.

Table 4. Absorbed Radiation Dose to Red Bone Marrow from Administered I-131. The Thyroid Radioiodine Uptake was 0%. Relative Exposure is (Rad/mCi)/(Rad/mCi) in Adults. Relative Dose is 1/Relative Exposure. This Table and Tables 5 and 6 are from JC Reynolds from the National Institutes of Health in the Reference Cited below.

		Child age in years			
Category	Adult	15	10	5	1
mCi/MBq	0.035	0.042	0.065	0.100	0.190
Rad/mCi	0.129	0.155	0.240	0.370	0.703
Relative Exposure	1.0	1.20	1.86	2.86	5.43
Relative Dose	1.0	0.830	0.538	0.350	0.184

Table 4 shows the absorbed radiation dose to the bone marrow from administered I-31 in children, and relates it to adult exposure. Table 5 shows the I-131 activity administered to a child that will give the same exposure as 1.0 mCi administered to an adult. The data in Table 5 also take into account thyroidal radioiodine uptake varying from 0% to 5%, which significantly changes tissue exposure to radiation. It shows that the I-131 activity administered to a 15 year-old child with 0% thyroidal uptake should be about 5/6 (83%) that of an adult. Table 6 lists values for body weight and body surface area of adults and children. Those in children are expressed in relation to the adult value, termed relative body surface area. These relative doses are also expressed in relation to the adult value both as relative body weight and relative body surface area. Figures 2, 3, 4 and 5 show the same data as they vary, respectively, with body weight, body surface area calculated by the DuBois Formula or by the Lissauer formula. The doses of I-131 administered to children based on surface area are larger than those based on body weight, and are slightly higher based on the Du Bois formula for body surface area.

There are limitations to the Reynolds method. The relative dose method can only be used to estimate safe I-131 doses for children when the adult dose is known. The comparisons shown in the Tables and Figures do not provide absolute or specific dosing rules, but show how the administrated I-131 activity can be adjusted for children. The Reynolds method cannot be used to estimate bone marrow radiation using the

Table 5. Relative Dose is I-131 Activity (mCi) Administered to a Child that will give the Same Exposure as 1.0 mCi Administered to an Adult. The Thyroid Radioiodine Uptake was Either 0% or 5%. Data Shown are MEAN and STD of 18 Organs and Tissues. This Table and Table 5 are from JC Reynolds from the National Institutes of Health in the Reference Cited Below.

		Child age in years			
Category	Adult	15	10	5	1
Relative Dose		**0.834**	**0.527**	**0.323**	**0.177**
0% Thyroid Uptake	1.0	± 0.046	± 0.032	± 0.022	± 0.012
Relative Dose		**0.817**	**0.520**	**0.331**	**0.179**
5% Uptake	1.0	± 0.062	± 0.036	± 0.027	± 0.022

Table 6. Weight (kgm) and Body Surface Area (m^2) of Adults and Children. The DuBois Formula is Body Surface Area (BSA) = 71.84 · 10^{-4}· Wt$^{0.4254}$· Ht$^{0.752}$. The Lissaur Formula is BSA = 0.1 · Wt$^{0.67}$. **Relative Body Weight** is Body Weight/70. **Relative Body Surface Area** is Body Surface Area/1.70.

		Child Age in Years			
Category	Adult	15	10	5	1
Body Weight (kgm)	70	55.2	32.0	18.2	9.8
Relative Body Weight	**1.0**	**0.789**	**0.457**	**0.260**	**0.140**
Body Surface Area (m^2) Du Bois	1.70	1.58	1.09	0.75	0.46
Relative Body Surface Area	**1.0**	**0.929**	**0.641**	**0.441**	**0.271**
Body Surface Area (m^2) Lissauer	1.70	1.45	1.01	0.69	0.46
Relative Body Surface Area	**1.0**	**0.853**	**0.594**	**0.406**	**0.271**

dosimetry method described by Benua et al. (1962) which must be less than 200 cGy during therapy, and cannot be used to administer doses calculated on a lesional basis as described by Maxon et al. (1983).

LUNG METASTASES THAT ARE DETECTED ON A POST-TREATMENT RADIOIODINE WHOLE BODY SCAN

In many patients, lung metastases are first detected on a post-treatment radioiodine whole body scan (RxWBS). The only situation in which the finding of lung metastases on the

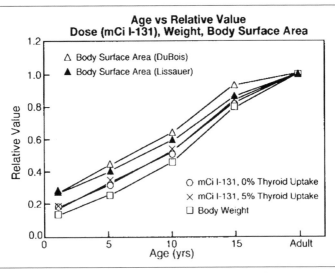

Figure 2. Estimate of I-131 dose given to children with lung metastases, based upon age. From Reynolds (1994).

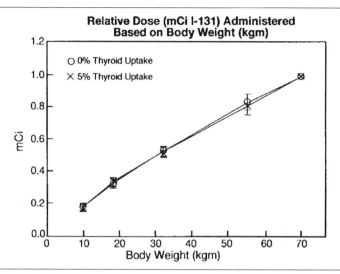

Figure 3. Estimate of I-131 dose given to children with lung metastases, based upon body weight. From Reynolds (1994).

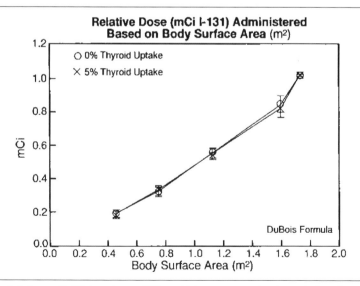

Figure 4. Estimate of I-131 dose given to children with lung metastases, based upon body surface area calculated by Du Bois Formula. From Reynolds (1994).

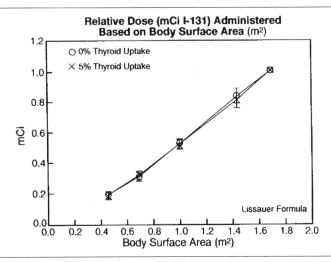

Figure 5. Estimate of I-131 dose given to children with lung metastases, based upon body surface area calculated by the Lissauer formula. From Reynolds (1994).

RxWBS affects the follow-up or treatment plan is when therapy consisted of 30 mCi I-131 given to ablate a thyroid remnant. In this setting we would deliver 200 mCi of I-131 after ablation of the thyroid remnant was confirmed.

In situations other than ablation of a large thyroid remnant with 30 mCi I-131, the finding of lung metastases on the RxWBS does not alter the follow-up or treatment plan. Radioiodine therapy with a dose of 150–200 mCi is capable of effectively treating patients with a small thyroid remnant and residual tumor in the neck and lungs. An RxWBS that shows lung metastases gives both physicians and patients information that additional treatment will likely be needed in the future. We treat patients with lung metastases that concentrate I-131 every 8-12 months with 200 mCi I-131 until no uptake is seen on the RxWBS. During this time we obtain periodic neck ultrasound examinations and pulmonary function tests if the patient has diffuse lung uptake of I-131. Although the complication rate of I-131 increases after large cumulative doses of I-131 are administered—this begins to occur with more than 800 mCi in adults and 500 mCi in children—treatment should be continued until the RxWBS is negative because lung metastases pose a more serious threat to the patient's life than the potential threat of late effects of I-131 therapy. On the other hand, once the RxWBS is negative (in a patient properly prepared for I-131 treatment), further I-131 therapy is not warranted.

LUNG METASTASES THAT ARE DETECTED > 3 MONTHS
FOLLOWING I-131 THERAPY

Lung metastases may be detected as part of the ongoing evaluation of a patient who is known to have residual cancer based on elevated thyroglobulin or imaging studies of the neck. When this occurs, the treatment is the same as that for patients with lung metastases and a small thyroid remnant.

SYMPTOMATIC LUNG METASTASES

Most patients have no symptoms from lung metastases at the time that they are diagnosed. The symptoms are the same as those from other malignancies: dyspnea, hemoptysis, dysphagia, and/or pain. Findings in addition to visualization of the metastases may include: obstructive pneumonia, pleural effusion, atelectasis, tracheal or bronchial compression, superior venocaval obstruction, esophageal compression, and chest wall invasion. Pleural effusion is a particularly ominous sign.

The guidelines in the previous sections of this chapter rarely apply to patients with bulky or symptomatic lung metastases because I-131 therapy almost never relieves the symptoms enough to produce a satisfactory result. External beam radiotherapy is usually the first step in trying to relieve symptoms from tumor compression. When metastases obstruct the trachea or major bronchus, laser therapy or internal bronchial stenting may be useful. The role of I-131 therapy is often limited in these cases, but when local therapies are successful and the tumor concentrates I-131, we frequently prescribe 200 mCi I-131 in the hope of slowing the progression of disease and occasionally producing a more prolonged remission.

LUNG DAMAGE FROM I-131 THERAPY FOR LUNG METASTASES

Pneumonitis and pulmonary fibrosis are potential complications of I-131 therapy that are specifically related to the presence of lung metastases. These terms are not defined or used precisely in the literature. Pneumonitis usually refers to an acute symptom complex consisting of dyspnea, cough, and pulmonary infiltrates. Pulmonary fibrosis is the general term for the end result of any process that results in permanent scaring or restriction in lung compliance. We use the term pneumonitis to include all forms of acute and chronic damage to the lung from radiation exposure.

Pneumonitis is rare if the dose per administration is < 250 mCi: The risk of pneumonitis probably increases with disease burden but this is not a clinically useful indicator of the likelihood of pneumonitis in patients who are known to have lung metastases unless both lungs are diffusely involved with tumor deposits. Pneumonitis is unusual even when metastases are visible on a chest radiograph. The most important factor in the development of symptomatic pneumonitis in patients with lung metastases is probably the amount of I-131 per administration. Specifically, there are reports of pneumonitis soon after administration of > 250 mCi I-131 over a wide range of total cumulative doses. More precise data are scarce. Some studies suggest that it is possible to identify patients who are at high risk for developing pneumonitis by measuring the whole body retention of I-131 at 48 hours. A guideline that appears repeatedly in the literature is that pneumonitis is rare if the whole body retention of I-131 at 48 hours is < 80 mCi.

We use spirometry and oxygen diffusion capacity to identify patients who are likely to be at high-risk for lung fibrosis: In our program we do not measure 48 hour I-131 retention or other dosimetric parameters to make the decision for ongoing I-131 treatment of a patient with diffuse lung metastases. In patients without pulmonary symptoms, which are the vast majority, we rarely perform additional testing to predict the risk of pneumonitis as long as the cumulative I-131 dose is ≤ 800 mCi with a maximum dose per administration of < 200 mCi. In patients who we retreated multiple times and have large cumulative amounts of I-131, we use the standard pulmonary function tests to make the decision about additional I-131 therapy. The most important parameter is the oxygen diffusion capacity (DLCO). We consider patients with an abnormal DLCO to be at risk for lung fibrosis to the point that we rarely deliver additional I-131 therapy in patients with a major decrease in this parameter.

As a practical matter, diffuse lung metastases usually stop taking up I-131 after three or four treatments because the entire I-131-sensitive tumor burden has been destroyed. In the large study of 28 children with lung metastases by Bal et al. (2004), the mean first dose and cumulative doses of administered 131-I were 75.4 ± 39.5 mCi and 352 ± 263 mCi, respectively. After an average number of 3.3 doses of I-131 and a mean duration of 33.2 ± 28.5 months, pulmonary lesions disappeared and thyroglobulin became undetectable in 70% of the children. In 4 other children, however, there was no radiologic or scinti-graphic (RxWBS) evidence of pulmonary metastasis, but the thyroglobulin was high in 2 patients in whom the disease persisted clinically.

We do not prescribe steroids prophylactically: Patients who develop pneumonitis must be watched closely as life-threatening problems can develop rapidly. When symptoms are progressive, or severe, steroid therapy is usually indicated. We do not advocate using steroids prophylactically prior to I-131 therapy as the withdrawal of steroids may precip-itate radiation pneumonitis in a patient who would otherwise not develop this problem.

REFERENCES

Bal, CS, A Kumar, P Chandra, SN Dwivedi, and S Mukhopadhyaya. 2004. Is chest x-ray or high-resolution computed tomography scan of the chest sufficient investigation to detect pulmonary metastasis in pediatric differentiated thyroid cancer? Thyroid **14(3):**217–225.

Benua, RS, NR Cicale, M Sonenberg, et al. 1962. The relation of radioiodine dosimetry to results and complications in the treatment of metastatic thyroid cancer. AJR **87:**171–178.

Brown, AP, WP Greening, VR McCready, HJ Shaw, and CL Harmer. 1984. Radioiodine treatment of metastatic thyroid carcinoma: the Royal Marsden Hospital experience. Br J Radiol **57:**323–327.

Maxon, HR, SR Thomas,VS Hertzberg, JG Kereiakes, IW Chen, MI Sperling, and EL Saenger. 1983. Relation between effective radiation dose and outcome of radioiodine therapy for thyroid cancer. N Engl J Med **309:**937–941.

Mazzaferri, EL, and RT Kloos. 2001. Current approaches to primary therapy for papillary and follicular thyroid cancer. J Clin Endocrinol Metab **86(4):**1447–1463.

Reynolds, JC. 1994. Comparison of I-131 absorbed radiation doses in children and adults: a tool for estimating therapeutic I-131 doses in children. In: Treatment of Thyroid Cancer in Childhood. Proceedings of a Workshop held September 10–11, 1992 at the National Institutes of Health, Bethesda, MD. Springfield, VA 22161. Available from the US Department of Commerce, Technology Administration, National Technical Information Service. pp. 127–135.

Ronga, G, M Filesi, T Montesano, AD Di Nicola, C Pace, L Travascio, G Ventroni, A Antonaci, and AR Vestri. 2004. Lung metastases from differentiated thyroid carcinoma. A 40 years' experience. Q J Nucl Med Mol Imaging **48(1):**12–19.

Schlumberger, MJ. 1999. Diagnostic follow-up of well-differentiated thyroid carcinoma: historical perspective and current status. J Endocrinol Invest **22(Suppl. 11):**3–7.

6.7. TREATMENT OF BONE METASTASES FROM DIFFERENTIATED THYROID CANCER

ROBERT J. AMDUR, MD AND ERNEST L. MAZZAFERRI, MD, MACP

The purpose of this chapter is to review the major principles that guide the management of patients with bone metastases from thyroid cancer. Table 1 summarizes the important points.

Metastases to bone are more common in patients over age 45 years, are usually symptomatic, and are often multicentric. In the large study of 146 patients with bone metastases reported by Pittas et al. (2000), almost half (47%) were present at the time of initial diagnosis. The most common sites of metastases were: vertebrae (29%), pelvis (22%), ribs (17%), and femur (11%). Multiple lesions were present in 53% of the cases.

Tickoo et al. (2000) found that bone metastases are usually from papillary thyroid carcinoma, most of which have poorly differentiated or undifferentiated features. Survival was not influenced by age at the time of diagnosis of bone metastases but was unfavorably affected by the histologic tumor type and degree of tumor differentiation.

Bone metastasis from thyroid cancer are usually well visualized on Technetium 99m bone scan and on FDG PET scan, regardless of their degree of differentiation (Fig. 1). FDG-PET scans may be the best way to identify bone metastases. Nakamoto et al. (2003) found that the most frequent pattern of detectable bone metastases with FDG PET imaging was multiple skeletal foci of intense uptake and that FDG-PET imaging revealed more lesions than did the standard bone scan, independent of the type of cancer or location of bone involvement. Lesions that concentrate radioiodine may also be visualized on I-123 or I-131 total body scan, but the sensitivity of radioiodine scan for the detection of bone metastases depends on tumor histology and avidity to concentrate iodine.

Table 1. Management of Bone Metastases From Thyroid Cancer.

Recognize the limitations of I-131 therapy:
I-131 therapy rarely alleviates symptoms from bone metastases, even when metastases are well visualized on radioiodine scan

Do not use I-131 therapy if tumor edema will cause neurologic problems:
Do not use I-131 therapy in patients with cord compression
Use external beam radiotherapy, or surgery, prior to I-131 when tumor is adjacent to important neurologic structures

Use surgical stabilization to prevent pathologic fracture:
Consult orthopaedic surgery in patients with long bone metastases with cortex invasion

Use external beam radiotherapy to relieve symptoms or prevent focal problems:
Use radiotherapy prior to I-131 when metastases are painful or if progression of a metastasis will cause a serious problem (e.g., pathologic fracture or neurologic compression)
External beam radiotherapy is usually indicated after surgical resection of a metastasis

Use I-131 therapy when metastases may concentrate radioiodine and there are no contraindications (as described above):
Give I-131 therapy alone or in addition to surgery and/or external beam radiotherapy whenever there is reason to believe that residual tumor concentrates iodine to a significant degree
With normal blood counts and renal function the I-131 dose for bone metastases is 200 mCi in adults and based on body surface area in children
We use lithium to potentiate radioiodine therapy for bone metastases unless there are medical contraindications to lithium use

Sumarium-153 or Strontium-89 when I-131 will not be beneficial:
We use Sm-153 (1 mCi/kg) when metastases are unlikely to respond to I-131
Check renal function and blood counts prior to prescribing Sm-153 or Sr-89

Consider bisphosphonate therapy in patients with bone metastases:
Pamidronate (90 mg) or zoledronate (4 mg) administered intravenously, usually every 4 weeks.

Management of the patient with bone metastases rests on several key issues that drive the therapeutic decisions: 1) the risk of pathologic fracture, particularly in weight bearing bones, 2) the risk of neurologic compromise, particularly cord compression by vertebral metastases, 3) the presence of bone pain, 4) tumor avidity to uptake radioiodine, and 5) the potential for significant bone marrow exposure from radiation arising from radioiodine-avid pelvic metastases (Fig. 2). Therapeutic options to manage the growth of bone metastases are I-131 therapy, complete surgical resection of tumor, and external beam radiotherapy (EBRT). Each has certain limitations and advantages.

THE ADVANTAGES AND LIMITATIONS OF RADIOIODINE THERAPY

Skeletal metastases from differentiated thyroid cancers frequently concentrate radioiodine. Several studies have found that radioiodine is an important therapeutic intervention that may improve survival. For example, Bernier et al. (2001) found that the independent factors that improved survival were the detection of symptomatic bone metastases, an absence of nonosseous metastases, the cumulative dose of radioiodine therapy, and complete resection of bone metastases. Pittas et al. (2000) also found that overall survival is best in patients whose metastases concentrate radioactive iodine and those who have no nonosseous metastases.

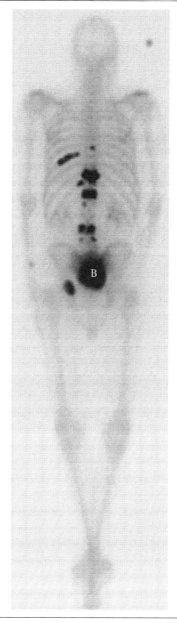

Figure 1. Posterior view of a Technetium 99m scan in a patient with metastases to vertebral bodies, ribs, and left acetabulum. The black structure in the pelvis is the bladder (B). Bone metastases from all types of thyroid cancer are usually well visualized on the standard technetium 99m bone scan and on 18-FDG PET scan. Lesions that concentrate radioiodine are also visualized on total body scan with I-123 or I-131.

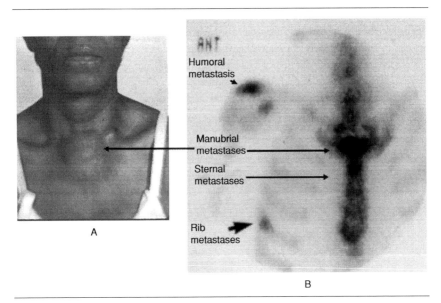

Figure 2. This is a post-treatment whole body scan of a 48 year-old woman with longstanding Graves' disease who developed widely metastatic follicular cell carcinoma. (A) tumor invading the sternum seen on physical examination. (B) Technetium-99m bone scan. She developed T3 toxicosis with this tumor and lived for about 10 years with widely metastatic disease.

Because radioiodine can deliver very high local radiation doses specifically targeted to metastatic lesions, it is the primary treatment modality employed for unresectable disease. Unfortunately, even though metastatic bone lesions often are clearly apparent on radioiodine imaging, I-131 therapy alone is very unlikely to entirely destroy them. Thyroid cancer in bone is often refractory to radioiodine therapy and mortality rates are high. Pittas et al. (2000) reported an overall 10-year survival rate of 13% from the time of diagnosis of bone metastasis, and Schlumberger et al. (1996) reported complete remission and 10-year survival rates of only 9% and 13%, respectively, for patients with bone as the only site of distant metastases from differentiated thyroid cancer.

For these reasons, radioiodine therapy should be viewed as only one aspect of therapy for the management of bone metastases that are likely to cause significant problems. The limitation of radioiodine in the management of bone metastases is discussed in detail in the articles by Tuttle et al. (2004), Schlumberger et al. (1996), and Wang et al. (2001).

SPINAL CORD COMPRESSION

Vertebral metastasis causing compression of the spinal cord is the subject of a separate chapter. The reason to mention it here is to remind the reader that radioiodine therapy may precipitate spinal cord compression in a previously asymptomatic patient with metastasis to the vertebral column. First-line therapy for patients with tumor close to the spinal cord is surgical decompression, external beam radiotherapy, or embolization.

SURGICAL STABILIZATION TO PREVENT PATHOLOGIC FRACTURE

Surgical resection of a metastatic bone lesion is the best way to manage tumor in weight-bearing bones and in acute compression syndromes or structurally unstable disease in the vertebrae or other bones. In many situations, surgical stabilization with internal fixation should be the first step in treating a metastasis that erodes a portion of a long bone in the arm or leg. Radiographic studies are done to quanitate the extent of cortex erosion from bone metastases. Pain with weight bearing in the case of a metastasis to the femur or tibia is a reliable sign of cortex erosion. Our policy is to consult an orthopaedic surgeon when a thyroid cancer patient is found to have a lytic lesion in a long bone of the arm or leg.

SURGICAL RESECTION OF METASTASES MAY IMPROVE SURVIVAL

A surgical procedure is usually the best way to relieve a cord compression or prevent pathologic fracture of a long bone. Zettinig et al. (2002) suggest that surgical resection of metastatic deposits (in addition to radioiodine and/or external beam radiotherapy) may improve survival in some groups of patients. Patients who are likely to benefit from surgical resection have a small number of lesions (preferably 1 or 2) and a reasonably long life expectancy. Many types of thyroid cancer have an indolent course to the point that even bone metastases should be treated with maximum aggressiveness.

EXTERNAL BEAM RADIOTHERAPY

External beam radiotherapy (EBRT) should be used when a bone metastasis is causing debilitating symptoms, or when it is likely to do so in the near future. When both radioiodine and EBRT are part of the treatment plan, EBRT should be given first if the metastasis is causing significant symptoms or impinging on important structures.

All types of thyroid cancer usually respond to conventional EBRT dose schedules. The degree and duration of response depends on the burden of disease and intensity of treatment. When life expectancy is more than a few years we recommend using protracted dose schedules that minimize the chance of late complications. In patients with differentiated thyroid cancer we will treat an isolated bone metastasis with 60 Gy at 2 Gy per treatment.

I-131 THERAPY

We use radioiodine therapy in addition to surgery and EBRT whenever there is reason to believe that residual tumor concentrates iodine to a significant degree. In patients who do not receive surgery or EBRT, we use radioiodine to delay tumor progression as long as toxicity is tolerable and the patient seems to be responding to the therapy.

Many series report outcomes following radioiodine in patients with distant metastases from differentiated thyroid cancer. The articles in the reference list with this chapter review the major studies. Radioiodine therapy for bone metastases brings up the controversy of how to determine the amount of radioiodine to be used in a specific situation.

A separate chapter in part VA discusses the three basic approaches to choosing radioiodine dose: Fixed dose categories, maximum blood dose, and quantitative tumor dosimetry.

The article by Tuttle et al. (2004) is a good example of the use of the maximum blood dose approach to prescribing radioiodine in patients with bone metastases. We use a fixed dose approach to prescribing I-131 in all situations. In an adult with normal renal function and normal peripheral blood counts we typically administer 200 mCi I-131 when our goal is to treat bone metastases. We use lithium to increase the potency of I-131 unless there are medical contraindications to the drug. We sometimes use recombinant human TSH to prepare patients with bone metastases, although this may cause intense bone pain in some patients (Vitale 2002).

SUMARIUM-153 OR STRONTIUM-89

I-131 therapy is not useful for tumor types that do not concentrate radioiodine (e.g., anaplastic carcinoma, medullary carcinoma) or progress in spite of positive post-treatment whole body scans. An option in these situations is to use a systemic radionuclide that is known to be effective at treating bone metastases. Sr-89 and Sm-153 have both been shown to be effective for bone metastases in clinical trials. Our preference is to use Sm-153 because symptoms respond quicker than with Sr-89. The approved dose for Sm-153 is 1 mCi/kg but some studies suggest that higher doses are more effective. Unlike radioiodine, Sm-153 (and Sr-89) is not concentrated in the saliva and lacrimal glands so many of the toxicities that are associated with high-dose radioiodine therapy are not seen with Sm-153 or Sr-89. The main toxicity with Sm-153 and Sr-89 is bone marrow suppression. This is often a problem if patients have previously received multiple treatments with I-131. It is important to check renal function and peripheral blood counts before giving a patient Sm-153 or Sr-89.

BISPHOSPHONATES

Bisphosphonates are a class of medications that inhibit bone resorption by a variety of mechanisms. Several drugs in this class have been shown to decrease the skeletal problems associated with osteoporosis, myeloma, and metastatic cancer. There is evidence that bisphosphonate therapy inhibits the development and progression of bone metastases.

We have limited experience using bisphosphonate therapy in patients with thyroid cancer. The articles by Tuttle et al. (2004) and Vitale et al. (2002) discuss the literature related to this subject. Tuttle and colleagues recommend treating patients with bone metastases from thyroid cancer with either pamidronate (90 mg) or zoledronate (4 mg). Both of these drugs are administered intravenously, usually at 4 week intervals.

REFERENCES

Bernier, MO, L Leenhardt, C Hoang, A Aurengo, JY Mary, F Menegaux, E Enkaoua, G Turpin, J Chiras, G Saillant, and G Hejblum. 2001. Survival and therapeutic modalities in patients with bone metastases of differentiated thyroid carcinomas. J Clin Endocrinol Metab **86(4)**:1568–1573.

Ceccarelli, C, F Bianchi, D Trippi, F Brozzi, F Di Martino, P Santini, R Elisei, and A Pinchera. 2004. Location of functioning metastases from differentiated thyroid carcinoma by simultaneous double isotope acquisition of I-131 whole body scan and bone scan. J Endocrinol Invest **27(9)**:866–869.

Nakamoto, Y, M Osman, and RL Wahl. 2003. Prevalence and patterns of bone metastases detected with positron emission tomography using F-18 FDG. Clin Nucl Med **28(4):**302–307.

Pittas, AG, M Adler, M Fazzari, S Tickoo, J Rosai, SM Larson, and RJ Robbins. 2000. Bone metastases from thyroid carcinoma: clinical characteristics and prognostic variables in one hundred forty-six patients. Thyroid **10(3):**261–268.

Schlumberger, M, C Challeton, F De Vathaire, JP Travagli, P Gardet, JD Lumbroso, C Francese, F Fontaine, M Ricard, and C Parmentier. 1996. Radioactive iodine treatment and external radiotherapy for lung and bone metastases from thyroid carcinoma. J Nucl Med **37(4):**598–605.

Tickoo, SK, AG Pittas, M Adler, M Fazzari, SM Larson, RJ Robbins, and J Rosai. 2000. Bone metastases from thyroid carcinoma: a histopathologic study with clinical correlates. Arch Pathol Lab Med **124(10):**1440–1447.

Tuttle, MR, RJ Robbins, SM Larson, and HW Strauss. 2004. Challenging cases in thyroid cancer: a multi-disciplinary approach. Eur J Nucl Med Mol Imaging **31:**605–612.

Vitale, G, GA Lupoli, A Ciccarelli, F Fonderico, M Klain, G Squame, M Salvatore, and G Lupoli. 2002. The use of recombinant human TSH in the follow-up of differentiated thyroid cancer: experience from a large patient cohort in a single centre. Clin Endocrinol (Oxford) **56(2):**247–252.

Wang, W, SM Larson, RM Tuttle, H Kalaigian, K Kolbert, M Sonenberg, and RJ Robbins. 2001. Resistance of [18F]-fluorodeoxyglucose-avid metastatic thyroid cancer lesions to treatment with high-dose radioactive iodine. Thyroid **11(12):**1169–1175.

Zettinig, G, BJ Fueger, C Passler, K Kaserer, C Pirich, R Dudczak, and B Niederle. 2002. Long-term follow-up of patients with bone metastases from differentiated thyroid carcinoma—surgery or conventional therapy? Clin Endocrinol **56:**377–382.

6.8. TREATMENT OF SPINAL CORD COMPRESSION FROM METASTATIC THYROID CANCER

ROBERT J. AMDUR, MD AND ERNEST L. MAZZAFERRI, MD, MACP

Spinal cord compression may occur from invasion of the primary tumor into the spinal canal or from growth of a vertebral metastasis. As described in the article by Ginsberg et al. (1982), spinal cord compression from extension of tumor from the primary site has been reported in patients with thyroid cancer. The subject of this chapter is the management of patients with spinal cord compression from growth of metastatic disease in a vertebral body or posterior element (Fig. 1). In general the management of spinal cord compression from metastatic thyroid cancer is the same as that for other types of cancer. Table 1 summarizes the important points from this chapter.

HIGH DOSE CORTICOSTEROIDS

First line therapy for spinal cord compression from metastatic cancer is high–dose corticosteroids to decrease tumor edema. Corticosteroid therapy should begin at diagnosis and be continued at full dose until symptoms are clearly responding. In the inpatient or emergency room setting we prescribe dexamethasone intravenously, 10 mg for the initial dose followed by 4 mg every 6 hours thereafter. In the outpatient setting we prescribe dexamethasone 4 mg by mouth every 6 hours. To decrease the chance of gastritis, we prescribe a proton pump inhibitor, such as Omeprazole 20 mg by mouth each day, as long as patients are on corticosteroids.

RADIOIODINE THERAPY

Radioiodine should not be used to treat spinal cord compression from thyroid cancer. Cord compression is an oncologic emergency in which the goal is to relieve compression

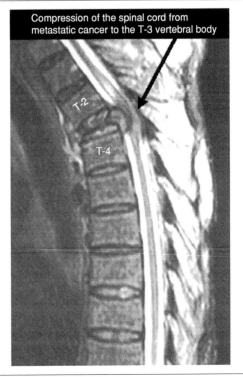

Figure 1. T2-weighted Magnetic Resonance image in the saggital plane demonstrating compression of the spinal cord from metastatic cancer to the T-3 vertebral body.

as soon as possible–preferably within hours or days of diagnosis. Radioiodine does not shrink metastatic deposits as rapidly or as reliably as the other treatment options. Radioiodine may actually cause tumor edema that may exacerbate neurologic problems.

Table 1. Treatment of Spinal Cord Compression from Metastatic Thyroid Cancer.

Start corticosteroids immediately:
Intravenous: Dexamethasone 10 mg loading dose then 4 mg every 6 hours
Oral: Dexamethasone 4 mg every 6 hours

Do not treat cord compression with radioiodine:
Time to response from radioiodine is too long
Radioiodine may initially cause tumor edema and exacerbate cord compression

Surgical decompression followed by external beam radiotherapy is the preferred treatment for patients with a single area of cord compression:
Patchell et al., A randomized trial of direct decompressive surgical resection in the treatment of spinal cord compression caused by metastases. Abstract presented May 2003

In patients who do not undergo surgical decompression, external beam radiotherapy should begin ASAP:
We use 30 Gy at 3 Gy per treatment in most patients

SURGICAL DECOMPRESSION VERSUS RADIOTHERAPY

Historically, the standard treatment for cord compression from metastatic cancer has been external beam radiotherapy based on studies that show no improvement in outcome with surgical decompression. Radiotherapy is usually started within 24 hours of diagnosis. The radiotherapy dose and technique varies with the extent of disease, the functional status of the patient, and the ability of the patient to travel daily for therapy.

In May 2003, Patchell et al. reported the results of a prospective, randomized trial comparing radiotherapy alone to surgical decompression followed by radiotherapy in patients with a single area of cord compression from metastatic carcinoma. The chance of regaining or retaining the ability to walk was higher in patients treated with surgery to the point that the trial was stopped early. This study has not been published in a peer-reviewed journal at the date of the writing of this chapter but already it has changed the management of patients with cord compression from metastatic cancer in many communities. In our institution surgical decompression followed by external beam radiotherapy is now the preferred treatment for patients with limited areas of cord compression. In patients where surgical decompression is not feasible because of extent of disease or underlying medical problems, we deliver external beam radiotherapy.

EMBOLIZATION

Endovascular embolization has been used to shrink tumor and metastatic deposits. This approach works best in highly vascular tumors. A paper by Smit et al. (2000) describes excellent results using embolization to relieve spinal cord compression from metastatic thyroid cancer. We do not have experience with this treatment but mention it as a reasonable alternative to surgical decompression and external beam radiotherapy in selected patients.

REFERENCES

Ginsberg, J, JD Pedersen, C von Westarp, and AB McCarten. 1982. Cervical cord compression due to extension of a papillary thyroid carcinoma. Am J Med **1987(1):**156–158.

Patchell, R, PA Tibbs, WF Regine, et al. 2003. A randomized trial of direct decompressive surgical resection in the treatment of spinal cord compression caused by metastases. In : Program/Proceedings of the 39th Annual Meeting of the American Society of Clinical Oncology, Chicago, IL, May 31–June 3, Abstract 2.

Smit, JW, GJ Vielvoye, and BM Goslings. 2000. Embolization for vertebral metastases of follicular thyroid carcinoma. Clin Endocrinol Metab **85(3):**989–994.

6.9. TREATMENT OF BRAIN METASTASIS FROM DIFFERENTIATED THYROID CANCER

ROBERT J. AMDUR, MD, ILLONA M. SCHMALFUSS, AND ERNEST L. MAZZAFERRI, MD, MACP

The purpose of this chapter is to explain important issues related to the diagnosis and management of brain metastases from differentiated thyroid cancer. Table 1 summarizes the main points from this chapter.

RADIOIODINE THERAPY IS CONTRAINDICATED IN PATIENTS WITH A BRAIN METASTASIS

In any patient where there is concern about the possibility of brain metastasis it is important to image the brain prior to administering radioiodine therapy. Radioiodine crosses the blood-brain barrier and affects a metastasis in a manner similar to that of the primary tumor. Tumor cell destruction in a metastatic deposit often results in hemorrhage and edema, which may cause serious neurologic problems. The general rule is to destroy brain metastases with either surgery or external beam radiotherapy prior to delivering radioiodine therapy for other sites of disease. If radioiodine therapy is given to a patient with brain metastases, we recommend treating the patient with dexamethasone 4 mg every 6 hours for a minimum of 5 days following radioiodine administration.

ELEVATED SERUM THYROGLOBULIN MAY INDICATE A BRAIN METASTASIS

The usual sign of a brain metastasis is a neurologic problem such as weakness, sensory loss, cognitive impairment, or seizure. In patients with thyroid cancer another important sign may be an unexplained elevation in the serum level of thyroglobulin. Brain metastases produce thyroglobulin to a degree that is similar to that of the primary tumor. Thyroglobulin produced in a brain metastasis contributes to the concentration

Table 1. Summary of Major Points About the Management of Brain Metastasis.

Radioiodine therapy is contraindicated in patients with a brain metastasis
Elevated serum thyroglobulin may indicate a brain metastasis
Magnetic Resonance imaging is the best way to screen for brain metastases
The Magnetic Resonance scan should include T2 gradient echo sequences

First line (intial) management of brain metastases:
- Dexamethasone 4 mg every 6 hours to decrease mass effect symptoms
- Phenytoin (usually start with 300 mg per day) to prevent seizures
- First line therapy for a metastasis > 3 cm is surgical resection
- First line therapy for a patient with 1–3 metastases, each < 3 cm, is radiosurgery alone or whole brain radiotherapy followed by radiosurgery to areas of residual disease
- Whole brain radiotherapy is indicated in a patient with > 3 metastases
- Selected patients will benefit from resection of lesions > 3 cm and/or from radiosurgery to lesions that do not completely respond to radiotherapy
- In patients with a life expectancy > 6 months, lesions that do not completely respond to fractionated radiotherapy should be treated with radiosurgery

of thyroglobulin in the serum. It is therefore important to consider the possibility of a brain metastasis when the serum thyroglobulin level is unexpectedly high. We image the brain in any patient with a neurologic sign or symptom that suggests a brain metastasis or when serum thyroglobulin is higher than what we expect from the extent of disease on whole body iodine scan.

MAGNETIC RESONANCE IMAGING

The best imaging study to identify the presence or extent of brain metastasis from thyroid cancer is a Magnetic Resonance (MR) scan. MR is much more sensitive than Computed Tomography or nuclear medicine studies for detecting brain metastases.

When evaluating a patient with thyroid cancer, it is important that the MR scan include T2* gradient echo sequences (TR/TE ~500/30 ms) which is sensitive in detecting small hemorrhagic foci. Thyroid cancer metastases are often hemorrhagic to the point that blood products make small metastases difficult to visualize on T1 sequences, even when the scan is done with intravenous contrast. Hemorrhagic metastases are well visualized as hypointense lesions with the proper T2* gradient echo sequence. Representative images are shown in Fig. 1. See the article by Murata et al. (2004) for further details.

MANAGEMENT OF BRAIN METASTASES

The articles by Nguyen and Deangelis (2004) are excellent reviews of the literature related to the management of brain metastases. The concepts discussed in these papers are applicable to patients with thyroid cancer.

All patients with symptoms of mass effect receive corticosteroids (we use Dexamethasone 4 mg every six hours). All patients with a history of seizure receive antiepileptic therapy (we start with Phenytoin 300 mg per day). We do not prescribe antiepileptic medications in patients who have not had a seizure but it is reasonable to do this prior to treatment of brain metastases.

Surgical resection, fractionated -meaning multiple treatments- radiotherapy, and single treatment radiosurgery are the main options for destroying brain metastases. The

Table 2. University of Florida Guidelines for Managing Brain Metastases from Thyroid Cancer.

<hr>

FIRST LINE (INITIAL) THERAPY:

Solitary metastasis < 3 cm:
- Radiosurgery alone

Solitary metastasis > 3 cm:
- Surgical resection followed by radiosurgery or fractionated radiotherapy
- Patients who are not good candidates for surgery because of the location of the metastasis or underlying medical problems receive radiosurgery or fractionated radiotherapy

1–3 metastases, each < 3 cm:
- Radiosurgery alone

1–3 metastases with a metastasis > 3 cm:
- Surgical resection of metastases > 3 cm followed by radiosurgery or fractionated radiotherapy to resection cavities, unresectable disease, and remaining lesions

> 3 metastases:
- Whole brain radiotherapy
- In a patient with a good functional status and a life expectancy of > 6 months, we evaluate response with an MR scan 4 weeks after the completion of whole brain radiotherapy
- If 1–5 lesions are still visible, and each is < 3 cm, we treat the lesions that have not completely responded with radiosurgery

SURVAILLIANCE PROTOCOL FOLLOWING TREATMENT:

Brain MR scan every 3 months × 4 then every 4 months × 3, then every 6 months × 2

SECOND LINE THERAPY FOR NEW OR RECURRENT METASTASES:

Recurrent metastasis in an area treated initially with radiosurgery:
- Surgical if the morbidity of resection is likely to be low
- Fractionated radiotherapy if this has not been previously used
- If surgical resection is not advisable, and fractionated radiotherapy has previously been given to this area, therapy is limited to supportive care

New or recurrent metastasis in an area not previously treated with radiosurgery:
- Radiosurgery for lesions < 3 cm
- Surgery for lesions > 3 cm when the morbidity of resection is likely to be low
- Supportive care when aggressive treatment of recurrent disease is not appropriate

RADIOSURGERY AND RADIOTHERAPY DOSE SCHEDULES:

Radiosurgery in the absence of fractionated radiotherapy:
- 20–22.5 Gy for lesions < 3 cm
- 10–15 Gy if radiosurgery is used to treat a lesion > 3 cm
- The dose is prescribed to the periphery of the tumor as visualized on a contrast enhanced T1 sequence MR scan

Radiosurgery in addition to fractionated radiotherapy:
- 10–15 Gy depending on target size and the dose of radiotherapy
- The dose is prescribed to the periphery of the tumor as visualized on a contrast enhanced T1 sequence MR scan

Fractionated radiotherapy:
- 45 Gy at 1.8 Gy/treatment or 30 Gy at 3 Gy/treatment
- When there is only one lesion the target volume is the resection cavity, or area of visible disease, plus a 1 cm margin
- The target volume is the entire brain when fractionated radiotherapy is used in a patient with multiple lesions

<hr>

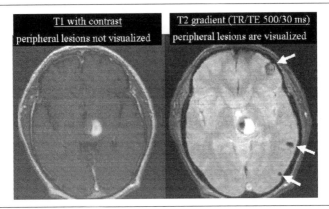

Figure 1. Magnetic resonance images from the same scanning session in a patient with follicular carcinoma. This patient has a large central metastasis and multiple smaller peripheral metastases. Hemorrhage makes the smaller lesions difficult to visualize on T1 echo sequences, even when the scan is done with intravenous contrast. Hemorrhagic metastases are easily visualized on the T2* weighted gradient echo sequence. [From Murata, Y., Itoh, S., Morio, K., Sasaki, T., Mizobuchi, H., Shimizu, K., and Yoshida, S. Hemorrhagic cerebral metastases from thyroid cancer on T2*-weighted gradient echo MRI. Magn Reson. Imaging 22(3), 435–439. 2004. Reproduced with permission from Elsevier, Inc.]

indication for each of these modalities is currently controversial to the point that there are major differences in treatment philosophy among recognized experts. The review article by Nguyen and Deangelis (2004) discusses the major issues. Our basic approach is summarized in Table 2.

REFERENCES

Deangelis, LM. 2001. Brain tumors. N Engl J Med **344(2)**:114–123.
Murata, Y, S Itoh, K Morio, T Sasaki, H Mizobuchi, K Shimizu, and S Yoshida. 2004. Hemorrhagic cerebral metastases from thyroid cancer on T2*-weighted gradient echo MRI. Magn Reson Imaging **22(3)**:435–439.
Nguyen, T, and, LM Deangelis. 2004. Treatment of brain metastases. J Support Oncol **2(5)**:405–410.

PART 7. DIFFERENTIATED THYROID CANCER DURING PREGNANCY, IN A THYROGLOSSAL DUCT, AND UNFAVORABLE HISTOLOGIC SUBTYPES OF DTC

7.1. MANAGEMENT OF DIFFERENTIATED THYROID CANCER DURING PREGNANCY

ROBERT J. AMDUR, MD AND ERNEST L. MAZZAFERRI, MD, MACP

Management of a patient with a thyroid nodule, or confirmed thyroid cancer, during pregnancy is controversial. The purpose of this chapter is to explain this controversy and make treatment recommendations. The paper by Moosa & Mazzaferri (1997) cites the major studies of this issue. Table 1 summarizes the main points from this chapter.

THE CONTROVERSY

Controversy about the management of pregnant patients with a thyroid nodule or thyroid cancer is based on disagreement about the effects that the hormonal changes of pregnancy have on the growth rate of thyroid cancer. Clinicians who believe that thyroid cancer is more aggressive during pregnancy take the position that the diagnosis of a thyroid nodule and, if necessary, thyroidectomy should be pursued during pregnancy and view termination of the pregnancy or premature delivery as necessary considerations. However, this is an older view of the problem, mainly based on isolated case reports or personal experiences in which pregnant women with thyroid cancer did not fare well (Kobayashi 1994). The contemporary view is that pregnancy has no major influence on the prognosis of thyroid cancer during pregnancy and that surgery and I-131 therapy can be delayed until after delivery in patients with well differentiated tumors (Herzon 1994; Moosa & Mazzaferri 1997; Driggers 1998; Vini 1999).

PREGNANCY STIMULATES THE GROWTH OF THYROID CANCER

A few case studies report aggressive features of differentiated thyroid cancers diagnosed during pregnancy. No prospective study demonstrates a difference in outcome compared

Table 1. Management of Thyroid Cancer During Pregnancy.

There is controversy about the prognosis of thyroid cancer during pregnancy:
- Some clinicians think that thyroid cancer behaves more aggressively during pregnancy
- Other clinicians think that pregnancy has no effect on the prognosis of thyroid cancer

There are data that suggest pregnancy may affect thyroid cancer behavior:
- There are reports that solitary nodules are more likely to be malignant during pregnancy
- There are in-vitro data that pregnancy hormones may cause neoplastic transformation of follicular cells, or stimulate proliferation of thyroid cancer

Data suggesting that pregnancy does not have an important effect on the behavior of thyroid cancer:
- Multiple clinical series with age-matched control groups find that the prognosis of differentiated thyroid cancer is the same in pregnant and nonpregnant women

Our policy:
- We recommend neck ultrasound and fine-needle aspiration at any stage of pregnancy for patients with a thyroid mass or adenopathy that is suspicious for cancer
- We do not recommend diagnostic studies that involve ionizing radiation as part of the evaluation of a patient with thyroid pathology during pregnancy
- In the absence of a history of rapid tumor growth or signs of problems that require immediate intervention (e.g., airway compromise), we do not recommend open biopsy or thyroidectomy if fine needle aspiration does not establish a diagnosis
- When thyroid cancer is diagnosed during pregnancy, we recommend delaying additional workup and treatment until after the completion of pregnancy as long as the tumor does not have anaplastic features or a history of rapid growth, metastases or other aggressive features
- In a patient with a large primary tumor or extensive adenopathy, we suggest completing the pregnancy as soon as the risk of premature delivery is low, otherwise we recommend letting the pregnancy take its normal course
- We recommend that the diagnostic workup be completed, and the appropriate treatment initiated, soon after the completion of the pregnancy

to a control group. Concern about rapid growth of thyroid cancer during pregnancy is based on several observations:

Malignant nodules may be more common during pregnancy: There are reports that a solitary thyroid nodule during pregnancy is more likely to be malignant than a solitary nodule in a woman of similar age who is not pregnant (Rosen 1986.) and a weak association between parity and risk of thyroid cancer was found in an epidemiologic study (Galanti 1995). Ascertainment bias is likely a problem in all of these studies. Most contemporary opinions of the risk of thyroid cancer in thyroid nodules do not consider pregnancy to be a risk factor for thyroid cancer in an isolated thyroid nodule. This is summarized in the recent study by (Hegedus 2004) and in Chapter 1.

Pregnancy hormones may stimulate thyroid cell proliferation: There is good evidence that human chorionic gonadotropin binds to the TSH receptor of normal and neoplastic cells of follicular origin and that it may stimulate their growth (Hershman 1999). There is also evidence that malignant thyroid tissue may bind endogenous estrogens, but this finding has not been confirmed in all studies and its significance in patients with thyroid cancer has never been demonstrated.

THE DATA THAT PREGNANCY HAS NO SIGNIFICANT EFFECT ON THE PROGNOSIS OF THYROID CANCER

There are now several studies that use age-matched controls to evaluate the effect of pregnancy on the prognosis of patients with differentiated thyroid cancer (Herzon 1994; Moosa & Mazzaferri 1997; Driggers 1998; Vini 1999). These studies demonstrate that the prognosis of differentiated thyroid cancer is the same in pregnant and nonpregnant women of the same age.

OUR APPROACH TO PREGNANT WOMEN WITH THYROID NODULES OR THYROID CANCER

In our opinion delaying the diagnosis or treatment of a thyroid nodule in patient with an early stage, well differentiated thyroid cancer until pregnancy takes its natural course does not compromise the outcome to a degree that warrants interventions that increase the risk of a pregnancy complication. Neck ultrasound and fine needle aspiration are low-risk procedures. We attempt to obtain a diagnosis using fine needle aspiration at any stage of pregnancy in patients who present with a thyroid mass or adenopathy. In the absence of a history of rapid tumor growth, or signs of problems that require immediate intervention—such as airway compromise—we do not recommend open biopsy or thyroidectomy if fine needle aspiration biopsy is not able to establish a diagnosis.

When thyroid cancer is diagnosed during pregnancy, we recommend delaying additional workup and treatment until after delivery as long as the tumor does not have anaplastic features or a history of rapid growth. In a patient with a large primary tumor or extensive adenopathy, we recommend premature delivery as soon as the risk is low. Otherwise, we recommend that the pregnancy take its normal course.

At some point, delaying the treatment of a patient with differentiated thyroid cancer will compromise outcome. A separate chapter presents data on the effect of delay in diagnosis and treatment of differentiated thyroid cancer. To minimize the delay caused by pregnancy, we recommend a diagnostic workup and appropriate treatment within two months following delivery. Radioiodine therapy, and to a lesser degree diagnostic studies, disrupt family life because they require that the mother be isolated from her baby and often eliminate the possibility of breast feeding.

REFERENCES

Driggers, RW, JN Kopelman, and AJ Satin. 1998. Delaying surgery for thyroid cancer in pregnancy—a case report. J Reprod Med **43**:909–912.

Galanti, MR, M Lambe, A Ekbom, P Sparen, and B Pettersson. 1995. Parity and risk of thyroid cancer: a nested case-control study of a nationwide Swedish cohort. Cancer Causes Control **6**:37–44.

Hegedus, L. 2004. Clinical practice. The thyroid nodule. N Engl J Med **351**:1764–1771.

Hershman, JM. 1999. Human chorionic gonadotropin and the thyroid: hyperemesis gravidarum and trophoblastic tumors. Thyroid **9**:653–657.

Herzon, FS, DM Morris, MN Segal, G Rauch, and T Parnell. 1994. Coexistent thyroid cancer and pregnancy. Arch Otolaryngol Head Neck Surg **120**:1191–1193.

Kobayashi, K, Y Tanaka, S Ishiguro, and T Mori. 1994. Rapidly growing thyroid carcinoma during pregnancy. J Surg Oncol **55**:61–64.

Moosa, M, and EL Mazzaferri. 1997. Outcome of differentiated thyroid cancer diagnosed in pregnant women. J Clin Endocrinol Metab **82(9):**2862–2866.

Rosen, IB, and PG Walfish. 1986. Pregnancy as a predisposing factor in thyroid neoplasia. Arch Surg **121:**1287–1290.

Vini, L, S Hyer, B Pratt, and C Harmer. 1999. Management of differentiated thyroid cancer diagnosed during pregnancy. Eur J Endocrinol **140(5)**:404–406.

7.2. THYROID CANCER ORIGINATING IN A THYROGLOSSAL DUCT REMNANT

ROBERT J. AMDUR, MD AND ERNEST L. MAZZAFERRI, MD, MACP

In is sometimes difficult to be confident about management decisions in patients with carcinoma in a thyroglossal duct remnant. This is an uncommon event with no large series on patient outcome. The articles that we include in the reference list present a review of the literature related to the epidemiology, diagnosis, and management of patients with carcinoma in a thyroglossal duct remnant. The purpose of this chapter is to present guidelines for managing patients with thyroid carcinoma in a thyroglossal duct remnant, which is usually a thyroglossal duct cyst.

BACKGROUND INFORMATION

During gestation, the thyroid gland descends from the foramen cecum to the usual adult location below the thyroid cartilage. The path of the thyroid gland during this migration is marked by an epithelial structure called the thyroglossal tract (or duct). In most people, the thyroglossal duct disappears by the tenth gestational week. In approximately 10% of people, however, some portion of the thyroglossal duct persists after birth. A thyroglossal duct remnant may be a cyst, a duct, a fistula, or a combination of these structures. Ectopic thyroid tissue may or may not be present in a thyroglossal duct remnant. Figures 1 and 2 are Computed Tomography images of a benign and a malignant thyroglossal duct cyst.

Thyroglossal duct carcinoma is usually a thyroid carcinoma, but squamous cell carcinoma may develop from the cells lining the thyroglossal duct. All types of carcinoma that arise from follicular thyroid cells have been reported in a thyroglossal duct remnant (papillary, follicular, insular, Hürthle cell, anaplastic) but 90% are papillary carcinoma

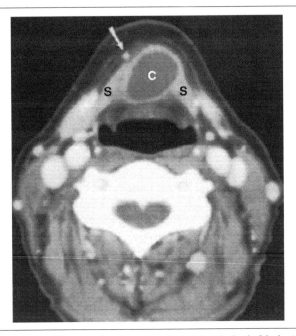

Figure 1. Benign thyroglossal duct cyst. Contrast-enhanced CT below the level of the hyoid bone reveals a cystic mass (c) inseparable from the strap muscles (s). The mass has a thin, smooth rim, and the contents are of fluid density. No calcifications are identified within the mass. The anterior jugular vein (arrow) is displaced by the mass. [Reproduced with permission from Branstetter BF, Weissman JL, Kennedy TL, Whitaker M. The CT appearance of thyroglossal duct carcinoma. Am J Neuroradiol **21**:1547–1550, 2000.]

(Falconieri 2001). Medullary carcinoma does not arise in a thyroglossal duct remnant because C cells are rare in the median thyroid.

In the general population the mean age at presentation of thyroglossal duct carcinoma is approximately 38 years with a slight female predominance. In the pediatric age group, the mean age at presentation is approximately 13 years (Peretz 2004).

THE THYROIDECTOMY CONTROVERSY

The most common procedure for excising benign and malignant thyroglossal duct remnants is the Sistrunk procedure. This procedure involves excision of the thyroglossal duct remnant, the central portion of the hyoid bone, and usually a core of tissue around the area where the thyroglossal duct would open in the oral cavity at the foramen cecum.

All patients with a thyroid cancer in a thyroglossal duct remnant should have the neck imaged to look for adenopathy and evidence of carcinoma in the thyroid gland. The need to perform thyroidectomy in patients with no evidence of tumor in the thyroid, based on imaging, is controversial (Luna-Ortiz 2004; Mazzaferri 2004; Miccoli 2004; Patel 2002). Thyroid cancer is sometimes a multifocal disease and a carcinoma arising in the

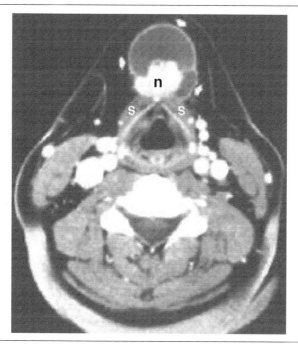

Figure 2. Papillary thyroid carcinoma of the thyroglossal duct. Contrast-enhanced CT at the level of the thyroid cartilage reveals a cystic mass in the anterior neck (arrows), inseparable from the strap muscles (s), with septation and a lobular mural nodule (n). [Reproduced with permission from Branstetter BF, Weissman JL, Kennedy TL, Whitaker M. The CT appearance of thyroglossal duct carcinoma. Am J Neuroradiol **21**:1547–1550, 2000.]

thyroid gland may occur simultaneously in a thyroglossal duct remnant. However, one must be particularly careful not to mistake thyroid carcinoma metastatic to a Delphian lymph node (overlying the laryngeal cartilage) for a thyroglossal duct carcinoma.

The published incidence of cancer in the thyroidectomy specimen in patients with thyroglossal duct carcinoma is 11–40% in adults and 0% in children. The arguments for and against making total thyroidectomy a routine part of the treatment in patients with thyroglossal duct carcinoma are the same as those discussed in other chapters for patients who appear to have carcinoma localized to one side of the thyroid gland. Total thyroidectomy increases the efficacy of radioiodine therapy, increases the sensitivity of radioiodine scans, and makes it possible to use the serum level of thyroglobulin as a sensitive marker of tumor status.

TREATMENT GUIDELINES

All patients with a diagnosis of thyroid cancer in a thyroglossal duct remnant should undergo comprehensive imaging of the neck to look for adenopathy and a tumor in the thyroid gland. Our preference is to use ultrasonography for these evaluations. We prefer

Table 1. Treatment Guidelines for Thyroid Cancer in a Thyroglossal Duct Remnant.

Sistrunk procedure alone (no thyroidectomy):
All of these factors must be present:
- Papillary microcarcinoma (≤1 cm)
- No history of radiation exposure
- No adenopathy by ultrasound
- No tumor in the thyroid by ultrasound
- No evidence of extension of tumor beyond thyroglossal duct cyst
- No unfavorable histologic features (e.g., tall cell, insular or anaplastic carcinoma)

Sistrunk procedure plus total thyroidectomy followed by radioiodine therapy:
If any of these factors are present:
- Age > 45 years
- History of radiation exposure
- Adenopathy by ultrasound (perform neck dissection also)
- Tumor in the thyroid by ultrasound
- Tumor > 1 cm
- Extension of tumor beyond thyroglossal duct cyst
- Unfavorable histologic features (e.g., tall cell, insular or anaplastic carcinoma)

External beam radiotherapy in addition to the treatment described above:
- Use the same indications as for carcinoma originating in the thyroid

to avoid Computed Tomography because iodinated contrast will decrease the efficacy of radioiodine studies and scanning for months. Table 1 presents management guidelines. Most patients are women and it is difficult to justify a total thyroidectomy for a papillary microcarcinoma confined to the thyroglossal duct cyst in a woman who may want to get pregnant in the future. Thyroid hormone replacement therapy during pregnancy causes a unique- and potentially serious-group of problems for mother and fetus.

REFERENCES

Branstetter, BF, JL Weissman, TL Kennedy, and M Whitaker. 2000. The CT appearance of thyroglossal duct carcinoma. Am J Neuroradiol **21**:1547–1550.
Falconieri, G, LD Della, and M Zanella. 2001. Papillary thyroid carcinoma of the thyroglossal duct cyst: comparative cytohistologic and immunochemical study of 2 new cases and review of the literature. Int J Surg Pathol **9(1)**:65–71.
Luna-Ortiz, K, LM Hurtado-Lopez, JL Valderrama-Landaeta, and A Ruiz-Vega. 2004. Thyroglossal duct cyst with papillary carcinoma: what must be done? Thyroid **14(5)**:363–366.
Mazzaferri, EL. 2004. Thyroid cancer in thyroglossal duct remnants: a diagnostic and therapeutic dilemma. Thyroid **14(5)**:335–337.
Miccoli, P, MN Minuto, D Galleri, M Puccini, and P Berti. 2004. Extent of surgery in thyroglossal duct carcinoma: reflections on a series of eighteen cases. Thyroid **14(2)**:121–123.
Patel, SG, M Escrig, AR Shaha, B Singh, and JP Shah. 2002. Management of well-differentiated thyroid carcinoma presenting within a thyroglossal duct cyst. J Surg Oncol **79(3)**:134–139.
Peretz, A, E Leiberman, J Kapelushnik, and E Hershkovitz. 2004. Thyroglossal duct carcinoma in children: case presentation and review of the literature. **14(9)**:777–785.

7.3. TALL AND COLLUMNAR VARIANTS OF PAPILLARY CARCINOMA

ROBERT J. AMDUR, MD AND ERNEST L. MAZZAFERRI, MD, MACP

The purpose of this chapter is to explain the classification and management of patients with Tall and Columnar cell variants of papillary carcinoma. Most references classify these tumors as unfavorable variants of well-differentiated papillary carcinoma. This assignment is somewhat arbitrary. These are relatively rare tumors and the criteria for diagnosis is controversial. With additional study of the outcome of the uncommon subtypes of thyroid carcinoma, it may be more appropriate to consider tumors with Tall or Columnar cell features as a subtype of poorly differentiated thyroid carcinoma.

TALL CELL VARIANT OF PAPILLARY CARCINOMA

The tall cell variant maintains the papillary architecture and the cytologic (nuclear) features of the usual type of papillary carcinoma, but in addition, the cells have abundant oxyphilic cytoplasm to the point that they are approximately twice as tall as they are wide. Unlike the usual type of papillary carcinoma, the tall cell variant usually has mitoses. A photomicrograph of a Tall Cell carcinoma is presented in the classification chapter in part 1 of this book.

Focal tall cell features may be a component of any of the subtypes of thyroid carcinoma. There has been controversy in the literature about the percent of the tumor that must have tall cell features to classify the tumor as a tall cell variant. The two most common recommendations in the literature are a 30% and 70% minimum tall cell component. Our preference is to follow the recommendation of LiVolsi et al. to use a minimum of 70% tall cells to classify the tumor as a tall cell variant of papillary carcinoma.

Table 1. Prognosis of Tall Cell Variant Papillary Carcinoma*.

	Tall cell variant (n = 148)	Classic differentiated (n = 1355)
Disease-free survival	∼ 45%	∼ 65%
Death from cancer	∼ 20%	∼ 10%

* The figures in this table are adapted from a review by Ringel and colleagues (2000) that includes data from multiple published series.

In most series, this tumor accounts for approximately 5% of all thyroid cancer cases. It may occur at any age but the mean age at diagnosis is higher than that for the classic form of papillary carcinoma (mean 52 years for tall cell versus 36 for classic histology). As with most forms of differentiated thyroid cancer, there is a slight female predominance in the tall cell variant. Tall cell carcinoma usually concentrates radioiodine well enough to be visualized on a total body radioiodine scan and usually produces thyroglobulin to the point that this marker is useful for monitoring tumor status following ablation of the thyroid remnant.

Prognosis

Most series support the concept that the tall cell variant has a worse prognosis than the classic form of well differentiated papillary carcinoma. At the time of diagnosis, older age, large tumor size, extrathyroidal extension, nodal and distant metastases are more likely in patients with tall cell tumors. Table 1 summarizes outcome data.

The controversy in the literature is the relative prognosis of the tall cell variant in young patients. This controversy exists because there are series that report that the clinical outcome of patients under 50 years of age with tall cell carcinoma is the same as that of age-matched patients with classic forms of well differentiated carcinoma (data summarized in the review chapter by Ringel 2000). Contradicting this concept is a recent study by Machens and colleagues (2004) that used multivariate analysis to evaluate prognostic variables in patients with the tall cell variant of papillary carcinoma. They found that after controlling for other major prognostic variables, the risk of distant metastasis was four times greater in patients with tall cell carcinoma than in patients with well differentiated tumors.

In our opinion, the chance of curing a tumor that is > 70% tall cell carcinoma is worse by approximately 20% compared to a patient of similar stage and age with a classic histology papillary carcinoma. The prognosis will likely be even worse if the tumor contains foci of poorly differentiated or undifferentiated (anaplastic) carcinoma in addition to the tall cell component.

COLUMNAR CELL VARIANT OF PAPILLARY CARCINOMA

Columnar cell variant is an extremely rare subtype of papillary carcinoma that occurs in less than 1% of thyroid cancer cases. This variant is characterized by elongated tumor cells with scant cytoplasm that often lack the nuclear features of papillary carcinoma. The growth pattern usually shows striking nuclear stratification with papillary architecture. Mitoses are common. As with Tall cell carcinoma, columnar cell carcinoma may by occur in tumors with other patterns of differentiation and there are multiple reports of tumors with mixed Tall and Columnar cell features. There are few data to direct the discussion about the percent of the tumor that must have columnar cells to classify the tumor as a separate subtype of papillary carcinoma. Our preference is to use the same criterion as for the tall cell variant (minimum 70% variant component).

The mean age of patients with columnar cell variant tumors is approximately 47 years and most series report a female predominance. While this variant probably can occur at any age, it has not been reported below age 16 years. Columnar cell carcinomas usually concentrate radioiodine well enough to be visualized on a total body radioiodine scan and usually produce thyroglobulin enough that this marker is useful for monitoring tumor status following ablation of the thyroid remnant.

Prognosis

The major report of outcome in patients with columnar cell variants of papillary carcinoma is that of Wenig and colleagues (1998). There are only 16 patients in this series. Patients were managed in the standard fashion with total thyroidectomy and radioiodine therapy. Only two patients had extrathyroid tumor extension. One of these patients died of cancer and the other was alive with pulmonary metastases, 9 years after diagnosis. In the 14 patients with disease limited to the thyroid, the disease-free survival was 88% with a mean follow-up of almost 6 years. The authors conclude that columnar cell features have little prognostic significance when the stage of disease is taken into account. There are several other series and case reports that include patients with locally aggressive or metastatic tumors at diagnosis. In the Ringel review (2000), 38% of 24 patients with columnar cell carcinoma died of uncontrolled cancer. They conclude that the prognosis of columnar cell variant is similar to that of the tall cell variant.

TREATMENT OF TALL AND COLUMNAR CELL VARIANTS

Our approach to patients with tall or columnar cell variant papillary carcinoma is the same as for poorly differentiated thyroid carcinomas, such as insular carcinoma. While these variants probably concentrate radioiodine less well that the classic form of papillary carcinoma, the management strategy is to use radioiodine therapy until it is clear that this is not a useful approach. This means that the treatment guidelines throughout this book for well-differentiated thyroid cancer apply to patients with tall and columnar cell variant papillary carcinoma.

As with insular carcinoma, the only aspect of management that should be different for patients with tall and columnar cell variant papillary carcinoma is that the threshold should be low for using a CT, MR, or PET scan to rule out the presence of recurrent disease following ablation of the thyroid remnant. The chance that tall or columnar cell carcinoma will concentrate radioiodine is low enough that that imaging that does not involve radioiodine should be done whenever it is important to rule out gross tumor recurrence. In patients with tall or columnar cell variants, we obtain a CT, MR, or

PET scan if symptoms suggest the possibility of a distant metastasis, or in a patient with markedly elevated thyroglobulin.

REFERENCES

Machens, A, HJ Holzhausen, C Lautenschlager, and H Dralle. 2004. The tall-cell variant of papillary thyroid carcinoma: a multivariate analysis of clinical risk factors. Langenbecks Arch Surg **389(4):**278–282.

Ringel, MD, KD Burman, and BM Shmookler. 2000. Clinical aspects of miscellaneous and unusual types of thyroid cancers. In: Thyroid Cancer: A Comprehensive Guide to Clinical Management. Totowa NJ: Humana Press Inc. (Wartofsky L, ed) 428–433 (Chapter 49).

Wenig, BM, LD Thompson, CF Adair, B Shmookler, and CS Heffess. 1998. Thyroid papillary carcinoma of columnar cell type: a clinicopathologic study of 16 cases. Cancer **82:**740–753.

7.4. DIFFUSE SCLEROSING VARIANT OF PAPILLARY CARCINOMA

ROBERT J. AMDUR, MD AND ERNEST L. MAZZAFERRI, MD, MACP

Diffuse sclerosing variant of papillary carcinoma accounts for approximately 5% of papillary carcinomas. Histologically, the tumor is characterized by extensive sclerosis, lymphocytic infiltration and psammoma body formation. Most reports suggest that the mean age at presentation is younger than for other differentiated thyroid carcinomas, with approximately 20% of cases presenting in the pediatric age range. This variant of papillary carcinoma appears to concentrate radioiodine, and produce thyroglobulin, as well as the classic form of well differentiated papillary carcinoma.

PROGNOSIS

Most reviews classify the diffuse sclerosing variant of papillary carcinoma as an aggressive histology because it frequently presents with extrathyroidal extension and/or metastases. However, when treated appropriately, the prognosis of patients with diffuse sclerosing tumors appears to be the same as similarly staged patients with the classic form of papillary carcinoma. We include the major studies in the reference list at the end of this chapter.

TREATMENT

We treat the diffuse sclerosing variant of papillary carcinoma the same way as the classic type of papillary carcinoma. The treatment and surveillance guidelines throughout this book for well–differentiated thyroid cancer apply to patients with the diffuse sclerosing variant of papillary carcinoma.

7.5. HÜRTHLE CELL CARCINOMA

ROBERT J. AMDUR, MD AND ERNEST L. MAZZAFERRI, MD, MACP

Hürthle (oxyphille) cell carcinomas comprise about 4% of all thyroid cancers. Hürthle cells are follicular epithelial cells that are larger than normal, with a large amount of granular, eosinophilic cytoplasm that is filled with mitochondria. These cells are found in a wide range of both non-neoplastic and neoplastic processes, including Hashimoto's disease, as well as benign and malignant Hürthle cell tumors. To be classified as a Hürthle cell neoplasm, at least 75% of the tumor must be composed of oxyphille cells. Hürthle cell carcinoma is distinguished from a benign Hürthle cell tumor in the same way the follicular carcinoma is distinguished from a follicular adenoma: by the finding of neoplastic cells invading the tumor capsule or blood vessels within the tumor capsule. Hürthle cell tumors are usually classified as a subtype of follicular adenoma or carcinoma by the World Health Classification of tumors, but a few are Hürthle cell variants of papillary carcinoma.

HÜRTHLE CELL VARIANT FOLLICULAR CARCINOMA

Hürthle cell variant follicular carcinoma constitutes approximately 3% of thyroid cancers and approximately 20% of follicular carcinomas. The mean age at the time of diagnosis is about 55 years with a slight female predominance.

A comprehensive review of the literature prior to 1997 related to the prognosis of Hürthle cell variant follicular carcinoma is presented in the book chapter by Ain that is cited in the reference section of this chapter. Multiple reports claim that the Hürthle cell variant has a worse prognosis than classic histology follicular carcinoma based on a higher risk of distant metastasis (~30% versus ~20%) and a higher diseases specific mortality (35–40% in some series). However, two more recent studies contradict the concept that Hürthle cell carcinoma has a worse prognosis when other variables are taken into account.

In a study by Hundahal et al. (1998), the 10-year cancer-specific mortality rates for patients operated on between 1985 and 1995 in the U.S. were 15% for follicular cancer and 25% for Hürthle cell carcinoma but outcome was similar when these two groups where matched for age and tumor stage. Similarly, the studies by Sanders and Silverman (1998) and Bhattacharyya et al. (2003) report no difference in outcome of patients with Hürthle cell carcinoma with low or high risk features compared to classic histology follicular carcinoma when patient age and tumor stage were taken into account. Bhattacharyya used a national database and multivariate analysis to compare the overall survival of 555 patients with nonmetastatic Hürthle cell carcinoma to a group of patients with classic follicular carcinoma matched for age, sex, tumor size, and local disease extension. Overall survival for Hürthle cell carcinoma was similar to that of comparably staged follicular cell carcinoma. Increasing age, male sex, and increasing tumor size substantially diminish survival in patients with Hürthle cell carcinoma.

Hürthle cell carcinoma can be a very aggressive tumor. In a recent large recent study by Lopez-Penabad et al. (2003), about 8% of 89 cases of Hürthle cell carcinoma were complicated by concurrent anaplastic thyroid carcinoma. Patients with Hürthle cell carcinoma tended to be older (51.8 vs 43.1 years) and to have larger tumors (4.3 cm vs. 2.9 cm) than those with Hürthle cell adenoma. Forty percent of the patients with Hürthle cell carcinoma died of tumor during follow-up and the authors found no improvement in disease-specific mortality in the past 5 decades for patients with these neoplasms. They found that older age and larger tumor size predicted reduced survival, and that I-131 therapy conferred a survival benefit when it was used for adjuvant ablation therapy, but not when residual disease was present. The authors could not demonstrate a survival benefit for the use of extensive surgery, external beam radiation therapy, or chemotherapy.

Hürthle cell carcinomas usually produce thyroglobulin but are generally less likely to concentrate radioiodine than follicular carcinoma. There are reports that the rate of radioiodine concentration in Hürthle cell carcinoma metastases is as low as 10%, while others report that 30% to 40% of distant metastases take up radioiodine.

HÜRTHLE CELL VARIANT PAPILLARY CARCINOMA

Many publications do not distinguish between the Hürthle cell variant of papillary carcinoma and the more common Hürthle cell variant of follicular carcinoma. The article by Berho and Suster (1997) is one of the classic references on the pathologic features of Hürthle cell variant papillary carcinoma.

A survey of the literature suggests that this variant accounts for approximately 3% of papillary carcinomas. The mean age at the time of diagnosis is about 50 years and there is a female predominance. As with Hürthle cell variant follicular carcinoma, there is controversy about the prognostic importance of Hürthle cell features in a papillary carcinoma. The largest series on this subject is that by Herrera et al. (1992) in which the tumor recurrence rate at 10 years was almost three times higher for patients with the Hürthle cell variant papillary thyroid carcinoma than with classic papillary carcinoma (28% versus 10%). There is no series with age or stage-matched comparisons limited to the Hürthle cell variant of papillary carcinoma.

A "WARTHOLIN-LIKE" SUBTYPE OF HÜRTHLE CELL VARIANT PAPILLARY CARCINOMA

An unusual subtype of the Hürthle cell variant of papillary carcinoma was first described in 1995 by Apel et al. The distinguishing feature of this Hürthle cell tumor was a papillary carcinoma growth pattern with lymphoid aggregates in the tumor stroma. The histologic features are similar to that of the Wartholin's tumor that commonly occurs in the salivary glands. The 13 patients in this series where free of disease 3 months to 9 years after treatment, which suggests that the prognosis is similar to that of classic papillary carcinoma.

TREATMENT OF HÜRTHLE CELL VARIANTS OF FOLLICULAR AND PAPILLARY CARCINOMA

Our approach to patients with the Hürthle cell variant of follicular or papillary carcinoma is the same as for poorly differentiated thyroid carcinomas, such as insular carcinoma. While these variants probably concentrate radioiodine less well that the classic form of papillary carcinoma, the management strategy is to use radioiodine therapy until it is clear that this is not a useful approach. This means that the treatment guidelines that we present throughout this book for well-differentiated thyroid cancer apply to patients with Hürthle cell variant carcinomas.

The only aspect of management that is different for patients with Hürthle cell variant carcinomas is that the threshold should be low for using a CT, MR, or PET scan to rule out the presence of recurrent disease following ablation of the thyroid remnant. The chance that Hürthle cell variant carcinoma will not concentrate radioiodine is high enough that imaging that does not involve radioiodine should be done whenever it is important to rule out gross tumor recurrence. In patients with Hürthle cell variant variant carcinomas, we obtain a CT, MR, or PET scan if symptoms suggest the possibility of a distant metastasis, or in a patient with markedly elevated thyroglobulin.

As we do for other forms of differentiated thyroid cancer, we give external beam radiotherapy to patients with Hürthle cell carcinoma when local-regional control cannot be achieved with I-131 therapy alone. The study by Foote et al. (2003) documents the efficacy of external beam radiotherapy for Hürthle cell carcinoma.

REFERENCES

Ain, KB. 1998. Rare forms of thyroid cancer. In: Thyroid Cancer. Norwell, MA: Kluwer Academic Publisher (Fagin JA, ed) 322–323 (Chapter 13).

Apel, RL, SL Asa, and VA LiVolsi. 1995. Papillary Hürthle cell carcinoma with lymphocytic stroma: "Warthin-like tumor" of the thyroid. Am J Surg Pathol **19:**810–814.

Berho, M, and S Suster. 1997. The oncocytic variant of papillary carcinoma of the thyroid: a clinicopathologic study of 15 cases. Hum Pathol **28:**47–53.

Bhattacharyya, N. 2003. Survival and prognosis in Hurthle cell carcinoma of the thyroid gland. Arch Oto-laryngol Head Neck Surg **129(2):**207–210.

Foote, RL, PD Brown, YI Garces, B McIver, and JL Kasperbauer. 2003. Is there a role for radiation therapy in the management of Hurthle cell carcinoma? Int J Radiat Oncol Biol Phys **56(4):**1067–1072.

Herrera, MF, ID Hay, PS-C Wu, et al. 1992. Hurthle cell (oxyphilic) papillary thyroid carcinoma: a variant with more aggressive biologic behavior. World J Surg **16:**669–675.

Lopez-Penabad, L, AC Chiu, AO Hoff, P Schultz, S Gaztambide, NG Ordonez, and SI Sherman. 2003. Prognostic factors in patients with Hürthle cell neoplasms of the thyroid. Cancer **97:**1186–1194.

Sanders, LE, and M Silverman. 1998. Follicular and Hürthle cell carcinoma: predicting outcome and directing therapy. Surgery **124:**967–974.

7.6. INSULAR AND OTHER POORLY DIFFERENTIATED THYROID CARCINOMAS

ROBERT J. AMDUR, MD AND ERNEST L. MAZZAFERRI, MD, MACP

Poorly differentiated thyroid carcinoma refers to the group of follicular cell neoplasms that are intermediate between differentiated and undifferentiated (anaplastic) carcinoma, both in terms of histologic appearance and biologic behavior. Solid, trabecular, and insular are some of the terms that describe variants of poorly differentiated thyroid carcinoma but the boundaries of this histologic category are ambiguous. For example, some experts consider the columnar cell variant of papillary carcinoma to be a subtype of poorly differentiated thyroid carcinoma whereas others view it as an unfavorable variant of differentiated carcinoma. The purpose of this chapter is to discuss the management of patients with poorly differentiated thyroid carcinoma. The focus of discussion will be insular carcinoma because this is the most common and well-defined subtype in this category. The behavior and management of insular carcinoma is the same as for other forms of poorly differentiated thyroid carcinoma.

INSULAR CARCINOMA

Insular carcinoma is the most well defined subtype of poorly differentiated thyroid cancer. Under low power microscopy, insular carcinoma has a distinct appearance in which the tumor cells are arranged in discrete nests (islands) separated by fibrous stroma. The term "insular" comes from the Latin word for island. Histologic images of insular carcinoma are presented in part 1 of this book.

Insular carcinoma accounts for approximately 2% of thyroid cancers, may occur in any age group (median age 45–55 years in most series), and occurs in both males and females. Insular carcinomas frequently concentrate radioiodine on nuclear medicine scans but it

Table 1. Results from Falvo et al. (2004) The American Surgeon. 70: 461–466, 2004.

	Insular*	Papillary and Follicular
Overall survival	66%	100%
Disease-free survival	22%	~95%
Lymph Node relapse	44%	5%
Distant relapse (lung and brain)	67%	0%
Radioiodine uptake	100%	—

* All patients had > 70% Insular carcinoma. All comparisons are statistically significant

is not possible to determine when the degree of concentration is adequate to produce tumor cure. Insular carcinomas usually produce thyroglobulin to the point that this is a useful marker for tumor recurrence.

PROGNOSIS

Most series suggest that the prognosis of insular carcinoma is significantly worse than a well differentiated tumor of similar stage, but not nearly as bad as an anaplastic carcinoma. Two recently published studies (Falvo 2004; Volante 2004) document the prognosis of patients with poorly differentiated carcinoma in general, and insular carcinoma in particular. The discussion sections of these papers review the literature on this subject.

The effect of insular histology on prognosis is most clearly demonstrated in studies that are limited to patients in whom the great majority (> 70%) of the tumor is insular carcinoma. The study by Flavo et al. is a case-controlled analysis of three groups of patients: insular carcinoma in > 70% of the tumor, 100% well differentiated follicular carcinoma, and 100% well differentiated papillary carcinoma. Patients in each group were similar in terms of age, tumor size, treatment approach (total thyroidectomy usually followed by radioiodine) and follow-up time (mean 33 months in the insular carcinoma group and 43 months in the groups with follicular and papillary carcinoma). Table 1 summarizes the major findings from this study.

A more detailed evaluation of outcome in patients with poorly differentiated thyroid cancer is the study by Volante and colleagues. The main point of this study was to identify prognostic factors in 183 patients with poorly differentiated carcinoma but it also contains a comparison to patients with well-differentiated carcinoma. Half of the 183 poorly differentiated tumors were insular carcinomas. Table 2 summarizes the major findings from this study.

Both the Flavo and Volante studies show that most patients with insular carcinoma have a prognosis that is substantially worse than patients with well-differentiated tumors (long-term survival ~65% versus ~95%, respectively). However, the prognosis of poorly differentiated thyroid carcinoma is much better than that of an undifferentiated tumor (anaplastic carcinoma) where most patients die of cancer within a few years of diagnosis.

The take-home message from the Volante study is that mitotic index, age, and necrosis are the major factors that determine prognosis of patients with poorly differentiated

Table 2. Results from Volante et al. (2004) Cancer 100: 950–7, 2004.

	10-year Overall Survival
All poorly differentiated carcinomas	67% (disease-free survival ~50%)
Prognostic factors at the p < 0.05 level on multivariate analysis:	
Mitotic index (≤ or > 3 per high power field)	71% vs 40% (p < 0.05)
Age (≤ or > 45 years)	83% vs 62% (p < 0.05)
Necrosis (absent or present)	81% vs 50% (p < 0.05)
Comparisons that were not significantly different:	
Extent of poorly differentiated component (< 50%, 50–75%, > 75%)	100% vs 54% vs 68% (p = NS)
Tumor size (≤ or > 4 cm)	66–67% in both groups
Vascular invasion (focal or extensive)	72% vs 62% (p = NS)

tumors, with mitotic index being the most important of these three variables. Other studies suggest that the prognosis is better when insular carcinoma comprises a minority of a tumor that is otherwise well differentiated. The Volante series suggests that prognosis is better with a minor insular component (100% survival when < 50% of the tumor was poorly differentiated) but the comparisons were not statistically significant.

TREATMENT

The treatment guidelines throughout this book for well differentiated thyroid cancer apply to patients with poorly differentiated thyroid cancer. Although most poorly differentiated carcinomas concentrate radioiodine poorly, the management strategy is to use radioiodine therapy until it is clear that this is not a useful approach.

The only aspect of management that should be different for patients with poorly differentiated thyroid carcinoma is that the threshold should be low for using a CT, MR, or PET scan to rule out the presence of recurrent disease following ablation of the thyroid remnant. The chance that poorly differentiated tumor will concentrate radioiodine is low enough that imaging that does not involve radioiodine should be done whenever it is important to rule out gross tumor recurrence. In patients with poorly differentiated thyroid carcinoma, we obtain a CT, MR, or PET scan if symptoms suggest the possibility of a distant metastasis, or in a patient with markedly elevated thyroglobulin.

REFERENCES

Flavo, L, A Catania, V D'Andrea, P Grilli, C D'Ercole, and E De Antoni. 2004. Prognostic factors of insular versus papillary/follicular thyroid carcinoma. Am Surgeon **70**:461–466.

Volante, M, S Landolfi, L Chiusa, N Palestini, M Motta, A Codegone, B Torchio, and MG Papotti. 2004. Poorly differentiated carcinomas of the thyroid with trabecular, insular, and solid patterns: a clinicopathologic study of 183 patients. Cancer **100(5)**:950–957.

7.7. ANAPLASTIC CARCINOMA

ROBERT J. AMDUR, MD AND ERNEST L. MAZZAFERRI, MD, MACP

The purpose of this chapter is to review the major issues that relate to the management of patients with anaplastic thyroid carcinoma. The discussion sections of the two articles that we include in the reference list at the end of this chapter contain a comprehensive literature review.

OVERVIEW OF THE ISSUES

Three main concepts dominate discussions about the managemeament of patients with anaplastic thyroid carcinoma:

- Anaplastic carcinoma is almost never curable
- Local extent of disease has almost no effect on prognosis
- Optimal therapy involves hyperfractionated radiotherapy and concurrent chemotherapy

In our opinion, these concepts are not accurate to the degree that they are often presented in the literature. The issue of local staging is especially misleading in view of the implications this has for treatment planning.

OVERALL PROGNOSIS

In the great majority of patients, anaplastic thyroid carcinoma is an extremely virulent disease. When all patients who are diagnosed over a specific time are analyzed together, most studies report an overall median survival of 3–6 months and there are multiple series in which no patient survived 2 years from the time of diagnosis.

The concept that anaplastic thyroid cancer is an incurable disease has important implications for treatment. When long-term tumor control is not possible, the goal of therapy is palliation of symptoms. In this setting, treatments that are likely to cause morbidity, such as aggressive combinations of surgery, radiotherapy, and chemotherapy, are rarely indicated. For this reason it is important to determine if there are any pretreatment characteristics that identify a subset of patients that are have a reasonable chance of long-term survival.

A SUBSET OF PATIENTS WITH A RELATIVELY FAVORABLE PROGNOSIS

In the American Joint Committee on Cancer System of staging thyroid cancer, local and regional tumor extent does not affect the classification of anaplastic carcinoma. All anaplastic carcinomas are stage T4 and overall stage group IV. According to this staging system, an anaplastic carcinoma confined to the thyroid has a similar prognosis to one that extensively infiltrates the soft tissues of the neck or has distant metastases. This aspect of the staging system underestimates the value of aggressive treatment in this disease.

There are now multiple series that report long-term relapse free survival in 10–50% of patients with anaplastic carcinoma that is limited to the thyroid and nearby tissues. With a microscopically positive margin, but no gross residual disease, the 2-year relapse-free survival (and probably cure rate) is approximately 10%. A 10% chance of success is clearly not a good situation, but it is much better than zero. For patients with disease confined to the thyroid, the chance of cure is likely to be closer to 50%. In most of the series that report a more favorable outcome, the long-term survivors also received aggressive radiotherapy and chemotherapy.

In our opinion, staging systems and treatment guidelines for anaplastic thyroid carcinoma should distinguish between patients who do, and do not, have unresectable disease with the standard thyroidectomy and neck dissection procedure. The select group of patients with tumor confined to the thyroid has an especially favorable prognosis. Patients with a focus of anaplastic carcinoma in a differentiated thyroid cancer or benign adenoma make up the majority of "favorable prognosis" anaplastic carcinoma cases in our practice.

TERMINOLOGY: HYPERFRACTIONATED AND ACCELERATED RADIOTHERAPY

A "fraction" is the term for a radiation therapy treatment. Standard fractionation radiation therapy is given once-a-day, five days per week, at a dose of 1.8–2.0 Gy per treatment. Hyperfractionation means that the dose of each treatment is lower than 1.8 Gy and that treatments are given two or three times per day. In a purely hyperfractionated regimen, the fraction size is small (for example, 1.0 Gy) so that the total dose and overall treatment time are similar to standard fractionation.

The term "accelerated fractionation" describes any regimen that gives the total dose over a shorter time than a standard fractionation schedule. There are two ways to shorten (accelerate) the overall treatment time: treat more than five days per week or treat multiple times per day (hyperfractionate). Most accelerated fractionation schedules shorten overall treatment time by giving an intermediate dose treatment (1.2–1.6 Gy) twice-a-day, five days per week. However, most fractionation schedules in use today are not purely hyperfractionated or accelerated. Most twice-a-day regimens both hyperfractionate and accelerate dose delivery with fraction sizes of 1.2–1.6 Gy.

There are now multiple articles that report encouraging results for anaplastic thyroid cancer with aggressive radiation therapy fractionation schedules. Some of these articles describe the dose schedule as hyperfractionation while others use the term "accelerated fractionation". In all cases, the regimen uses twice-a-day treatments to deliver a conventional dose in a shorter time. For this reason, these schedules are both hyperfractionated and accelerated. We explain fractionation terminology here so that the reader will not be confused when evaluating papers on this subject. In the remainder of this chapter, we use the term hyperfractionation to refer to all of the twice-a-day fractionation schedules that have been reported to produce favorable results in patients with anaplastic thyroid carcinoma.

HYPERFRACTIONATED RADIOTHERAPY AND CHEMOTHERAPY

Beginning in the mid 1980s, several groups reported encouraging results in patients with locally advanced anaplastic thyroid carcinoma using combinations of hyperfractionated radiotherapy and concomitant chemotherapy. The most influential publications are those from Sweden by Tennvall and colleagues (2002). The most recent report from this group describes a series of prospective trails that escalated the intensity of the radiotherapy regimen given concurrently with doxorubicin (20 mg IV weekly). Surgical resection was performed when complete resection appeared likely. The rate of local control was 60% and 9% of patients where long-term survivors with no evidence of disease.

Because of reports from the Swedish group and other centers, some clinicians now consider hyperfractionated radiotherapy and concomitant doxorubicin-based chemotherapy to be optimal therapy in otherwise healthy patients with anaplastic thyroid carcinoma. The radiotherapy program that we use to treat anaplastic thyroid carcinoma aggressively involves accelerated therapy and hyperfractionation (Table 1).

We are currently undecided about the value of cytotoxic chemotherapy in patients with anaplastic thyroid carcinoma. The reported regimens increase the toxicity and complexity of therapy. In several of the largest series, chemotherapy (doxorubicin in the Swedish trials and cisplatin in an Italian trial) produced almost no response in distant metastases. Because of these factors, we are reluctant to use chemotherapy routinely in patients with anaplastic carcinoma.

RADIOIODINE THERAPY

Anaplastic thyroid carcinoma does not concentrate radioiodine. Some physicians use radioiodine with the idea that concentration of radioiodine in thyroid tissue, or differentiated thyroid cancer cells in the case of a mixed cancer, will deliver a lethal dose or radiation to anaplastic cells nearby. We do not have confidence in this "bystander effect" and therefore do not consider radioiodine as part of the treatment of anaplastic carcinoma in any setting. This philosophy becomes especially important in the patient with a potentially curable situation. When treating a patient aggressively, we deliver external

Table 1. Dose Schedules and Techniques for EBRT[1] for Thyroid Cancer.

Palliation of symptoms of terminal cancer		Curative intent	
Dose (Gy)	Technique	Dose (Gy)[3]	Technique
20 @ 10 /treatment (2 treatment days) 1–6 weeks between treatments	6 MV photons through opposed anterior and posterior fields	63–72 using the UF IMRT[2] schedule (30 treatment days)	IMRT[2]
20 @ 4/treatment (5 treatment days)	6 MV photons through opposed anterior and posterior fields	74.4 @ 1.2 /treatment with twice-a-day fractionation (31 treatment days)	Give 45.6 with opposed anterior and posterior fields using 6 MV photons and then avoid the spinal cord using 20 MV photons through opposed lateral fields with shoulder compensators
30 @ 3 /treatment (10 treatment days)	6 MV photons through opposed anterior and posterior fields	63–72 @ 1.8/treatment/day (35–40 treatment days)	Same as above with 45 given through anterior and posterior fields

[1] External Beam Radiotherapy.
[2] IMRT = Intensity Modulated Radiation Therapy.
[3] We use 72 @ 1.8, 74.4 @ 1.2, or 72 IMRT when there is a high-risk feature. If there are no high-risk features the prescribed dose is 63 @ 1.8 or 63 IMRT. High-risk features: gross residual disease, positive margin, invasion of normal tissues that define a stage T4 primary tumor, or nodal metastasis with extensive extracapsular tumor extension.

Table 2. Treatment Guidelines for Anaplastic Thyroid Carcinoma*.

Massive neck disease or widespread distant metastases or medical problems that preclude an aggressive approach:
• Consider palliative radiotherapy (see table below for dose schedule)
• Supportive care
• Referral to hospice program

Disease limited to the neck and complete resection (no gross residual) is likely:
• Total thyroidectomy and resection of adjacent structures as indicated. Level II–V neck dissection if clinically positive nodes
• External beam radiotherapy (see table below for dose schedule)

Disease limited to the neck but complete resection is unlikely:
• External beam radiotherapy (see table below for dose schedule)
• Consider concomitant chemotherapy (doxorubicin 20 mg IV each week)
• Evaluate response 2–4 weeks after the completion of radiotherapy. Operate 4–6 weeks after radiotherapy if complete resection is likely

Distant metastases requiring palliation of symptoms:
• Analgesics for pain
• Localized radiotherapy to relieve pain or relieve compression**
• Surgical stabilization for certain long bone lesion**
• Resection and/or radiotherapy for brain metastasis**

* Note: these guidelines refer only to adults. Due to the toxicity of radiotherapy in children, we consider radiotherapy only as a last resort for the palliation of life-threatening symptoms in children < 11 years of age. In children 11–18 years old, we consider using radiotherapy with curative intent in select situations.
** See the chapters on the management of bone and brain metastasis.

beam radiotherapy (preceded or followed by surgery) as soon as possible following diagnosis. Delaying external beam radiotherapy to deliver radioiodine therapy is likely to compromise outcome in this rapidly growing neoplasm.

FUTURE TRIALS

Activation of tyrosine kinase has an important pathophysiologic role in thyroid cancer. There is a high frequency of BRAF mutations in anaplastic thyroid carcinomas, which is further evidence that these tumors arise from more differentiated thyroid carcinomas and indicates that there may be benefits of anti-BRAF therapy. We plan to enroll patients with anaplastic carcinoma in clinical trials that use drugs that block tyrosine kinase activation when these trials become available.

TREATMENT GUIDELINES FOR ANAPLASTIC CARCINOMA

Tables 1 and 2 summarize our guidelines for the management of patients with anaplastic thyroid carcinoma.

REFERENCE

Tennvall, J, G Lundell, P Wahlberg, A Bergenfelz, L Grimelius, M Akerman, A-L Hjelm Skog, and G Wallin. 2002. Anaplastic thyroid carcinoma: three protocols combining doxorubicin, hyperfractionated radiotherapy, and surgery. Br J Cancer **86**:1848–1853.

PART 8. MEDULLARY THYROID CANCER

8.1. DIAGNOSIS AND MANAGEMENT OF MEDULLARY THYROID CARCINOMA

ERNEST L. MAZZAFERRI, MD, MACP AND NICOLE A. MASSOLL, MD

Medullary thyroid carcinoma (MTC) arises from thyroid C cells that secrete calcitonin (CT). It accounts for only about 5% of thyroid carcinomas in the United States (Hundahl 1998), but has aroused considerable interest because of its distinctive biochemical, genetic and clinical features. Although this is usually a sporadic tumor, some are familial tumors that occur as a result of autosomal dominant genetic mutations in the RET protooncogene that produce unique clinical syndromes (Dunn 1993). The explication of the genetic basis of MTC has revolutionized management of the familial form of this tumor and has provided insight into its pathogenesis and clinical behavior. In this chapter we review the important clinical characteristics, hereditary and sporadic forms of the disease, and its biochemical and molecular diagnosis, treatment and follow-up. Several recent publications summarize the major advances in this field, (Eng 1996; Machens 2003b; Massoll 2004) and the Seventh International Workshop on Multiple Endocrine Neoplasia held in Gubbio, Italy in 1999 provides some consensus on the diagnosis and therapy of familial MTC (Brandi 2001), although major questions remain concerning the timing of thyroidectomy in certain gene carriers.

PATHOLOGY

C-cell Hyperplasia and MTC

RET germ-line mutations in humans affect four major types of tissues that originate from neural crest cells: thyroid C cells, parathyroid cells, chromaffin cells of the adrenal medulla, and enteric autonomic plexus (Eng 1996). MTC, which arises from thyroid

C cells, is mainly found in the upper third of the thyroid lobes. In familial disease, this is the site of its first identifiable manifestation: C cell hyperplasia (CCH), which is a precursor of familial MTC that progresses to microscopic MTC (Modigliani 1998). The progression of CCH to MTC occurs at different rates depending on the RET mutation (Machens 2003b). Hereditary MTC is thus bilateral and multicentric, whereas sporadic MTC is generally manifest as a single thyroid tumor (Beressi 1998; Bachelot 2002).

A wide spectrum of histologic patterns may be seen with MTC. Although lymph node metastases are rarely present when MTC is diagnosed early by genetic screening (Wells Jr 1994), they are almost always present when the tumor is palpable, whether it is sporadic or familial MTC. The tumor typically metastasizes to lymph nodes in the central and lateral cervical compartments, to mediastinal lymph nodes, or to the lung, liver or bone.

In fine-needle aspiration (FNA) cytology samples, MTC cells may appear cuboidal, spindled or plasmacytoid. MTC tends to be over-diagnosed by cytology because it may mimic a variety of benign and malignant entities and should therefore be confirmed by immunohistochemical staining for CT.

CCH is usually diagnosed when more than 6 C-cells are seen per thyroid follicle and/or more than 50 intrafollicular CT-positive cells are seen in at least one low-power (100x) field. CCH can be confirmed by a immunohistochemical reaction for CT and can range in appearance from mild to diffuse CCH, which can develop into nodules that replace preexisting follicular epithelium (Hinze 1998). The transition from benign CCH to invasive MTC is marked by disruption of the follicular basement membrane by C-cells. Familial tumors undergo a transition from a RET mutation that leads to early clonal C-cell expansion, which then proceeds to transformation from neoplastic CCH to MTC, and eventually to lymph node and distant metastases, all proceeding at strikingly different rates with different RET mutations (Machens 2003a, 2003b).

HORMONAL ACTIVITY OF MTC

MTC secretes several proteins in addition to CT, including ACTH, CEA, histamines and vasoactive peptides, but clinically the most important is CT, which serves as the major clinical marker for the tumor. In fact, plasma CT levels correlate closely with MTC size (Engelbach 2000), especially in familial cases, and preoperative CT levels <50 pg/mL predict postoperative normalization of CT (Cohen 2000).

SURVIVAL RATE OF PATIENTS WITH MTC

The 10-year survival rate of patients with MTC ranges from about 50% to 80%, and averaged 75% in over 2,000 cases of MTC in a national cancer database with 53,856 cases of thyroid carcinoma treated in the US between 1985–1995 (Hundahl 1998). Survival rates are tightly linked to early diagnosis and tumor stage, and vary significantly among patients with sporadic and familial MTC (Cohen 2000; Brandi 2001). Early thyroidectomy has lowered the mortality rate of hereditary MTC to less than 5%, well below that in sporadic cases; however, the longest follow-up period of survival with MTC, done well before current screening methods, is less than 25 years (Gagel 1988).

SPORADIC MTC

Clinical Presentation

Sporadic MTC tends to be unifocal without prominent CCH, and is not associated with other endocrine tumors. Dense tumor calcifications may be apparent on ultrasound or other imaging studies (Tokuue 1990; Yokozawa 1996). Sporadic MTC usually presents at about 55 years of age, and at a more advanced stage than familial MTC (Beressi 1998). The tumor is usually palpable in sporadic MTC, and up to 80% is metastatic to cervical lymph nodes and in 20% of the cases to distant sites (Moley 1999). Advanced stage tumors may be rapidly growing and associated with hoarseness, dysphagia or other symptoms of invasion or may present with systemic symptoms of diarrhea, flushing and bone pain (Kebebew 2000; Dolan 2000). Most patients, however, do not have these symptoms, but simply present with a long-standing multinodular goiter or an asymptomatic thyroid nodule.

Diagnosis of CCH and MTC

Sporadic MTC is usually diagnosed by FNA of a palpable thyroid nodule or lymph node; whereas CCH is usually apparent only on histochemical staining of the permanent surgical pathology sections (Aulicino 1998). In some situations accurate FNA diagnosis requires a more objective method than cytological examination alone. RET somatic mutations at codon 918, which occur only in the tumor and are not present in peripheral blood cells, can sometimes be detected in the tumor cells rinsed from the needle after preparing slides from an FNA of a malignant nodule (Russo 1997), establishing a diagnosis of MTC before surgery. Plasma CT or CEA mRNA can also be used for this purpose (Takano 1999). Routine preoperative plasma CT measurements may be the only clue to a diagnosis of MTC in a multinodular goiter (Elisei 2004), although normal CT levels do not rule out MTC (Redding 2000). European endocrinologists widely advocate routinely measuring plasma CT in all patients who undergo FNA for multinodular goiter (Henry 1996; Ozgen 1999; Bonnema 2000; Elisei 2004) but most American endocrinologists do not do this for a variety of reasons (Hodak 2004), but mainly because patients without MTC often have high plasma CT levels and the diagnosis often must be confirmed by pentagastrin injection, which stimulates plasma CT to rise only in CCH and MTC, but the drug is not available in the U.S.A.. Still, the index case of an MTC kindred may be identified by measuring plasma CT levels in a patient with an isolated thyroid nodule in which MTC is not suspected (Mayr 1999). This is a major conundrum (Hodak 2004).

Factors Affecting Mortality Rates with Sporadic MTC

In some cases survival with MTC is prolonged, even with distant metastases, whereas others die within a few years of diagnosis. A French study (Cohen 1996) of 119 deceased patients with MTC showed that the tumor was usually the cause of death (87%). Prognosis depends on the clinical form of the disease (sporadic or familial), the patient's age at the time of diagnosis, the tumor stage at the time of surgery, including size, the presence of local tumor invasion, lymph node and distant metastases, and the extent of surgery (Hyer 2000). Although 10-year mortality rates average about 75%, when sporadic MTC presents with systemic symptoms of diarrhea, bone pain, or flushing and is widely metastatic, 33% die within 5 years (Kebebew 2000).

Initial Management of Sporadic MTC

Surgery is the only completely effective form of therapy. Total thyroidectomy and central neck dissection is the minimum surgical procedure that should be performed (Wells Jr 1994; Kebebew 2000; Hyer 2000). Preoperative staging and the extent of previous surgery determine the need for further neck dissection, and if metastases are identified in the lateral neck, compartment-oriented lymphadenectomy is advised (Kebebew 2000; Weber 2001; Franc 2001). Modified radical neck dissection provides the best outcomes in patients with lateral lymph nodes metastases (Kebebew 2000; Hyer 2000; Weber 2001). Preoperative plasma CT levels predict tumor size and postoperative normalization of CT (Pentagastrin-stimulated CT < 10 pg/mL) (Cohen 2000) but this does not always predict freedom from recurrence (Franc 2001), and long-term follow-up is always necessary.

External beam radiotherapy (EBRT), which is effective in eradicating foci of residual tumor, is indicated when surgical excision is incomplete (Rougier 1983; Sarrazin 1984). It significantly reduces local relapse in those with ipsilateral lymph node metastases (Rougier 1983; Hyer 2000). Chemotherapy has little effect on MTC. Although some have advocated I-131 therapy, there are neither data nor enthusiasm to support its use (3).

FAMILIAL MTC: MULTIPLE ENDOCRINE NEOPLASIA TYPE2 (MEN2) SYNDROMES

The MEN2 syndromes comprise a clinical framework to conceptualize the manifestations of the familial RET protooncogene mutations, thus providing clinicians the basis for an approach to patients with these disorders.

Classification of MEN2 Syndromes (Table 1)

Nearly 40% of MTC cases are inherited as one of several autosomal dominant syndromes, which affect about 1,000 kindreds around the world (Eng 1996; Brandi 2001). The familial MTC syndromes occur either as part of multiple endocrine neoplasia (MEN) type 2A or 2B syndromes or as familial MTC without other endocrine tumors (FMTC, Table 1). Different RET germ-line mutations are responsible for each these syndromes, but the specific mutations and clinical features of the syndromes differ substantially among affected families (Phay 2000).

MTC is the main tumor manifested in these syndromes, but its expression is variable. MTC appears at different times during life and displays different growth rates according to the specific RET mutation. Sill, the penetrance of MTC is high enough that 90% of the carriers eventually develop a palpable tumor or blood CT abnormality if the trait is

Table 1. Clinical Syndromes Associated with MTC and the Exons with Mutations Involved.

	MEN2A	FMTC	MEN2B	Sporadic MTC
MTC Incidence	100%	100%		100%
Multicentricity		100%		Rare
Bilaterality		100%		Rare
C-Cell Hyperplasia		100%		
Age of Onset (years)	20–30	40–50	0–20	>40
Clinical Features	MTC Pheochromocytoma (50%) Parathyroid hyperplasia (20%–30%)	MTC	MTC Pheochromocytoma (50%) Mucosal Neuromas (100%) Marfanoid habitus (100%) Ganglioneuromas	MTC
Inheritance	Autosomal Dominant	Autosomal Dominant	Autosomal Dominant	Sporadic
Affected gene	RET	RET	RET	RET
Exons	G* 10,11	G* 13,14,15	G* 16,15	S† 10,11,13,14,15,16
Codons	609‡, 611‡, 618‡, 620‡, 630‡, 634, [take out‡ after 634] 635, 637, 790‡, 791 and 804‡, 891‡	532¶, 609‡, 611‡, 618‡, 620‡, 630‡, 790‡ 768¶, 791¶ val804met, 844§, A891S	918, 833	S† 918 (25%) 664, or A833F (rare)

* G = Germline mutations.
† S = Somatic mutations.
‡ Mutations that may be found in families with either MEN2A or FMTC phenotypes. Accordingly, all patients with these mutations should be screened for pheochromocytoma.
¶ Mutations associated exclusively with FMTC.
§ 844 mutation, see footnotes 1 & 2 in text.

not identified early in life by genetic testing (Brandi 2001). MTC appears earlier or at the same time as pheochromocytoma and hyperparathyroidism (HPT), which are the other two neoplasms associated with the MEN2 syndromes.

MEN2A comprises over 75% of the MEN2 cases (Eng 1996; Brandi 2001). Other less common variants of MEN2 are:

1) FMTC (Siggelkow 2001)
2) MEN2A with cutaneous lichen amyloidosis (Pacini 1993)
3) MEN2A or FMTC with Hirschsprung's disease (Blank 1996; Eng 1996)

MEN2A CARRIERS HAVE:

1) Bilateral MTC thyroid tumors before age 10
2) Pheochromocytomas (about 50% develop unilateral or bilateral tumors) (Melvin 1972; Gagel 1988; Schuffenecker 1998b; Brandi 2001)
3) Multiple parathyroid tumors that produce HPT (about 30%) (Melvin 1972; Gagel 1988; Schuffenecker 1998a; Schuffenecker 1998b)

MEN2B is the most distinctive and aggressive form of familial MTC. Only few MEN2B children undergoing thyroidectomy for MTC after the first several years of life are cured; many experience recurrence or death within several decades of initial surgery (Carney 1978; Skinner 1996). The causes of MEN2B deaths in one study (Carney 1978) were MTC (15 deaths), pheochromocytoma (10 deaths) and alimentary tract complications (2 deaths). Children with MEN2B commonly develop microscopic MTC, sometimes with metastases, during the first year of life (Smith 1999; Sanso 2002).

This syndrome can be recognized at the bedside. Persons affected with MEN2B have:

1) Long bones, ribs, and skull, which results in a marfanoid habitus with a decreased upper/lower body ratio, and increased laxity of joint ligaments.
2) Thickened corneal nerves.
3) Mucosal neuromas.
4) Ganglioneuromas in the lips, tongue and conjunctiva and digestive tract, conjunctiva, lips and tongue (Fig. 1), and also in the salivary glands, pancreas, gallbladder, upper respiratory tract and urinary bladder.
5) Pheochromocytoma (half the carriers).
6) None have HPT.

FMTC is not associated with pheochromocytoma or HPT.

1) MTC has a high penetrance in all MEN2 syndromes but is manifest at an older age and is clinically more indolent in FMTC than it is in sporadic tumors or in other MEN2 syndromes.

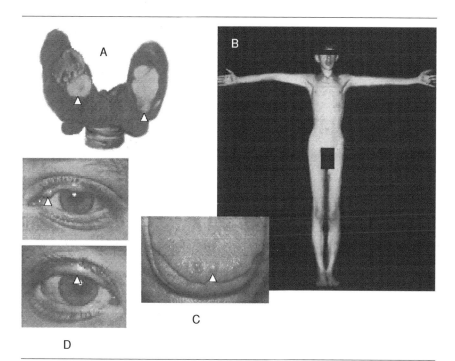

Figure 1. Features of MEN2B. A) Bilateral MTC (arrows), B) Marfanoid habitus (without the cardiovascular abnormalities of Marfan's syndrome), with long arm and leg span giving a reduced upper segment to lower segment ratio or arm span to height ratio >1.05, C) multiple tongue neuromas (arrows), D) Eyelid neuromas and thickening of the tarsal plates (arrows). Not shown in the figure is corneal nerve thickening, which is also found in these patients.

2) MTC is usually is the initial neoplastic manifestation in MEN2 syndromes, often before pheochromocytoma develops, and it is easy to mistake a small MEN2A kindred for an FMTC kindred, with the resulting danger that the diagnosis of pheochromocytoma may not be considered prior to surgery (Brandi 2001).

Categorization of an MEN kindred as FMTC, according to the 1999 International Multiple Endocrine.

Neoplasia meeting in Gubbio, Italy (Brandi 2001), requires fulfillment of all of the following criteria:

1) More than 10 carriers in the kindred.
2) Multiple carriers or affected members over age 50 years.
3) An adequate medical history, particularly in older kindred members.

These conservative criteria deliberately categorize small FMTC kindreds as MEN2A to avoid missing occult pheochromocytomas. Others (Moers 1996) suggest that MEN2

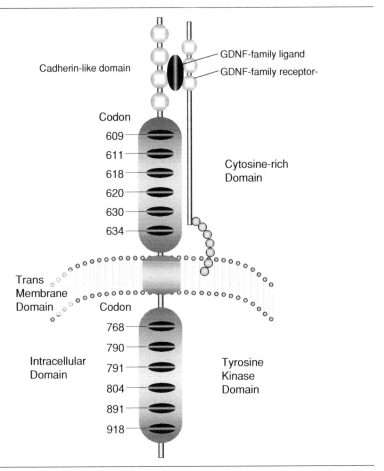

Figure 2. Schematic representation of the membrane-associated RET tyrosine kinase receptor, modified from Massoll (2004).

should not be subclassified as MEN2A or FMTC, but rather should be subclassified according to their specific RET mutation because the difference in outcome among kindreds with different RET mutations is so unique, which is important in making decisions about prophylactic thyroidectomy in children with a RET mutation.

RET Mutations

RET, the predisposing gene for inherited MTC, is located in the pericentric region of chromosome 10q11.2 and consists of 21 exons encoding a plasma membrane-bound tyrosine kinase enzyme termed ret. This membrane-associated protein contains an extracellular domain, a transmembrane domain and an intracellular domain (Fig. 2). Familial

MTC results from single RET point mutations that change one amino acid that activates the ret tyrosine kinase receptor. Activating germline mutations of the RET protooncogene are found in 98% of families with MEN2A and FMTC (Table 1) (Brandi 2001). There is a close relationship between genotype and phenotype expression (Eng 1996).

FMTC is the most difficult of the MEN2 kindreds to identify. By 2001 (3) pheochromocytoma had been found in kindreds with all RET mutations except those in codons 609, val804met and 891, suggesting that these are the only mutations causing FMTC. At present, RET mutations in FMTC are thought to occur at exon 13 in codons 609 and at exon 14 in codons 804 (Bartsch 2000; Siggelkow 2001), 844 (Bartsch 2000) and/or with S836S polymorphism. families have a less virulent form of MEN2A that can be mistaken for FMTC (Table 1) (Machens 2001; Gimm 2002; Fitze 2002). This is important because operative deaths can occur from hypertensive crises in MEN2A patients mistakenly thought to have FMTC.

Over 95% of MEN2B cases are due to a single germline point mutation in the intracellular tyrosine kinase region of the RET protooncogene, which is frequently a *de novo* mutation located on an allele inherited from the patient's father and is associated with advanced paternal age (Carlson 1994). A few cases have been reported with other mutations (Table 1) In comparison with mutations in exon 11, those with mutations in exons 13 and 14 or with MEN2B phenotypic syndrome have MTC that occurs earlier in life and behaves more aggressively (Carlson 1994; Bolino 1995; Eng 1996).

Genotype-phenotype Correlations in MTC Kindreds

Correlations between tumor behavior in MEN2 kindreds and the RET mutation causing the syndrome provide powerful insight into the clinical management—screening, surveillance, and prophylaxis paradigms—of individuals with familial MTC (Eng 1996) and are more likely than CT testing to identify the correct selection and timing of patients for surgery. The clinically relevant features of specific RET mutations that induce unique clinical manifestations in large MTC kindreds provides and prognostic information that bears directly on the selection and timing of prophylactic thyroidectomy in children and young adults.

MTC WITH HIRSCHSPRUNG'S DISEASE. The rare cases of Hirschsprung's disease with exon 10 germline mutations identical to those found in hereditary MTC (Blank 1996) has resulted in an international consensus recommendation that germline (blood) testing for RET mutations be done at exon 10 in codons 609, 618 and 620 in all children with Hirschsprung's disease.

PHEOCHROMOCYTOMA is an important cause of morbidity and mortality in MEN2 carriers. In the past when MTC was identified late in its course with CT testing, sudden death often occurred from pheochromocytoma, perhaps as often as that from MTC (Gagel 1988). One large study (Modigliani 1995a) found that in about 25% of the cases, the manifestations of pheochromocytoma occurred 2 to 15 years before the diagnosis of MTC and were identified simultaneously with MTC in 35% and 2 to 11 years after MTC in 40%; about 68% of the pheochromocytomas were bilateral and 4% were malignant. In a more recent prospective study (Modigliani 1995b) in which MTC was identified by genetic testing, pheochromocytomas were identified simultaneously with the MTC in half the cases but the other half was detected during follow-up after MTC had been identified. The same was true for bilaterality: adrenal tumors were initially found to be bilateral in almost 80% while bilaterality became manifest in the others during follow-up. The presentation of pheochromocytoma is thus highly variable and unpredictable necessitating regular long-term clinical and biological monitoring.

SCREENING FOR PHEOCHROMOCYTOMA. Plasma free metanephrine, which is the best test for excluding or confirming pheochromocytoma (Lenders 2002), should be done in all MEN2A and MEN2B patients and should be done as follows:

1) In carriers with high-risk codons for pheochromocytoma, screening should begin at the age when thyroidectomy would be considered or by the age of 5 to 7 years, whichever is earlier, and should be done annually thereafter (Skinner 1996).
2) In families at less risk for pheochromocytoma, especially those with codons 609, 768, val804met, and 891, screening may be initiated at an older age, depending on the familial pattern of the pheochromocytoma. There is no consensus on the best imaging studies for pheochromocytoma, although most use abdominal CT (Skinner 1996).

TREATMENT OF PHEOCHROMOCYTOMA With high metanephrine levels or symptoms consistent with pheochromocytoma, a retroperitoneal imaging study (Computed tomography or MR) should be performed, although many also use MIBG (meta-iodo benzyl guanidine) scanning for preoperative localization. All patients with evidence of excessive catecholamine production should receive appropriate medical therapy with α-adrenergic antagonist before adrenal surgery Laparoscopic adrenalectomy is now the procedure of choice for patients with unilateral pheochromocytoma with bilateral or unilateral adrenal tumors. However, adrenal insufficiency remains a major problem.

HYPERPARATHYROIDISM (HPT) IN MEN2A HPT occurs in 20-30% of MEN2A patients (Melvin 1972). It is found with the highest frequency in those with any codon 634 mutation. Most patients are asymptomatic, although hypercalciuria and renal calculi may occur. HPT is milder in MEN2A than it is in MEN1.

SCREENING FOR AND TREATMENT OF HPT IN MEN2A Since MEN2A carriers are more likely to have HPT if they have a mutation causing any amino acid substitution in RET codon 634 (Eng 1996; Schuffenecker 1998b), they should be screened annually. Those with mutations at codons 609, 611, 618, 620, 790, and 791, which are less often associated with HPT, require less frequent screening for HPT, perhaps every 2 years (Skinner 1996). Screening for HPT is done with plasma PTH and calcium.

TREATMENT OF HPT IN MEN2A The diagnosis of HPT and indications for parathyroid surgery are similar to those for sporadic HPT (O'Riordain 1993; Raue 1995; Kraimps 1996; Bilezikian 2002). Although fewer than four parathyroid glands may be enlarged, the consensus is that all four glands should be identified at parathyroid surgery (Brandi 2001). The indications and operations—resection of only enlarged glands, subtotal parathyroidectomy, and parathyroidectomy with autotransplantation—should be similar to those in other patients with a potential for multiple parathyroid tumors (Brandi 2001). If the surgeon encounters one or more parathyroid tumors during surgery for MTC in a patient with MEN2, they should be excised as would be done if there is biochemical evidence of mild HPT (Brandi 2001).

DIAGNOSIS AND MANAGEMENT OF FAMILIAL MTC

Studies of MEN2 families have demonstrated a direct correlation between early diagnosis of MTC and outcome (Tashjian 1968; Melvin 1972; Jackson 1973; Gagel 1975; Gagel 1987; Lips 1994; Niccoli-Sire 1999; Brandi 2001). Prevention or cure of MTC is mainly dependent upon the adequacy and success of the initial operation, which in turn is dependent on early diagnosis and low tumor stage (Wells Jr 1994).

RET Testing

Early detection and intervention alters the clinical course of MTC (Gagel 1988; Gagel 1995). This can only be done with RET testing. Potential carriers at risk for a specific RET mutation can be identified by direct DNA blood testing, providing an opportunity for prophylactic thyroidectomy before MTC develops. In an international workshop in 1997 (Lips 1998), a consensus was reached that the decision to perform thyroidectomy in MEN2 carriers should be based predominantly on the result of a RET mutation rather than CT testing. This was reaffirmed at the Seventh International Workshop on Multiple Endocrine Neoplasia held in Gubbio, Italy in 1999 (Brandi et al, 2001). This recommendation stems from several unique features of MEN2:

1) Children operated upon in their teenage years in the era of provocative CT testing usually experienced long-term cure, but many were identified only after MTC had developed. In one long-term study, for example, when surgery was recommended for any elevation in annual provocative CT testing of MEN2 kindred, 77% of the children already had MTC at the time of surgery, some of which were macroscopic tumors; moreover, recurrent disease developed in 24% (Iler 1999).
2) Provocative CT testing of select patients for thyroidectomy is associated with an incidence of false positive tests as high as 10%, which may result in unnecessary thyroidectomy (Lips 1994; Brandi 2001).
3) RET testing has a higher true positive rate and a lower false negative rate than any other test, thus facilitating earlier thyroidectomy in carriers (Wells Jr 1998; Van Heurn 1999; Heptulla 1999; Niccoli-Sire 1999).
4) Nearly every index case has an identifiable RET mutation (Wells Jr 1994; Komminoth 1995; Niccoli-Sire 2001).

Table 2. Indications for RET Testing.

RET Testing is Indicated in:
Patients with presumed sporadic MTC
Members of known MTC kindreds
All patients with pheochromocytoma
Children with Hirschsprung's disease

RET Testing is not Recommended in:
Patients with apparently sporadic hyperparathyroidism

Indications for RET Mutation Testing (Table 2)

To properly manage kindred with MEN2A or FMTC, a RET

1) RET analysis should always be first performed on the index case, even if the MTC appears to be sporadic (Olson 1992; Komminoth 1995; Fink 1996).
2) A RET analysis should always be done in patients with sporadic MTC, even when the family history appears to be negative, because such patients often have germline RET mutations identifying them as an index case for an unrecognized MEN2 kindred (Fitze 2002). The likelihood of a RET germline mutation in an individual with a supposedly sporadic MTC is between 1% and 7% (Brandi 2001). Certain RET mutations frequently present as MTC in a long-standing multinodular goiter (Niccoli-Sire 2001).
3) All patients with ostensibly sporadic pheochromocytoma or Hirschsprung's disease should be tested for germline MEN2 RET mutations (Brandi 2001; Neumann 2002).

Method of RET Testing

TESTING THE INDEX CASE The leukocytes of suspected carriers should be tested for MEN2-associated germline mutations by polymerase chain reaction amplification of the appropriate RET gene exons and direct DNA sequencing, which is a practical means of identifying the mutation since all known mutations are found in exons 10,11,13,14,15 and 16 (Table 1). If these exons prove to be negative, the other 15 should be sequenced, which is only available in research laboratories (Brandi 2001). It is particularly important to examine exons 13, 14 and 15 because mutations in these exons are likely to cause MTC with a low prevalence of pheochromocytoma that is likely to escape recognition as a familial disorder (Brandi 2001).

TESTING FAMILY MEMBERS When a RET mutation is found in an index case:

1) All first degree relatives must be screened to determine which individuals carry the gene. This is performed twice and on separate blood samples to exclude errors.
2) Theoretically, half of first degree relatives do not carry the mutated gene and their risk of developing the disease is similar to that of the general public.

A small risk of hereditary MTC remains if no germline mutation is found. The probability that a first-degree relative will inherit an autosomal dominant gene for MTC from an individual with sporadic MTC in whom no germline mutation is found is 0.18% (Brandi 2001).

ANALYSIS FOR RET MUTATIONS IN TUMOR TISSUE from ostensibly sporadic cases of MTC has limited value in identifying an index case, but may provide a substitute if peripheral blood from an affected person is not available. However, somatic mutations in RET, predominantly at codon 918, and very rarely at codon 883 have been found in nearly 90% of the thyroid tumors of sporadic MTC cases in which case the peripheral blood tests are negative for germline RET mutations (Eng 1998; Gimm 1999). Somatic codon 918 mutations, which can be identified by RET immunohistochemical staining, (Eng 1998), are more aggressive and may metastasize earlier and be more lethal than other somatic MTC tumors (Eng 1998); however, whether identifying this somatic mutation will enhance management is unclear.

Calcitonin Testing

This peptide hormone is secreted by the C cells of both CCH and MTC, which in the past was used to detect MEN2 carriers. Although RET testing identifies carriers much earlier and more reliably (Lips 1994), there still are some indications for CT testing for CCH or MTC; however, affected individuals often have normal basal plasma CT levels, and it is necessary to use intravenous pentagastrin,[1] calcium[2], or both[3] to stimulate CT secretion from MTC or hyperplastic C-cells. Omeprazole may be used for this purpose when pentagastrin is contraindicated, unavailable, or refused because of its unpleasant side effects, but pentagastrin produces a significantly greater rise in CT (Vitale 2002). The indications for CT testing are as follows:

1) Screening MEN2 family members in which the RET mutation has not been identified.
2) Testing carriers from MEN2 kindred with MTC that has displayed an indolent course presenting later in life, so children can undergo thyroidectomy when they are in the second decade of life.
3) Pre- and postoperative CT correlates with the extent of tumor and may distinguish between macroscopic and microcarcinoma MTC or identify CCH (Cohen 2000) or may suggest metastases (Pomares 2002).

Prognosis of Familial MTC

Prognosis is related to tumor stage (Modigliani 1998) and the plasma CT level (Pomares 2002). When plasma CT is used preoperatively to identify indolent forms of MTC, surgery is usually indicated when the pentagastrin-stimulated CT rises >10 pg/ml (Niccoli-Sire 1999). Preoperative CT levels are predictive of postoperative

---

[1] Pentagastrin peptide for testing is currently not available in the USA. Give 0.5 μg/Kg IV push, measure plasma calcitonin at 1, 2, 5, 10 minutes. Normal response in men is < 210 pg/mL, women <105 pg/mL.

[2] Calcium 2 mg/kg IV push, measure plasma calcitonin at 1, 2, 5, 10 minutes. Normal response in men is < 265 pg/mL, women <120 pg/mL.

[3] Combined test use calcium immediately followed by Pentagastrin, measure plasma calcitonin at 1, 2, 5, 10 minutes. Normal response is <300 pg/ml for men and women.

CT normalization. The French Calcitonin Tumor Study Group (Cohen 2000) found that a preoperative plasma CT level <50 pg/mL was predictive of postoperative CT <10 pg/mL although a higher level did not necessarily mean that the postoperative CT would not fall to <10 pg/mL. Postoperatively, any rise in plasma CT may be indicative of persistent MTC, but false-positive CT measured by RIA is common (Lips 1994; Scheuba 1999).

INITIAL MANAGEMENT OF MEN2 SYNDROMES BASED UPON CLASSIFICATION OF FAMILIAL SYNDROMES

The Goal of Management

The goal is to prevent or cure MTC in all MEN2A carriers by performing genetic testing and thyroidectomy during early childhood (Brandi 2001). Total thyroidectomy including the posterior capsule will usually remove all normal and malignant C-cells and will prevent MTC from developing (Bachelot 2002).

Timing of Surgery

GENERAL RECOMMENDATIONS BASED UPON MEN2 STRATIFICATION The timing of surgery in MEN2 carriers continues to be refined, because genotype-phenotype correlations and gene penetration are not always predictable, but is different among MEN2 kindreds (Fig. 3). Differing recommendations among groups, mainly on the timing of surgery, are summarized below.

MEN2A. MTC associated with any RET mutation in codon 634 commonly appears before the age of 10and has been reported to occur in children as young as 17 months but is rarely metastatic before the age of 14 years (Fig. 4) (Machens 2003b). According to recent consensus guidelines (Brandi 2001), thyroidectomy should be done before age 5 years for children with MEN2A.

FMTC MTC usually becomes manifest in the third or fourth decade of life and has an indolent course (Fugazzola 2002). Pentagastrin testing has been recommended every other year in gene carriers identified by genetic testing, usually starting around 10 years of age (Brandi 2001). Thyroidectomy should be performed only after the pentagastrin test becomes positive (CT>10 pg/mL) or during the third or fourth decade of life when the disease is known to progress, whichever comes first (Bachelot 2002). This may be modified depending on the genotype and the clinical behavior of MTC in affected families (Oriola 1998; Siggelkow 2001; Fitze 2002).

MEN2B. Carriers have more advanced tumor than those with MEN 2A, in spite of presenting at a younger age (O'Riordain 1994). Children with a MEN2B with RET mutations at codons 918 or 883 are at highest risk for having aggressive MTC (O'Riordain 1994; Sanso 2002) and should ideally undergo routine total thyroidectomy, including the posterior thyroid capsule, within the first 6 months of life (Brandi 2001; Leboulleux 2002) and preferably within the first month of life (Brandi 2001). This is justified in infants regardless of serum CT levels because microscopic MTC in the first year of life is common and is sometimes associated with metastases. Still, this is difficult surgery that can be done safely in only a few centers. In a study (Leboulleux 2002) of MEN2B patients, aged 2 to 27 years in which most had a 918 mutation in exon 16 and the

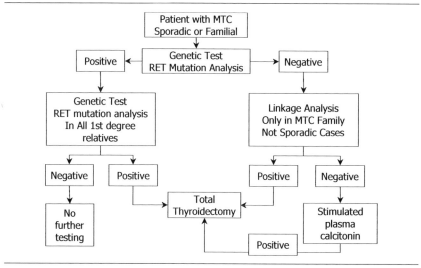

Figure 3. Algorithm for testing patients for familial MTC RET mutations.

identification of MTC was based on the presence of a thyroid nodule or involved neck lymph nodes or on dysmorphic features of MEN2B, most had Stage 3 or 4 tumors at surgery, further confirming the need for early treatment of MTC.

THYROID MANAGEMENT BASED ON STRATIFIED GENETIC INFORMATION Machens et al. (2001) on the basis of careful follow-up of a cohort of 63 patients recommended a more individualized approach to the timing and extent of prophylactic surgery. They devised three MTC risk groups according to genotype:

1) **High risk** (codons 634 and 618) with the youngest ages being 3 and 7 years at MTC diagnosis.
2) **Intermediate risk (**codons 790, 620, and 611) with ages of 12, 34, and 42 year at diagnosis.
3) **A low risk** (codons 768 and 804) with ages of 47 and 60 yr, at diagnosis, respectively.

THE SEVENTH INTERNATIONAL WORKSHOP ON MULTIPLE ENDOCRINE NEOPLASIA RECOM-MENDATIONS The conference held in Gubbio, Italy (Brandi 2001) advocates prophylactic total thyroidectomy before the age of five years in patients with mutations in RET codon 611, 618, 620, or 634 (Table 3). However, the participants in this workshop failed to reach an agreement on the approach to children with codon 609, 768, 790, 791, 804, or 891 mutations; the recommended age for prophylactic total thyroidectomy ranged from 5 to 10 years. Moreover, they did not reach a consensus on the need for prophylactic dissection of the central cervical lymph node compartment in patients with MEN2A, with differences of opinion ranging between surgeons and internists regarding

Table 3. Recommendations for Prophylactic Testing and Surgery According to RET Mutations.

RET mutation	Affected exon	International workshop on multiple endocrine neoplasia recommendations for prophylactic thyroidectomy*	EUROMEN recommendations for prophylactic thyroidectomy	Earliest reported age of MTC
609	10	Before age 5-10 years†	Yes but not before age 10 years¶	5 years
611	10	Before age 5 years	Not before age 5 years	7 years
618	10	Before age 5 years	Not before age 5 years	7 years
620	10	Before age 5 years	Not before age 5 years	11 years
630	11	No recommendation§	Yes but not before age 10 years¶	15 years
634	11	Before age 5 years	Before age 5 years	15 months
768	13	Before age 5–10 years†	Yes but not before age 10 years¶	>20 years
790	13	Before age 5–10 years†	Yes but not before age 10 years¶	12 years
791	13	Before age 5–10 years†	Yes but not before age 10 years¶	13 years
804	14	Before age 5–10 years†	No explicit recommendation	6 years
891	15	Before age 5–10 years†	Not before age 10 years¶	13 years
918‡MEN2B	16	Before age 1 years (preferable) Before age 5 years (minimum)	No explicit recommendation	9 months

* Total thyroidectomy including the posterior thyroid capsule. No consensus was reached regarding the need for prophylactic dissection of the central lymph nodes.
** Plasma free metanephrine is the best test for pheochromocytoma and should always be done preoperatively. It should be done in all MEN2A and 2B patients. In carriers with high-risk codons for pheochromocytoma, screening should begin at the age when thyroidectomy would be considered or by the age of 5 to 7 years, whichever is earlier, and should be done annually thereafter. In families at less risk for pheochromocytoma, especially those with codons 609, 768, val804met, and 891, screening may be initiated at an older age, depending on the familial pattern of the pheochromocytoma. There is no consensus on the best imaging studies for pheochromocytoma, although most use abdominal CT (56).
† There was consensus that this group should undergo prophylactic thyroidectomy, but there was little consensus regarding the timing of surgery. Some opted for a strategy similar to the high risk group, others suggested thyroidectomy at age 10 and still others opted for periodic pentagastrin-stimulated CT testing. These patients should undergo thyroidectomy when the pentagastrin test becomes positive (CT>10 pg/mL) or during the third or fourth decade of life, whichever comes first (28).
§ A rare mutation at exon 11 in codon 630 (Bachelot 2002) is often associated with a late appearance of MTC.
‡ Includes mutations in RET codons 883 or 922 with or without somatic manifestations of MEN2B, or MTC with MEN2B phenotype.
¶ The authors conclude that their data do not support the need for prophylactic thyroidectomy in asymptomatic carriers with this mutation before the age of 10 years or from central lymph node dissection before the age of 20 years.
**** All patients should be tested for pheochromocytoma prior to surgery using plasma metanephrine levels.

whether central neck dissection should be done during the primary operative procedure. Most surgeons favored a central lymph node dissection during the primary operation because of the higher morbidity associated with reentry into the central compartment during a second procedure; whereas, internists were more concerned with the higher rate of permanent hypoparathyroidism and permanent laryngeal nerve damage associated with primary central node dissection (Brandi 2001). The consensus was to stratify management of hereditary MTC into three levels on the basis of genetic information (Table 3) (Brandi 2001).

Level 1 (lowest risk): Children with RET codon 609, 768, 790, 804, and 891 mutations have the least high risk among the three RET codon mutation stratifications (Shan 1998; Bartsch 2000). There was consensus that this group should undergo prophylactic thyroidectomy, but there was little consensus on the management of these mutations. Some opted for a strategy similar to the high risk group, others suggested thyroidectomy at age 10 and still others opted for periodic pentagastrin-stimulated CT testing. These patients should undergo thyroidectomy when the pentagastrin test becomes positive (CT>10 pg/mL) or during the third or fourth decade of life, whichever comes first (Bachelot 2002).

Level 2 (intermediate risk): Children with any RET codon 611, 618, 620 or 634 mutation are classified as having high risk for MTC and should undergo thyroidectomy, including removal of the posterior capsule, before the age of 5 years.

Level 3 (highest risk): Children with MEN2B and/or RET codon 918 or 883 mutation should have a total thyroidectomy within the first 6 months of life, preferably within the first month of life. Thyroid surgery should include a central neck dissection. If metastases are identified, more extensive neck dissection is appropriate.

EUROPEAN MULTIPLE ENDOCRINE NEOPLASIA (EUROMEN) STUDY GROUP RECOMMENDATIONS
A 2003 report (Machens 2003b) by the EUROMEN Study Group gives another opinion on the selection of patients for surgery and management of familial MTC. This group collected data from several European countries on 207 carriers of a RET mutation who were under age 20 years and who had undergone total thyroidectomy for MTC ≤ 10 mm confined to the thyroid. The most common RET codon was 634 (62.8%) followed by codon 618 (9.2%), codons 620 and 790 (6.8% each), codon 791 (2.4%), codons 609, 611, 804, and 918 (1.9% each), and codon 630 (0.5%).

There was a significant age-related progression from CCH to MTC, and eventually, to nodal metastases in patients whose RET mutations were grouped according to the extracellular- and intracellular-domain codons affected (Fig. 4). The mean age at the time of diagnosis was 8.3 years among patients who had CCH and extracellular-domain mutations and was 11.2 years among those with intracellular-domain mutations (P = 0.01). Among patients with node-negative MTC, the mean age at diagnosis was 10.2 years in those with extracellular-domain mutations and 16.6 years in those with intracellular-domain mutations (P = 0.002). The mean age at diagnosis among patients with node-positive MTC was 17.1 years in those with extracellular-domain mutations, and none of the patients with MTC and intracellular-domain mutations had nodal metastases during the first two decades of life. Still, they found that grouping the rare RET mutations as extracellular- and intracellular-domain mutation is not a useful way of identifying the optimal age at which asymptomatic carriers should undergo prophylactic thyroidectomy. The authors opine that as more clinical information emerges, some of the rare RET mutations may need to be reclassified if they turn out to behave differently from the others in that group. The EUROMEN report demonstrates the following:

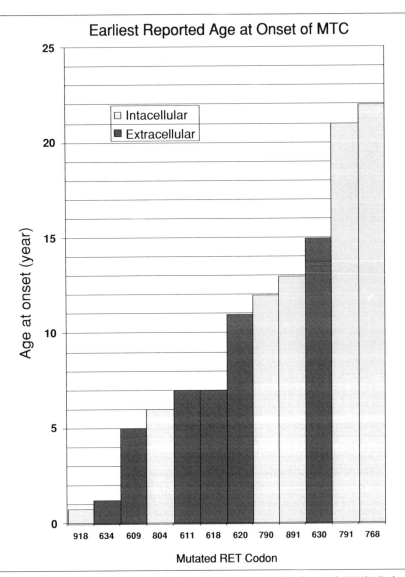

Figure 4. Earliest reported age at onset of familial MTC. From the data of Machens et al. (2003b). Dark bars represent extracellular codons and light bars intracellular codons of RET (see Fig. 2).

WITH ANY CODON 634 MUTATION, REGARDLESS OF THE AMINO ACID SUBSTITUTION (FIG. 4)

1) MTC commonly appears before the age of 10 years but perhaps of greatest importance, it may occur in children as young as 17 months.
2) MTC is rarely metastatic before the age of 14 years, regardless of the amino acid substitution.
3) Nodal metastases were found an average of 6.6 years after MTC had appeared.
4) These observations support the recommendation for prophylactic thyroidectomy at least by 5 years if not earlier for carriers of the 634 RET mutation.

AMONG ASYMPTOMATIC CARRIERS OF MUTATIONS IN CODON 611, 618, OR 620

1) None had evidence of MTC before the age of 5 years, suggesting early thyroidectomy is not **necessary.**

AMONG ASYMPTOMATIC CARRIERS OF MUTATIONS IN CODON 609, 630, 768, 790, 791, OR 891

2) The data do not support the need for prophylactic thyroidectomy before the age of 10 years or for central lymph-node dissection before the age of 20 years.

Summary of Timing of Surgery for MTC

While these data are reassuring, they are somewhat in conflict with prior studies. A slightly different perspective is gained by combing results among the studies and showing the earliest age at which MTC has been reported for a particular RET mutation (Fig. 4), which was suggested by Cote and Gagel (2003). For example, the recommendation made at the Gubbio consensus conference of performing thyroidectomy by the age of 5 years for children with a 634 codon mutation would have missed the window of opportunity to operate on the patient before the MTC had appeared according to the data shown in Figure 4 from EUROMEN group (Machens 2003b), which shows that occasionally a child may develop MTC as young as 17 months of age. Cote and Gagel (2003) suggest that a broader experience will be required before specific recommendations can be made for each mutation, but for now, the question is whether the decision regarding thyroidectomy should be based on the average behavior of MTC in MEN-2 kindreds, or on the earliest reported age at which metastasis occurs. Cote and Gagel (2003) advise that for now physicians must chart a course that balances the risks of early metastases and the small risks and sequelae of surgery in young children against the biologic behavior of MTC in other family members. The EUROMEN recommendation and the Gubbio Workshop recommendation are thus the same for 634 carriers for surgical intervention before age 5; however, they differ and for most of the other less common RET mutations (Table 3) often beginning at 10 years of age, although such an approach would likely be associated with metastases at the time of treatment in a small number of children (Fig. 4).

SUMMARY

Successful treatment of MTC depends heavily upon early diagnosis and treatment. Although this is not usually possible for sporadic MTC, it is achievable in MTC carriers who have genetic testing and undergo surgery before their C cells undergo malignant transformation. The following represents the highlights of management of patients with this disease:

1) All patients with MTC should be tested for RET mutations, including putative sporadic cases.

2) The leukocytes of suspected carriers and sporadic MTC cases should be tested for MEN2-associated germline mutations by polymerase chain reaction amplification of the appropriate RET gene exons including 10,11,13,14,15 and 16 (Table 1).

3) When a RET mutation is found, all first degree relatives must be screened to determine which individuals carry the gene. If these exons are negative, the other 15 should be sequenced but this is only available in research laboratories.

4) There is a 0.18% probability that a first-degree relative will inherit an autosomal dominant gene for MTC from an individual with ostensibly sporadic MTC in whom no germline mutation is found.

5) Patients with MEN2B and/or RET codon 883 or 918 mutation should have a total thyroidectomy within the first 6 months of life, preferably within the first month of life.

6) Patients with 634 mutations, which comprise about 70% of all MTC mutations, should undergo thyroidectomy by age 5 years or younger; children with this mutation as young as 17 months are reported with MTC.

7) The recommendations for the timing of prophylactic thyroidectomy are not consistent for less common mutations (Table 3, Fig. 3). There is a balance between performing prophylactic thyroidectomy earlier than the youngest age at with MTC has been reported to occur for a specific RET mutation and the high risk of complications, mainly permanent hypoparathyroidism and laryngeal nerve damage, that occur when thyroidectomy is done on very young children.

8) Initial treatment of MTC is total thyroidectomy, regardless of its genetic type or putative sporadic nature, because surgery offers the only chance for a cure.

9) Treatment with I-131 has no place in the management of MTC.

10) Plasma CT measurements provide an accurate estimate of tumor burden, and are especially useful in identifying patients with residual tumor.

11) Pentagastrin-or calcium-stimulated plasma CT testing is useful in identifying CCH or early MTC in carriers of RET mutations associated with late onset MTC, but Pentagastrin in not available in the USA.

12) Pheochromocytoma may occur before or after MTC, and is an important cause of mortality, even in young patients.

13) When a diagnosis of familial MTC has been made, preoperative measurement of plasma free metanephrine should always be done, even in FMTC kindreds.
14) HPT is an important aspect of MEN2A and requires surgery according to current guidelines for the management of primary HPT.

REFERENCES

Aulicino, MR, AH Szporn, RB Dembitzer, J Mechanick, N Batheja, IJ Bleiweiss, and DE Burstein. 1998. Cytologic findings in the differential diagnosis of c-cell hyperplasia and medullary carcinoma by fine needle aspiration—a case report. Acta Cytol **42**:963–967.

Bachelot, A, F Lombardo, E Baudin, JM Bidart, and M Schlumberger. 2002. Inheritable forms of medullary thyroid carcinoma. Biochimie **84**:61–66.

Bartsch, DK, C Hasse, C Schug, P Barth, M Rothmund, and W Hoeppner. 2000. A RET double mutation in the germline of a kindred with FMTC. Exp Clin Endocrinol Diabetes **108**:128–132.

Beressi, N, JM Campos, JP Beressi, B Franc, P Niccoli-Sire, B Conte-Devolx, A Murat, P Caron, L Baldet, JL Kraimps, R Cohen, JC Bigorgne, O Chabre, P Lecomte, and E Modigliani. 1998. Sporadic medullary microcarcinoma of the thyroid: a retrospective analysis of eighty cases. Thyroid **8**:1039–1044.

Bilezikian, JP, JT Potts Jr, G Fuleihan, M Kleerekoper, R Neer, M Peacock, J Rastad, SJ Silverberg, R Udelsman, and SA Wells. 2002. Summary statement from a workshop on asymptomatic primary hyperparathyroidism: a perspective for the 21st century. J Clin Endocrinol Metab **87**:5353–5361.

Blank, RD, CA Sklar, A Dimich, MP LaQuaglia, and MF Brennan. 1996. Clinical presentations and RET protooncogene mutations in seven multiple endocrine neoplasia type 2 kindreds. Cancer **78**:1996–2003.

Bolino, A, I Schuffenecker, Y Luo, M Seri, M Silengo, T Tocco, G Chabrier, C Houdent, A Murat, and M Schlumberger. 1995. RET mutations in exons 13 and 14 of FMTC patients. Oncogene **10**:2415–2419.

Bonnema, SJ, FN Bennedbaek, WM Wiersinga, and L Hegedus. 2000. Management of the nontoxic multinodular goitre: a European questionnaire study [in process citation]. Clin Endocrinol (Oxford) **53**:5–12.

Brandi, ML, RF Gagel, A Angeli, JP Bilezikian, P Beck-Peccoz, C Bordi, B Conte-Devolx, A Falchetti, RG Gheri, A Libroia, CJ Lips, G Lombardi, M Mannelli, F Pacini, BA Ponder, F Raue, B Skogseid, G Tamburrano, RV Thakker, NW Thompson, P Tomassetti, F Tonelli, SA Wells Jr, and SJ Marx. 2001 CONSENSUS: guidelines for diagnosis and therapy of men type 1 and type 2. J Clin Endocrinol Metab **86**:5658–5671.

Carlson, KM, J Bracamontes, CE Jackson, R Clark, A Lacroix, SA Wells Jr, and PJ Goodfellow. 1994. Parent-of-origin effects in multiple endocrine neoplasia type 2B. Am J Hum Genet **55**:1076–1082.

Carney, JA, GW Sizemore, and AB Hayles. 1978. Multiple endocrine neoplasia, type 2b. Pathobiol Annu **8**:105–153.

Cohen, R, B Buchsenschutz, P Estrade, P Gardet, and E Modigliani. 1996. Causes of death in patients suffering from medullary thyroid carcinoma: report of 119 cases. Presse Medicale **25**:1819–1822.

Cohen, R, JM Campos, C Salaun, HM Heshmati, JL Kraimps, C Proye, E Sarfati, JF Henry, P Niccoli-Sire, and E Modigliani. 2000. Preoperative calcitonin levels are predictive of tumor size and postoperative calcitonin normalization in medullary thyroid carcinoma. Groupe d'Etudes des Tumeurs a Calcitonine (GETC). J Clin Endocrinol Metab **85**:919–922.

Cote, GJ, and RF Gagel. 2003. Lessons learned from the management of a rare genetic cancer. N Engl J Med **349**:1566–1568.

Dolan, SJ, and CF Russell. 2000. Medullary thyroid carcinoma in Northern Ireland, 1967–1997. Ann R Coll Surg Engl **82**:156–161.

Dunn, JM, and JR Farndon. 1993. Medullary thyroid carcinoma. Br J Surg **80**:6–9.

Elisei, R, V Bottici, F Luchetti, G Di Coscio, C Romei, L Grasso, P Miccoli, P Iacconi, F Basolo, A Pinchera, and F Pacini. 2004. Impact of routine measurement of serum calcitonin on the diagnosis and outcome of medullary thyroid cancer: experience in 10,864 patients with nodular thyroid disorders. J Clin Endocrinol Metab **89**:163–168.

Eng, C. 1996a. The RET proto-oncogene in multiple endocrine neoplasia type 2 and Hirschprung's disease. N Engl J Med **335**:943–951.

Eng, C, D Clayton, I Schufenecker, G Lenoir, G Cote, RF Gagel, HKP Van Amstel, CJM Lips, I Nishisho, SI Takai, DJ Marsh, BG Robinson, K Frank-Raue, F Raue, F Xue, WW Noll, C Romei, F Pacini, M Fink, B Niederle, and J Zedenius. 1996b. The relationship between specific RET proto-oncogene mutations and disease phenotype in multiple endocrine neoplasia type 2: international RET mutation consortium analysis. J Am Med Assoc **276**:1575–1579.

Eng, C, GA Thomas, DS Neuberg, LM Mulligan, CS Healey, C Houghton, A Frilling, F Raue, ED Williams, and BA Ponder. 1998. Mutation of the RET proto-oncogene is correlated with RET immunostaining in subpopulations of cells in sporadic medullary thyroid carcinoma. J Clin Endocrinol Metab 83:4310–4313.

Engelbach, M, R Gorges, T Forst, A Pfutzner, R Dawood, S Heerdt, T Kunt, A Bockisch, and J Beyer. 2000. Improved diagnostic methods in the follow-up of medullary thyroid carcinoma by highly specific calcitonin measurements. J Clin Endocrinol Metab 85:1890–1894.

Fink, M, A Weinhäusel, B Niederle, and OA Haas. 1996. Distinction between sporadic and hereditary medullary thyroid carcinoma (MTC) by mutation analysis of the RET proto-oncogene. Int J Cancer 69:312–316.

Fitze, G, M Schierz, J Bredow, HD Saeger, D Roesner, and HK Schackert. 2002. Various penetrance of familial medullary thyroid carcinoma in patients with RET protooncogene codon 790/791 germline mutations. Ann Surg 236:570–575.

Franc, S, P Niccoli-Sire, R Cohen, S Bardet, B Maes, A Murat, A Krivitzky, and E Modigliani. 2001. Complete surgical lymph node resection does not prevent authentic recurrences of medullary thyroid carcinoma. Clin Endocrinol (Oxford) 55:403–409.

Fugazzola, L, N Cerutti, D Mannavola, G Ghilardi, L Alberti, R Romoli, and P Beck-Peccoz. 2002. Multigenerational familial medullary thyroid cancer (FMTC): evidence for FMTC phenocopies and association with papillary thyroid cancer. Clin Endocrinol (Oxford) 56:53–63.

Gagel, RF, GJ Cote, MJGM Bugalho, AE Boyd III, T Cummings, H Goepfert, DB Evans, A Cangir, S Khorana, and PN Schultz. 1995. Clinical use of molecular information in the management of multiple endocrine neoplasia type 2A. J Intern Med 238:333–341.

Gagel, RF, KE Melvin, AH Tashjian Jr, HH Miller, ZT Feldman, HJ Wolfe, RA DeLellis, S Cerviskinner, and S Reichlin. 1975. Natural history of the familial medullary thyroid carcinoma-pheochromocytoma syndrome and the identification of preneoplastic stages by screening studies: a five-year report. Trans Assoc Am Physicians 88:177–191.

Gagel, RF, AH Tashjian Jr, T Cummings, N Papathanasopoulos, MM Kaplan, RA DeLellis, HJ Wolfe, and S Reichlin. 1988. The clinical outcome of prospective screening for multiple endocrine neoplasia type 2a. An 18-year experience. N Engl J Med 318:478–484.

Gagel, RF, AH Tashjian Jr, T Cummings, N Papathanasopoulos, and S Reichlin. 1987. Impact of prospective screening for multiple endocrine neoplasia type 2. Henry Ford Hosp Med J 35:94–98.

Gimm, O, DS Neuberg, DJ Marsh, PLM Dahia, HV Cuong, F Raue, R Hinze, H Dralle, and C Eng. 1999. Over-representation of a germline RET sequence variant in patients with sporadic medullary thyroid carcinoma and somatic RET codon 918 mutation. Oncogene 18:1369–1373.

Gimm, O, BE Niederle, T Weber, M Bockhorn, J Ukkat, M Brauckhoff, PN Thanh, A Frilling, E Klar, B Niederle, and H Dralle. 2002. RET proto-oncogene mutations affecting codon 790/791: a mild form of multiple endocrine neoplasia type 2A syndrome? Surgery 132:952–959.

Henry, JF, A Denizot, M Puccini, P Niccoli, B Conte-Devolx, and C de Micco. 1996. Early diagnosis of sporadic medullary cancer of the thyroid: contribution of routine calcitonin assay. Presse Medicale 25:1583–1588.

Heptulla, RA, RP Schwartz, AE Bale, D Flynn, and M Genel. 1999. Familial medullary thyroid carcinoma: presymptomatic diagnosis and management in children. J Pediatr 135:327–331.

Hinze, R, HJ Holzhausen, O Gimm, H Dralle, and FW Rath. 1998. Primary hereditary medullary thyroid carcinoma—C-cell morphology and correlation with preoperative calcitonin levels. Virchows Arch Int J Pathol 433:203–208.

Hodak, SP, and KD Burman. 2004. The calcitonin conundrum-is it time for routine measurement of serum calcitonin in patients with thyroid nodules? J Clin Endocrinol Metab 89:511–514.

Hundahl, SA, ID Fleming, AM Fremgen, and HR Menck. 1998. A National Cancer Data Base report on 53,856 cases of thyroid carcinoma treated in the US, 1985–1995. Cancer 83:2638–2648.

Hyer, SL, L Vini, R A'Hern, and C Harmer. 2000. Medullary thyroid cancer: multivariate analysis of prognostic factors influencing survival. Eur J Surg Oncol 26:686–690.

Iler, MA, DR King, ME Ginn-Pease, TM O'Dorisio, and JF Sotos. 1999. Multiple endocrine neoplasia type 2A: a 25-year review. J Pediatr Surg 34:92–96.

Jackson, CE, AH Tashjian Jr, and MA Block. 1973. Detection of medullary thyroid cancer by calcitonin assay in families. Ann Int Med 78:845–852.

Kebebew, E, PH Ituarte, AE Siperstein, QY Duh, and OH Clark. 2000. Medullary thyroid carcinoma: clinical characteristics, treatment, prognostic factors, and a comparison of staging systems. Cancer 88:1139–1148.

Komminoth, P, EK Kunz, X Matias-Guiu, O Hiort, G Christiansen, A Colomer, J Roth, and PU Heitz. 1995. Analysis of RET protooncogene point mutations distinguishes heritable from nonheritable medullary thyroid carcinomas. Cancer **76**:479–489.

Kraimps, JL, A Denizot, B Carnaille, JF Henry, C Proye, F Bacourt, E Sarfati, JL Dupond, B Maes, JP Travagli, A Boneu, P Roger, C Houdent, J Barbier, and E Modigliani. 1996. Primary hyperparathyroidism in multiple endocrine neoplasia type IIa: retrospective French multicentric study. World J Surg **20**:808–813.

Leboulleux, S, JP Travagli, B Caillou, A Laplanche, JM Bidart, M Schlumberger, and E Baudin. 2002. Medullary thyroid carcinoma as part of a multiple endocrine neoplasia type 2B syndrome: influence of the stage on the clinical course. Cancer **94**:44–50.

Lenders, JW, K Pacak, MM Walther, WM Linehan, M Mannelli, P Friberg, HR Keiser, DS Goldstein, and G Eisenhofer. 2002. Biochemical diagnosis of pheochromocytoma: which test is best? J Am Med Assoc **287**:1427–1434.

Lips, CJ. 1998. Clinical management of the multiple endocrine neoplasia syndromes: results of a computerized opinion poll at the Sixth International Workshop on Multiple Endocrine Neoplasia and von Hippel-Lindau disease. J Intern Med **243**:589–594.

Lips, CJM, RM Landsvater, JWM Höppener, RA Geerdink, G Blijham, JM Jansen-Schillhorn van Veen, APG Van Gils, MJ De Wit, RA Zewald, MJH Berends, FA Beemer, J Brouwers-Smalbraak, RPM Jansen, HKP Van Amstel, TJMV Van Vroonhoven, and TM Vroom. 1994. Clinical screening as compared with DNA analysis in families with multiple endocrine neoplasia type 2A. N Engl J Med **331**:828–835.

Machens, A, O Gimm, R Hinze, W Hoppner, BO Boehm, and H Dralle. 2001. Genotype–phenotype correlations in hereditary medullary thyroid carcinoma: oncological features and biochemical properties. J Clin Endocrinol Metab **86**:1104–1109.

Machens, A, HJ Holzhausen, PN Thanh, and H Dralle. 2003a. Malignant progression from C-cell hyperplasia to medullary thyroid carcinoma in 167 carriers of RET germline mutations. Surgery **134**:425–431.

Machens, A, P Niccoli-Sire, J Hoegel, K Frank-Raue, TJ van Vroonhoven, HD Roeher, RA Wahl, P Lamesch, F Raue, B Conte-Devolx, and H Dralle. 2003b. Early malignant progression of hereditary medullary thyroid cancer. N Engl J Med **349**:1517–1525.

Massoll, N, and EL Mazzaferri. 2004. Diagnosis and management of medullary thyroid carcinoma. Clin Lab Med **24**:49–83.

Mayr, B, G Brabant, and Mü Von zur. 1999. Incidental detection of familial medullary thyroid carcinoma by calcitonin screening for nodular thyroid disease. Eur J Endocrinol **141**:286–289.

Melvin, KE, AH Tashjian Jr, and HH Miller. 1972. Studies in familial (medullary) thyroid carcinoma. Recent Prog Horm Res **28**:399–470.

Modigliani, E, R Cohen, JM Campos, B Conte-Devolx, B Maes, A Boneu, M Schlumberger, JC Bigorgne, P Dumontier, L Leclerc, B Corcuff, I Guilhem, and The GETC Study Group. 1998. Prognostic factors for survival and for biochemical cure in medullary thyroid carcinoma: results in 899 patients. Clin Endocrinol (Oxford) **48**:265–273.

Modigliani, E, HM Vasen, K Raue, H Dralle, A Frilling, RG Gheri, ML Brandi, E Limbert, B Niederle, L Forgas, M Rosenberg-Bourgin, and C Calmettes. 1995a. Pheochromocytoma in multiple endocrine neoplasia type 2: European study. J Intern Med **238**:363–367.

Modigliani, E, HM Vasen, K Raue, H Dralle, A Frilling, RG Gheri, ML Brandi, E Limbert, B Niederle, L Forgas, M Rosenberg-Bourgin, and C Calmettes. 1995b. Pheochromocytoma in multiple endocrine neoplasia type 2: European study. J Intern Med **238**:363–367.

Moers, AMJ, RM Landsvater, C Schaap, JMJS Van Veen, IAJ De Valk, GH Blijham, JWM Höppener, TM Vroom, HKP Van Amstel, and CJM Lips. 1996. Familial medullary thyroid carcinoma: not a distinct entity? Genotype–phenotype correlation in a large family. Am J Med **101**:635–641.

Moley, JF, and MK DeBenedetti. 1999. Patterns of nodal metastases in palpable medullary thyroid carcinoma—recommendations for extent of node dissection. Ann Surg **229**:880–887.

Neumann, HP, B Bausch, SR McWhinney, BU Bender, O Gimm, G Franke, J Schipper, J Klisch, C Altehoefer, K Zerres, A Januszewicz, C Eng, WM Smith, R Munk, T Manz, S Glaesker, TW Apel, M Treier, M Reineke, MK Walz, C Hoang-Vu, M Brauckhoff, A Klein-Franke, P Klose, H Schmidt, M Maier-Woelfle, M Peczkowska, C Szmigielski, and C Eng. 2002. Germ-line mutations in nonsyndromic pheochromocytoma. New Engl J Med **346**:1459–1466.

Niccoli-Sire, P, A Murat, E Baudin, JF Henry, C Proye, JC Bigorgne, B Bstandig, E Modigliani, S Morange, M Schlumberger, and B Conte-Devolx. 1999. Early or prophylactic thyroidectomy in MEN 2/FMTC gene carriers: results in 71 thyroidectomized patients. The French Calcitonin Tumours Study Group (GETC). Eur J Endocrinol **141**:468–474.

Niccoli-Sire, P, A Murat, V Rohmer, S Franc, G Chabrier, L Baldet, B Maes, F Savagner, S Giraud, S Bezieau, ML Kottler, S Morange, and B Conte-Devolx. 2001. Familial medullary thyroid carcinoma with noncysteine ret mutations: phenotype–genotype relationship in a large series of patients. J Clin Endocrinol Metab **86:**3746–3753.

Olson, JE, J Hughes, and HD Alpern. 1992. Family members of patients with sporadic medullary thyroid carcinoma must be screened for hereditary disease. Surgery **112:**1074–1079.

Oriola, J, C Páramo, I Halperin, RV García-Mayor, and F Rivera-Fillat. 1998. Novel point mutation in exon 10 of the RET proto-oncogene in a family with medullary thyroid carcinoma. Am J Med Genet **78:**271–273.

O'Riordain, DS, T O'Brien, CS Grant, A Weaver, H Gharib, and JA van Heerden. 1993. Surgical management of primary hyperparathyroidism in multiple endocrine neoplasia types 1 and 2. Surgery **114:**1031–1039.

O'Riordain, DS, T O'Brien, AL Weaver, H Gharib, ID Hay, CS Grant, and JA van Heerden. 1994. Medullary thyroid carcinoma in multiple endocrine neoplasia types 2A and 2B. Surgery **116:**1017–1023.

Ozgen, AG, F Hamulu, F Bayraktar, C Yilmaz, M Tuzun, E Yetkin, M Tuncyurek, and T Kabalak. 1999. Evaluation of routine basal serum calcitonin measurement for early diagnosis of medullary thyroid carcinoma in seven hundred seventy-three patients with nodular goiter. Thyroid **9:**579–582.

Pacini, F, L Fugazzola, G Bevilacqua, P Viacava, V Nardini, and E Martino. 1993. Multiple endocrine neoplasia type 2A and cutaneous lichen amyloidosis: description of a new family. J Endocrinol Invest **16:**295–296.

Phay, JE, JF Moley, and TC Lairmore. 2000. Multiple endocrine neoplasias. Semin Surg Oncol **18:**324–332.

Pomares, FJ, JM Rodriguez, F Nicolas, J Sola, M Canteras, M Balsalobre, M Pascual, P Parrilla, and FJ Tebar. 2002. Presurgical assessment of the tumor burden of familial medullary thyroid carcinoma by calcitonin testing. J Am Coll Surg **195:**630–634.

Raue, F, JL Kraimps, H Dralle, P Cougard, C Proye, A Frilling, E Limbert, LF Llenas, and B Niederle. 1995. Primary hyperparathyroidism in multiple endocrine neoplasia type 2A. J Intern Med **238:**369–373.

Redding, AH, SN Levine, and MR Fowler. 2000. Normal preoperative calcitonin levels do not always exclude medullary thyroid carcinoma in patients with large palpable thyroid masses. Thyroid **10:**919–922.

Rougier, P, C Parmentier, A Laplanche, M Lefevre, JP Travagli, B Caillou, M Schlumberger, J Lacour, and M Tubiana. 1983. Medullary thyroid carcinoma: prognostic factors and treatment. Int J Radiat Oncol Biol Phys **9:**161–169.

Russo, D, F Arturi, E Chiefari, D Meringolo, D Bianchi, B Bellanova, and S Filetti. 1997. A case of metastatic medullary thyroid carcinoma: early identification before surgery of an RET proto-oncogene somatic mutation in fine-needle aspirate specimens. J Clin Endocrinol Metab **82:**3378–3382.

Sanso, GE, HM Domene, R Garcia, EdMAK Pusiol, M Roque, A Ring, H Perinetti, B Elsner, S Lorcansky, and M Barontini. 2002. Very early detection of RET proto-oncogene mutation is crucial for preventive thyroidectomy in multiple endocrine neoplasia type 2 children: presence of C-cell malignant disease in asymptomatic carriers. Cancer **94:**323–330.

Sarrazin, D, F Fontaine, P Rougier, P Gardet, M Schlumberger, JP Travagli, H Bounik, C Parmentier, and M Tubiana. 1984. Role of radiotherapy in the treatment of medullary cancer of the thyroid. Bull Cancer (Paris) **71:**200–208.

Scheuba, C, K Kaserer, A Weinhaeusl, R Pandev, A Kaider, C Passler, G Prager, H Vierhapper, OA Haas, and B Niederle. 1999. Is medullary thyroid cancer predictable? A prospective study of 86 patients with abnormal pentagastrin tests. Surgery **126:**1089–1095.

Schuffenecker, I, M Virally-Monod, R Brohet, D Goldgar, C Conte-Devolx, L Leclerc, O Chabre, A Boneu, J Caron, C Houdent, E Modigliani, V Rohmer, M Schlumberger, C Eng, PJ Guillausseau, GM Lenoir, and Groupe Etud Tumerurs Calcitonine. 1998a. Risk and penetrance of primary hyperparathyroidism in multiple endocrine neoplasia type 2A families with mutations at codon 634 of the RET proto-oncogene. J Clin Endocrinol Metab **83:**487–491.

Schuffenecker, I, M Virally-Monod, R Brohet, D Goldgar, C Conte-Devolx, L Leclerc, O Chabre, A Boneu, J Caron, C Houdent, E Modigliani, V Rohmer, M Schlumberger, C Eng, PJ Guillausseau, GM Lenoir, and Groupe Etud Tumerurs Calcitonine. 1998b. Risk and penetrance of primary hyperparathyroidism in multiple endocrine neoplasia type 2A families with mutations at codon 634 of the RET proto-oncogene. J Clin Endocrinol Metab **83:**487–491.

Shan, L, M Nakamura, Y Nakamura, H Utsunomiya, NH Shou, XH Jiang, XF Jing, T Yokoi, and K Kakudo. 1998. Somatic mutations in the RET protooncogene in Japanese and Chinese sporadic medullary thyroid carcinomas. Jpn J Cancer Res (Amsterdam) **89:**883–886.

Siggelkow, H, A Melzer, W Nolte, K Karsten, W Hoppner, and M Hufner. 2001. Presentation of a kindred with familial medullary thyroid carcinoma and Cys611Phe mutation of the RET proto-oncogene demonstrating low grade malignancy. Eur J Endocrinol **144:**467–473.

Skinner, MA, MK DeBenedetti, JF Moley, JA Norton, and SA Wells Jr. 1996. Medullary thyroid carcinoma in children with multiple endocrine neoplasia types 2A and 2B. J Pediatr Surg **31**:177–182.

Smith, VV, C Eng, and PJ Milla. 1999. Intestinal ganglioneuromatosis and multiple endocrine neoplasia type 2B: implications for treatment. Gut **45**:143–146.

Takano, T, A Miyauchi, F Matsuzuka, G Liu, T Higashiyama, T Yokozawa, K Kuma, and N Amino. 1999. Preoperative diagnosis of medullary thyroid carcinoma by RT-PCR using RNA extracted from leftover cells within a needle used for fine needle aspiration biopsy. J Clin Endocrinol Metab **84**:951–955.

Tashjian Jr, AH, and EW Melvin. 1968. Medullary carcinoma of the thyroid gland. Studies of thyrocalcitonin in plasma and tumor extracts. N Engl J Med **279**:279–283.

Tokuue, K, and M Furuse. 1990. Usefulness of the 99mTc-MDP scan in the detection of calcified liver metastases. Nuklearmedizin **29**:231–233.

Van Heurn, LWE, C Schaap, G Sie, AAM Haagen, WJ Gerver, G Freling, HKP Van Amstel, and E Heineman. 1999. Predictive DNA testing for multiple endocrine neoplasia 2: a therapeutic challenge of prophylactic thyroidectomy in very young children. J Pediatr Surg **34**:568–571.

Vitale, G, A Ciccarelli, M Caraglia, M Galderisi, R Rossi, S Del Prete, A Abbruzzese, and G Lupoli. 2002. Comparison of two provocative tests for calcitonin in medullary thyroid carcinoma: omeprazole vs. pentagastrin. Clin Chem **48**:1505–1510.

Weber, T, T Schilling, K Frank-Raue, M Colombo-Benkmann, U Hinz, R Ziegler, and E Klar. 2001. Impact of modified radical neck dissection on biochemical cure in medullary thyroid carcinomas. Surgery **130**:1044–1049.

Wells Jr, SA, DD Chi, K Toshima, LP Dehner, CM Coffin, SB Dowton, JL Ivanovich, MK DeBenedetti, WG Dilley, and JF Moley. 1994. Predictive DNA testing and prophylactic thyroidectomy in patients at risk for multiple endocrine neoplasia type 2A. Ann Surg **220**:237–247.

Wells Jr, SA, and MA Skinner. 1998. Prophylactic thyroidectomy, based on direct genetic testing, in patients at risk for the multiple endocrine neoplasia type 2 syndromes. Exp Clin Endocrinol Diabetes **106**:29–34.

Yokozawa, T, S Fukata, K Kuma, F Matsuzuka, A Kobayashi, K Hirai, A Miyauchi, and M Sugawara. 1996. Thyroid cancer detected by ultrasound-guided fine-needle aspiration biopsy. World J Surg **20**:848–853.

PART 9. EXTERNAL BEAM RADIATION THERAPY

9.1. EXTERNAL BEAM RADIOTHERAPY DOSE SCHEDULES

ROBERT J. AMDUR, MD, SIYONG KIM, PhD, JONATHAN GANG LI, PhD, CHIRAY LIU, PhD, WILLIAM M. MENDENHALL, MD, AND ERNEST L. MAZZAFERRI, MD, MACP

Table 1 summarizes the dose schedules and basic techniques that we use to deliver radiotherapy for thyroid cancer. The options summarized in this table apply to all types of thyroid cancer. The technical details of our conventional and IMRT program is the subject of others chapters.

PALLIATIVE INTENT

When treating patients with palliative intent we use dose schedules that do not require field reductions to exclude the spinal cord. We give palliative radiotherapy with 6 MV photons through opposed anterior and posterior fields. The treatment isocenter is at the midplane depth and dose delivery is preferentially weighted to the anterior field. The next chapter describes field boundaries.

We have used the dose schedules of 20 Gy in 2 fractions (1 week between fractions), 20 Gy in 5 fractions, and 30 Gy in 10 fractions for many years to palliate advanced head and neck cancers. All of these schedules produce tumor shrinkage in the majority of patients with acceptable acute toxicity. To decrease mucosal toxicity, we start Dexamethasone (4 mg three times a day) the day prior to starting radiotherapy with rapid taper at the end of radiotherapy. Late complications are rare with these hypofractionated schedules because patients usually do not live for more than a year after treatment and because the total dose is relatively low. The expected lifespan of the patient, the ability of the patient to travel for outpatient therapy, and physician preference determine the dose schedule in this setting.

Table 1. External Beam Radiotherapy Dose Schedules and Techniques for Thyroid Cancer.

External beam radiotherapy dose schedules and techniques			
Palliation of symptoms of terminal cancer		Curative intent	
Doses	Technique	Doses[2]	Techniques
20 @ 10 /treatment (2 treatment days) 1-6 weeks between treatments	6 MV photons through opposed anterior and posterior fields	63–72 using the UF IMRT[1] schedule (30 treatment days)	IMRT[1]
20 @ 4 /treatment (5 treatment days)	6 MV photons through opposed anterior and posterior fields	74.4 @ 1.2 /treatment with twice-a-day fractionation (31 treatment days)	Give 45.6 with opposed anterior and posterior fields using 6 MV photons and then avoid the spinal cord using 20 MV photons through opposed lateral fields with shoulder compensators
30 @ 3 /treatment (10 treatment days)	6 MV photons through opposed anterior and posterior fields	63-72 @ 1.8/treatment/day (35–40 treatment days)	Same as above with 45 given through anterior and posterior fields

[1] IMRT = Intensity Modulated Radiation Therapy.
[2] With high-risk features we use: 72 @ 1.8/fraction, 74.4 @ 1.2/fraction BID, or IMRT 72 @ 1.8 and 1.5/fraction. If there are no high-risk features the prescribed dose is 63 @ 1.8 or IMRT to 63 Gy. High-risk features include gross residual disease, positive margin, invasion of normal tissues that define a stage T4 primary tumor, or nodal metastasis with extensive extracapsular tumor extension.

CURATIVE INTENT

We choose between two basic dose prescriptions based on the likely burden of residual disease. We prescribe 63 Gy in the absence of high-risk features and 72 or 74.4 Gy when a high-risk feature is present. The details of the conventional and IMRT techniques used at our institution are the subject of the next few chapters.

9.2. INDICATIONS FOR EXTERNAL BEAM RADIATION THERAPY FOR DIFFERENTIATED THYROID CANCER

ROBERT J. AMDUR, MD, WILLIAM M. MENDENHALL, MD, AND
ERNEST L. MAZZAFERRI, MD, MACP

In this chapter, we use the term External Beam Radiation Therapy (EBRT) to mean irradiation of the neck and upper mediastinum. EBRT for brain, bone, spine, or lung metastases are the subjects of other chapters.

There are no well-designed prospective randomized trials of EBRT in patients with Differentiated Thyroid Cancer (DTC). Retrospective series from multiple institutions suggest that EBRT improves the rate of tumor control in high-risk subgroups but most series do not report an improvement in overall survival. As the major prognostic variables (the presence of gross disease, history of I-131 therapy, patient age, irradiation dose, etc), length of follow-up, and endpoints of analysis (local control versus survival) differ markedly from one study to the next, it is no surprise that some authors recommend EBRT while others conclude that it is not beneficial.

Based on our clinical experience and review of the literature, our opinion is that there are situations where EBRT is likely to improve the length or quality of life of patients with DTC. The reference list at the end of this chapter includes most of the publications that study the role of EBRT in DTC. It is not useful to discuss the details of any specific study here. The two most widely quoted series to support the use of EBRT are those from Tubiana et al. (1985) and Farahati et al. (1996). Probably the most widely quoted study that concludes that EBRT is of no value is that of Samaan et al. (1992).

INDICATIONS FOR EBRT

Table 1 summarizes our indications for using EBRT in patients with Differentiated Thyroid Cancer, Hürthle Cell carcinoma, and Poorly Differentiated (Insular) thyroid

Table 1. Indications for External Beam Radiation Therapy (EBRT) for Differentiated Thyroid Cancer.

Indications for EBRT[1] for differentiated[2] thyroid cancer	
Child **Age ≤ 18 years**	• Give EBRT only when there is no other way to palliate symptoms or prevent normal tissue damage from tumor growth
Younger Adult **Age 19–45 years**	• **EBRT for visible disease that is resistant to I-131:** Give EBRT when tumor persists or recurs following thyroidectomy, ablation of the thyroid remnant with I-131, and at least one additional treatment with ≥ 100 mCi I-131 with optimal preparation[3] • Regardless of the risk of tumor recurrence or the results of imaging studies, we do not give EBRT in this age group when additional I-131 therapy may be curative • We do not give EBRT when the only evidence of disease is an elevated serum Tg level
Older Adult **Age > 45 years**	• **EBRT in addition to I-131 when the risk of local or regional recurrence is high:** In this age group we give EBRT (usually a few weeks after I-131) following initial thyroidectomy, or following surgical resection recurrent disease, when the surgical specimen demonstrates a positive margin, invasion of normal tissues that define a T4[4] primary tumor, or nodal metastasis with extensive extracapsular tumor extension **EBRT for disease that is visible and resistant to I-131:** Give EBRT when tumor persists or recurs following thyroidectomy, ablation of the thyroid remnant with I-131, and at least one additional treatment with ≥100 mCi I-131 with optimal preparation[3], is visible on an imaging study or the surgeon says that tumor was left behind, and there is no evidence of distant metastasis • We do not give EBRT when the only evidence of disease is an elevated serum Tg level

[1] In this table, the term External beam radiation Therapy (EBRT) means irradiation of the neck and upper mediastinum.
[2] These guidelines apply to differentiated forms of papillary and follicular thyroid cancer including tall cell, columnar cell, insular (poorly differentiated) variants of papillary carcinoma and to Hürthle cell carcinoma.
[3] Optimal preparation for I-131 therapy means: A two week low-iodine diet, a 24 hour urine iodine < 100μg when there is any question of iodine contamination from drugs or radiological studies, lithium pretreatment (unless there are contraindications to using lithium), thyroid hormone withdrawal sufficient to raise the serum TSH to above 30 mIU/L or preparation with rhTSH and 4 day withdrawl of thyroid hormone (see the chapter on preparation with rhTSH).
[4] 6th edition (year 2002) of the AJCC staging system (see text).

carcinoma. The guidelines in this chapter apply only to patients with a life expectancy of at least 5 years. Patients with a short life expectancy receive supportive care or palliative radiotherapy.

SEQUENCING OF EBRT AND I-131

In most situations, we recommend giving I-131 prior to EBRT. The sequencing issue is the subject of another chapter.

OPTIMAL PREPARATION FOR I-131 THERAPY

Thyroid cancer may not respond to I-131 therapy for three main reasons: Tumor cells are resistant to I-131, insufficient I-131 dose, or suboptimal preparation for I-131 therapy. Suboptimal preparation for therapy is usually the result of high dietary iodine intake prior to therapy, an insufficient TSH response to thyroid hormone withdrawal, or diagnostic studies involving iodinated contrast within a few months of I-131. Lithium (usually at 900 mg/day) for 5 days prior to, and 2 days after I-131 administration, is likely to increase the efficacy of I-131 therapy.

We reserve EBRT for situations where the risk of recurrent disease in the neck or mediastinum is high and I-131 therapy alone is unlikely to be curative. We consider persistent or recurrent tumor to be resistant to I-131 therapy to the point that we do not recommend additional I-131 therapy when disease has progressed following thyroidectomy, ablation of the thyroid remnant with I-131, and at least one additional treatment with ≥ 100 mCi I-131 with optimal preparation. We consider optimal preparation to be a two week low-iodine diet, a 24 hour urine iodine <100 μg when there is any question of iodine contamination from drugs or radiological studies, lithium pretreatment (unless there are contraindications to lithium use), thyroid hormone withdrawal sufficient to raise the serum TSH to above 30 mIU/L, or preparation with rhTSH and 4 day withdrawl of thyroid hormone.

Patients are referred to our program for treatment of metastases that have failed to respond to I-131 therapy at another facility. Regardless of the number of previous I-131 administrations, or cumulative I-131 dose, we are not comfortable concluding that additional I-131 treatments will not be effective when we do not have evidence that the patient has been optimally prepared for I-131 therapy. In patients with a diagnosis of refractory disease following I-131 therapy at another program, we usually administer one more I-131 treatment under optimal conditions to be certain that the tumor does not concentrate I-131.

INDICATIONS FOR EBRT TO THE NECK AND UPPER MEDIASTINUM

Surgery should be used to remove residual tumor whenever complete resection is likely and the risk of surgery is acceptable. The guidelines in this section apply only to situations where additional surgery is not likely to be beneficial. Table 1 and the text in the remainder of this section summarize our indications for EBRT to the neck and upper mediastinum in patients with DTC. The indications for EBRT depend mainly on the age of the patient, the likelihood that additional I-131 therapy will be curative, and the risk of residual disease in the neck or mediastinum:

Children ≤ 18 Years Old

- We avoid EBRT whenever possible in children. Even when there is gross residual disease, we use I-131 and TSH suppression in an attempt to delay tumor progression until skeletal and organ development is complete. We give EBRT only when there is no other way to palliate symptoms or prevent normal tissue damage from tumor growth.

Adults Age 19–45 Years

- In view of the risk of giving EBRT to young patients, and the lack of definitive evidence for a survival benefit from EBRT, we only give EBRT to young adults when:
  - The surgeon tells us that they did not remove all visible tumor or when we see residual tumor in the neck or mediastinum on an imaging study
  - There is no evidence of distant metastasis

- The tumor is resistant to I-131 therapy- meaning there is viable tumor following thyroidectomy, ablation of the thyroid remnant with I-131 and at least one additional treatment with ≥ 100 mCi I-131 with optimal preparation

- Regardless of the risk of tumor recurrence or the results of imaging studies, we do not give EBRT in this age group when additional I-131 therapy may be curative
- We do not give EBRT when the only evidence of disease is an elevated serum Tg level

Adults > 45 Years Old

We use EBRT (usually a few weeks after I-131 therapy) 1-3 months following thyroidectomy when there is a locally advanced tumor:

- Stage T4 primary tumor using the version of the AJCC staging system described in the 6th edition (2002) of the staging manual. In this version, T4 is defined as major tumor extension beyond the thyroid capsule to invade subcutaneous soft tissues, larynx, trachea, esophagus, recurrent laryngeal nerve, or prevertebral fascia, or tumor encasement of the carotid artery or mediastinal vessels. Extrathyroidal tumor extension that is limited to the sternothyroid muscle or perithyroidal soft tissue is stage T3
- Nodal metastasis with extension of tumor beyond the node capsule in multiple lymph nodes or complete obliteration of the node capsule in any single node.
- No major wound problems in the neck
- No evidence of distant metastasis

We use EBRT at the time of tumor recurrence when there is unresectable disease or the patient is at high risk for tumor recurrence in the neck or mediastinum following salvage surgery:

- No major wound problems in the neck
- No evidence of distant metastasis
- Unresectable tumor in the neck or mediastinum or the surgical specimen demonstrates a positive margin, extension of tumor into any of the structures that define a T4 primary tumor as described above, or extracapsular lymph nodal extension of tumor
- The patient's life expectancy is >2 years
- We do not give EBRT when the only evidence of disease is an elevated serum Tg level

We use EBRT when tumor recurrence in the neck or mediastinum is visible only on a nuclear medicine study and additional surgery or I-131 therapy is unlikely to be beneficial:

- In our program, the usual scenario where we encounter this situation is a positive FDG-PET scan in a part of the mediastinum that is not abnormal on CT or MR scan

- In most situations we require an elevated serum Tg level in addition to the abnormal nuclear medicine study before giving EBRT
- We only give EBRT when tumor is resistant to I-131 therapy- meaning there is viable tumor following thyroidectomy, ablation of the thyroid remnant with I-131, and at least one additional treatment with ≥ 100 mCi I-131 with optimal preparation.
- We do not give EBRT if there is evidence of distant metastasis or the patient's life expectancy is <2 years

REFERENCES

Farahati, J, C Reiners, M Stuschke, et al. 1996. Differentiated thyroid cancer: Impact of adjuvant external radiotherapy in patients with perithyroidal tumor infiltration. Cancer **77**:172–180.

Samaan, NA, PN Schultz, RC Hickey, H Goepfert, TP Haynie, DA Johnston, and NG Ordonez. 1992. The results of various modalities of treatment of well differentiated thyroid carcinomas: a retrospective review of 1599 patients. J Clin Endocrinol Metab **75**:714–720.

Tubiana, M, E Haddad, M Schlumberger, et al. 1985. External radiotherapy in thyroid cancers. Cancer **55**:2062–2071.

9.3. SEQUENCING OF I-131 AND EXTERNAL BEAM RADIATION THERAPY FOR DIFFERENTIATED THYROID CANCER

ROBERT J. AMDUR, MD AND ERNEST L. MAZZAFERRI, MD, MACP

When a patient is going to receive both I-131 and External Beam Radiotherapy (EBRT), we have to decide on the timing of these modalities. Our discussion of this topic will be brief because there are no data specific to this subject.

WE PREFER TO GIVE I-131 BEFORE EBRT

Many review articles and textbook chapters emphasize the importance of giving I-131 prior to EBRT to decrease the chance of thyroid stunning. Thyroid stunning is the subject of a previous chapter. Thyroid stunning refers to a decrease in the ability of a cell to concentrate I-131 as a result of prior radiation exposure.

We agree in general with this recommendation with some qualifications. First, there are no data evaluating the affect of EBRT on subsequent I-131 uptake. While it makes sense that EBRT may cause thyroid stunning, it is also possible that the hyperemia that occurs in tissues 2–6 weeks after EBRT could improve the delivery of I-131 to cancer deposits. The point is that EBRT may not influence I-131 uptake the same way that prior I-131 administration does.

The second qualification is that there are situations where delaying EBRT for months after surgery will decrease the chance of tumor cure. We know that delaying the initiation of EBRT following cancer surgery decreases the chance of cure in multiple kinds of cancer. The mechanism for this observation is "accelerated repopulation of malignant clonogens"—a term that describes the accelerated growth of the cancer cells that remain following subtotal resection. Studies in squamous cell carcinoma demonstrate that control rates drop significantly when the interval between surgery and radiotherapy is greater than 6–8 weeks. We do not know the kinetics of thyroid cancer repopulation but the relationship between overall treatment time and cure rate is likely to exist in all tumor systems.

MAKE IT A PRIORITY TO START EBRT WITHIN 8 WEEKS OF SURGERY

Our policy is to make it a priority to start EBRT within 8 weeks of surgery when there are no major wound problems in the neck. In patients who are also going to receive I-131, we try to deliver the I-131 within 6 weeks after surgery. As explained in other chapters, we are comfortable giving I-131 therapy with rhTSH stimulation. This makes it possible to shorten the overall I-131 treatment package to 2 weeks. Requiring the standard 6 weeks of T4 deprivation prior to I-131 makes it difficult to start EBRT within a few months of surgery.

WE USUALLY START EBRT 2 WEEKS AFTER I-131

Our goal is to keep the overall treatment time as short as possible. We schedule a whole body scan (RxWBS) 5–7 days following I-131 administration. We usually simulate the patient for EBRT the week following the RxWBS and start EBRT the week following simulation.

9.4. INDICATIONS FOR EBRT FOR MEDULLARY AND ANAPLASTIC THYROID CARCINOMA

ROBERT J. AMDUR, MD, WILLIAM M. MENDENHALL, MD, AND
ERNEST L. MAZZAFERRI, MD, MACP

The purpose of this chapter is to present indications for using external beam radiation therapy (EBRT) in patients with Medullary and Anaplastic thyroid cancer. Radiotherapy dose schedules and techniques are in the subject of other chapters in this section of this book.

MEDULLARY THYROID CANCER

The role of therapy other than surgical resection in patients with medullary carcinoma is controversial. These tumors do not concentrate radioiodine. We do not use radioiodine with the idea that radioiodine concentration in normal tissue will destroy nearby medullary carcinoma cells. There are data to suggest that postoperative EBRT increases the chance of cure of medullary cancer but all of these data come from retrospective series (see reference list at the end of this chapter). Some experts think that the only role for EBRT in medullary cancer is to palliate symptoms of terminal cancer.

Survival data on patients with medullary carcinoma suggest that cure is likely when tumor is confined to the thyroid gland and possible with metastatic disease in the neck. According to National Cancer Institute data from Hundahl et al. (1998), of 53,856 cases of thyroid carcinoma treated in the US between 1985-1995, 4% were medullary thyroid cancers, in which the 10-year relative survival was 75%. However, survival depends upon the disease stage at the time of diagnosis. According to the 6th edition of the AJCC staging manual (2002), the 5-year survival for patients with medullary carcinoma, relative to age-matched patients who do not have cancer, is approximately 95% for stage I-II disease, 75% for stage III and 25% for stage IV. These data suggest

Table 1. Indications for External Beam Radiation Therapy for Medullary Thyroid Cancer.

Indications for EBRT[1] for medullary thyroid cancer	
Child **Age ≤ 18 years**	Give EBRT only when there is no other way to palliate symptoms or prevent normal tissue damage from tumor growth
Adults **Age > 18 years**	Offer EBRT for unresectable disease or when the surgical specimen demonstrates a positive margin, invasion of normal tissues that define a T4[2] primary tumor, or nodal metastasis with extensive extracapsular tumor extension

[1] EBRT = External beam radiotherapy.
[2] High-risk features include: positive surgical margin, invasion of normal tissues that classify a tumor as stage T4 in the 6th edition (year 2002) of the AJCC staging system, or nodal metastasis with extensive extra capsular tumor extension.

that medullary cancer spreads in an orderly fashion from primary site to regional nodes and tissues immediately adjacent to the thyroid. Distant metastases are less common in patients with low volume disease in the neck.

Table 1 summarizes our guidelines for using EBRT in patients with medullary thyroid carcinoma. In our opinion, EBRT is likely to be curative in patients with low-volume residual disease following surgery and palliative in patients with incurable disease that is causing symptoms. We recognize the lack of data to support these assumptions and therefore do not consider EBRT in patients where the toxicity of EBRT is likely to be high or in patients with a short life expectancy due to other medical problems. For example, we do not recommend EBRT following surgical resection in children and young adults, even when we know that there is residual disease. In this age group, we prefer to let time pass and attempt to treat recurrences with additional surgery. In older adults with a life expectancy of at least 5 years, we are more aggressive about the use of EBRT.

ANAPLASTIC CARCINOMA

Anaplastic carcinoma has a terrible prognosis. The 6th edition of the AJCC staging manual (2002) classifies all anaplastic carcinomas as stage T4 and group IV regardless of tumor size or other factors. Cure is rare and the chance of five-year survival is approximately 10%.

It is not clear that any form of therapy improves the outcome of patients with anaplastic thyroid cancer if the tumor invades extrathyroidal tissues. When total resection of the tumor is surgically possible, this should be the goal of initial treatment. The potential for a gross total resection is important to consider because debulking procedures that leave gross tumor are rarely helpful.

Anaplastic carcinoma does not concentrate radioiodine. We do not use radioiodine with the idea that radioiodine concentration in normal tissue will destroy nearby carcinoma cells. EBRT is the standard treatment. In most cases, the goal of radiotherapy is temporary palliation of symptoms. There are now several reports that suggest that chemotherapy may improve the response rate of anaplastic carcinoma following radiotherapy. We include the major series that evaluate the role of EBRT or chemotherapy in the reference list at the end of this chapter.

With the exception of the rare case of a small anaplastic tumor found at the time of thyroidectomy, we are not convinced that anaplastic carcinoma extending beyond

Table 2. Indications for External Beam Radiation Therapy for Anaplastic Thyroid Cancer.

Indications for EBRT[1] for anaplastic thyroid cancer	
Age < 18 years	Anaplastic carcinoma rarely occurs in this age group
Age > 18 years	Always offer EBRT

[1] EBRT = External beam radiotherapy.

the thyroid gland is a curable disease and often see no palliative response to high-dose radiation therapy. For this reason, we do not push patients with anaplastic thyroid carcinoma to undergo EBRT therapy, especially if there are distant metastases and there is no threat of local disease invading the airway. When we think it is reasonable to offer EBRT, we explain the low likelihood of benefit and the potential for serious toxicity. We emphasize that it is reasonable for the patient to choose not to receive EBRT. We prefer to use chemotherapy only on a research protocol.

Table 2 presents our guidelines for offering EBRT to patients with anaplastic thyroid carcinoma. Each case is individualized. We offer EBRT to almost all adults with anaplastic thyroid cancer.

REFERENCES

American Joint Committee on Cancer. 2002. AJCC Cancer Staging Handbook From The AJCC Cancer Staging Manual, 6th edn. New York: Springer **22**:95–96.

Brierley, J, and HR Maxon. 1998. Radioiodine and external radiation therapy in the treatment of thyroid cancer. In: Thyroid Cancer. Boston/Dordrecht/London: Kluwer Academic Publishers (Fagin JA, ed) 285–317.

9.5. CONVENTIONAL RADIOTHERAPY TECHNIQUE FOR TREATING THYROID CANCER

ROBERT J. AMDUR, MD, SIYONG KIM, PhD, JONATHAN GANG LI, PhD, CHIRAY LIU, PhD, WILLIAM M. MENDENHALL, MD, AND ERNEST L. MAZZAFERRI, MD, MACP

The term "conventional radiotherapy" refers to techniques that do not involve segmental modulation of beam intensity. Intensity Modulation Radiation Therapy and Tomotherapy are examples of delivery systems that are not conventional radiotherapy.

The radiation oncology literature contains descriptions of many different conventional radiotherapy techniques for treating patients with thyroid cancer. The use of different techniques is not surprising because thyroid cancer presents the radiation oncology planning team with a difficult technical challenge. The basic problem is that the primary target volume (the thyroid bed) is in the midline of the body, extends both above and below the level of the shoulders, and requires a dose that exceeds spinal cord tolerance.

The standard approach to irradiating a midline target in the neck to a dose above spinal cord tolerance is to deliver a portion of the dose with opposed lateral fields that exclude the spinal cord. The problem with this approach for thyroid cancer is that a lateral field that extends above and below the shoulders will produce a high dose gradient across midline structures. Specifically, midline dose above the shoulders is too high when the dose is specified at midline below the plane of the shoulders and too low below the shoulders when the dose is specified in the neck.

There is no consensus within the radiation oncology community on how to manage the competing goals of target coverage, spinal cord shielding, and dose homogeneity in patients with thyroid cancer. Almost every textbook chapter and journal article on this subject describes a different radiotherapy technique. We include references at the end of this chapter that describe the range of conventional radiotherapy techniques for thyroid cancer. Every technique has advantages and disadvantages. At the University of Florida,

Table 1. Conventional Radiotherapy Dose Guidelines for Thyroid Cancer.

Conventional Radiotherapy Dose Guidelines for Thyroid Cancer

INITIAL FIELDS:

45 @ 1.8/treatment (25 treatment days) using 6 MV photons through opposed
anterior and posterior fields

PHOTON BOOST FIELDS:

Standard-risk subclinical disease: 18 @ 1.8/treatment (10 treatment days) using
20 MV photons through opposed lateral fields that exclude the spinal cord with tissue
compensators on the shoulders.

• Total dose: 63 @ 1.8/treatment (35 treatments over 7 weeks)

High-risk subclinical or gross disease: 25.2 @ 1.8/treatment (14 treatment days)
using 20 MV photons through opposed lateral fields that exclude the spinal cord with
tissue compensators on the shoulders. High-risk subclinical disease usually means a
positive surgical margin or nodal metastases with extensive extracapsular extension.

• Total dose: 70.2 @ 1.8/treatment (39 treatments over 8 weeks)

ELECTRON BOOST (POSTERIOR NECK STRIP) FIELDS:
(treated on the same days as the photon boost fields)

The level V nodes and soft tissue of the neck posterior to the plane of the spinal cord are
boosted to 50.4–70.2 at 1.8/treatment using 8–12 MeV electrons through lateral fields
that match to the posterior border of the photon boost fields above the shoulders.

• Total dose: 50.4–70.2 @1.8/treatment

We usually boost the posterior strip of a hemineck to 70.2 with pathologically positive
nodes in level V, a pathologically positive margin in the neck near the plain of the spinal
cord, or gross residual disease. Other situations receive 50.4 or 63.

our preference is to use Intensity Modulated Radiation Therapy (IMRT) in patients
with thyroid cancer. Our IMRT technique is the subject of the next chapter. When we
treat thyroid cancer with conventional radiotherapy, we use a technique that is so old
that it predates the era of CT treatment planning. Basically, we build tissue compensators
on the shoulders so that we can use standard lateral fields to treat the thyroid bed above
spinal cord tolerance.

TISSUE COMPENSATORS ON THE SHOULDERS

We deliver 45 Gy with 6 MV photons through opposed anterior and posterior fields
that cover most of the level II–VII nodes bilaterally (Fig. 1). After 45 Gy, we use opposed

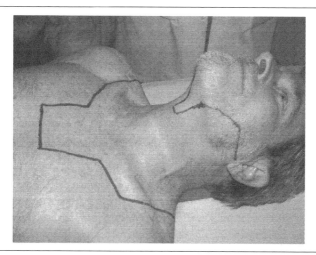

Figure 1. Usual borders of the anterior and posterior 6 MV photon fields that are used to deliver the first 45 Gy (prescribed at midplane) in patients with thyroid cancer.

lateral fields that exclude the spinal cord (Fig. 2). The posterior border of these lateral fields is near the middle of the vertebral bodies. The lateral fields are treated with 18–20 MV photons to the final prescription midline dose. Radiation therapists position the lateral fields each day using laser coordinates and field borders drawn on the skin.

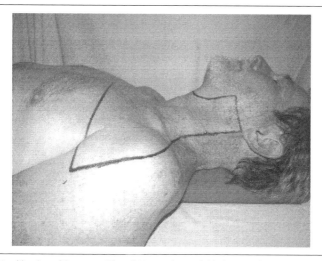

Figure 2. Usual borders of the opposed lateral 20 MV photon fields that start following the completion of therapy through opposed anterior and posterior fields. The posterior border of the lateral photon fields is located along the midline of the vertebral bodies.

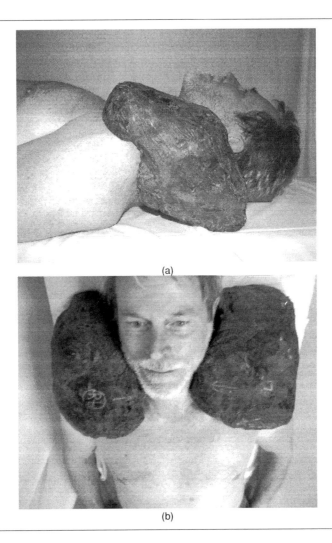

(a)

(b)

Figure 3. Lateral (A) and superior (B) direction view of the tissue compensators that are used to prevent large dose gradients at midline above and below the level of the shoulders. We use beeswax but commercial products are readily available that work well for this purpose (Radiation Products Design, Inc. at www.rpdinc.com).

When the patient is in the correct position, the therapists place tissue compensators on the shoulders (Fig. 3). These compensators must be made of a material that is easy to conform to the shape of the patients shoulder and has an electron density that is similar to tissue. We make the compensators out of beeswax that we buy from a local beekeeper. Super Stuff Bolus Material is a commercial product that is equally useful (Radiation

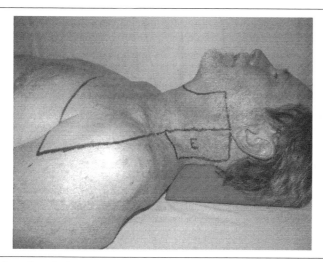

Figure 4. The nodes and soft tissue posterior to the lateral photon fields (and overlying the spinal cord) are boosted with 8-10 MeV electron beams. The photon fields are treated first with the tissue compensators in place. The posterior border of the photon fields is drawn on the skin each day. After removing the tissue compensators, the poster neck strips are treated with electrons. The anterior border of the electron field matches the posterior border of the lateral photon fields on the skin.

Products Design, Inc. at www.rpdinc.com). It is essential that the compensators extend to the edge of the shoulder laterally and beyond the field border superiorly.

The use of tissue compensators eliminates the skin sparing normally associated with high-energy photon beams. When treating patients to a total dose of 70.2-74.4 Gy, we see small areas of moist desquamation of the neck skin. Overall, the acute toxicity and frequency of late complications is similar to what we see with without tissue compensators. It is rare to see skin fibrosis or shoulder problems from radiotherapy.

We treat the tissue posterior to the posterior border of the lateral photon fields with 8-12 MeV electrons depending on the estimated depth of nodal tissue (Fig. 4). The therapists remove the compensators when treating electron fields. The anterior border of the electron field matches to the posterior border of the lateral photon field. The posterior border of the electron field is usually just posterior to the spinous process of the second cervical vertebra. The superior border is at the superior border of C-2 and the inferior border is at the junction of the neck and shoulder.

9.6. INTENSITY MODULATED RADIATION THERAPY FOR THYROID CANCER

ROBERT J. AMDUR, MD, SIYONG KIM, PhD, JONATHAN GANG LI, PhD, CHIRAY LIU, PhD, WILLIAM M. MENDENHALL, MD, AND ERNEST L. MAZZAFERRI, MD, MACP

Intensity Modulated Radiation Therapy (IMRT) is a technology that makes it possible to shape the radiation dose distribution in a way that is not possible with conventional delivery systems. The main rationale for using IMRT is to decrease normal tissue damage. However, there are people who talk about IMRT as if it were a fundamentally different kind of radiation therapy. This is not the situation. All of the hardware- meaning the machines that generate the radiation beam, the blocking devices, and the imaging equipment- used with IMRT is the same as that currently used for conventional radiotherapy. The unique thing about IMRT is the computer software that plans and directs radiation delivery. With IMRT, computer programs direct radiation blocking devices (multileaf collimators) to split a small number of conventional radiotherapy beams into a large number (sometimes hundreds) of small "beamlettes". The IMRT planning program is able to adjust the shape and intensity of each beamlette in a way that matches the radiation dose distribution to the shape of the target volume better than conventional radiation therapy systems. A more detailed explanation of IMRT is beyond the scope of this book and not necessary to understand the role of IMRT in treating patients with thyroid cancer.

THE ROLE OF IMRT FOR THYROID CANCER

At the University of Florida we have a large-volume IMRT program for head and neck cancer and are enthusiastic about its value in the right setting. In our opinion, conventional radiotherapy is just as good as IMRT for thyroid cancer when radiotherapy is planned and executed properly. However, as we explain in the previous chapter, there

Table 1. University of Florida IMRT Dose Schedule for Thyroid Cancer.

UF IMRT Dose Schedule for Thyroid Cancer (All doses are specified in Gray).

	PTV standard-risk	PTV high-risk
Plan #1 treated **MORNINGS** for 30 days	$1.65 \times 30 = 49.5$	$1.8 \times 30 = 54$
Plan #2 treated **AFTERNOONS** for 6 or 12 days	—	Usually: $1.5 \times 6 = 9$ High-risk*: $1.5 \times 12 = 18$
Total dose	49.5 @ 1.65/treatment once-a-day × 30 days (6 weeks)	Usually: 63 @ 1.8 and 1.5/treatment High-risk*: 72 @ 1.8 and 1.5/treatment 30 treatment days with 1.5 given as the second treatment of the day on the last 6 or 12 treatment days**

* High-risk means a positive surgical margin or nodal metastases with extensive extracapsular extension.
** 6 hours between 1.8 and 1.5 Gy treatments.

is no standard or simple conventional radiotherapy solution to the problem of a midline target volume that crosses the level of the shoulders, and must be treated to a dose that exceeds spinal cord tolerance.

We use IMRT to treat most patients with thyroid cancer because it is easier for us to manage the problem of a target volume that straddles the level of the shoulders with IMRT than it is with a conventional radiotherapy plan. We are familiar with, and have confidence in, our conventional radiotherapy technique but still find it demanding to implement properly. In our department, it takes more time and effort to treat a thyroid cancer patient with conventional radiotherapy than it does with IMRT. We are not critical of groups that use conventional radiotherapy to treat thyroid cancer as long as they plan and execute the therapy properly.

DOSE AND FRACTIONATION GUIDELINES

Table 1 summarizes the University of Florida dose and fractionation guidelines for thyroid cancer. There are two main differences between our IMRT program and that used at other institutions. The first difference is that we use two IMRT plans. We use two IMRT plans for the same reason that we make field reductions in conventional radiotherapy- it is difficult to get a large difference between the dose to different target volumes if a single plan is used for the entire treatment. Our initial IMRT plan treats both standard and high-risk target volumes. The second plan treats only high-risk areas. Guidelines for drawing target volumes are the subject of the next chapter.

The second unusual feature of our IMRT program is that it uses twice-a-day fractionation. Multiple studies show that accelerated and hyperfractionated dose schedules improve the therapeutic ratio of radiation therapy. To limit the number of twice-a-day treatments, we designed our IMRT program to duplicate the M.D. Anderson Hospital

Table 2. Technical Parameters of the UF IMRT Program for Thyroid Cancer.

Technical Parameters of the UF IMRT Program for Thyroid Cancer

Planning System	Pinnacle (version 7.06)	
Delivery Machine	Elekta SLI	
Collimation	80 Multileaf. Leaf width 1 cm	
Beam Energy	6 MV photon	
Plane of all beams	Axial (couch angle 0 degrees)	
5 Beam angles	Typically: 20, 70, 135, 225, 320 degree (12 O'clock = 0 degree)	
CTV expansion	PTV = CTV + 3mm	

	Plan #1 (Initial)	Plan #2 (Boost)
	PTV standard risk:	PTV high-risk:
Prescribed Dose	49.5 @ 1.65 Gy/treatment	9 or 18 @ 1.5 Gy/treatment
	PTV high-risk:	given in the afternoon of the last
	54 @ 1.8 Gy/treatment	6 or 12 days of treatment

Beam angle	Monitor Units	Segments	Beam angle	Monitor Units	Segments
20^0	103	20	20^0	42	8
70^0	111	11	70^0	115	12
135^0	181	17	135^0	118	12
225^0	156	12	225^0	149	12
320^0	94	17	320^0	48	8

concomitant boost schedule. Our IMRT fractionation schedule is the same as that used in the M.D. Anderson program except that we treat the standard-risk volume at 1.65 Gy per day as opposed to 1.8 Gy. The total prescribed dose in our IMRT program is either 63 or 72 Gy depending on the risk of recurrence. The only difference between these two dose schedules is the number of days in which the patient receives an afternoon treatment.

TECHNICAL PARAMETERS

Tables 2, 3, 4 and 5 present the technical parameters of our IMRT program for thyroid cancer. While many of these parameters will only be useful to groups that use the Pinnacle planning system, the main features of the program will be useful to anyone who is interested in optimizing IMRT for thyroid cancer.

Table 3. Target and Normal Tissue Goals for IMRT Plans.

Target and Normal Tissue Goals for IMRT Plans

Structure	Goals
Each PTV	95% of the PTV receives the prescription dose
	99% of the PTV receives $\geq$ 93% of the prescription dose
	20% of the PTV receives $\leq$ 110% of the prescription dose
Spinal cord + 3 mm	0.1 cc receives $\leq$ 50 Gy
Parotid glands + 3 mm	Mean dose to at least one gland is $\leq$ 26 Gy

Table 4. Optimization objectives for IMRT plan #1 (Initial).

| Optimization Objectives for IMRT Plan #1 (Initial) | | | | |
Region of interest	Type	Target cGy	% Volume	Weight
PTV 49.5 Gy	Uniform Dose	5198	—	1.0
PTV 49.5 Gy	Min DVH	5198	95	1.0
PTV 49.5 Gy	Min Dose	4600	—	1.5
PTV 54/72 Gy	Uniform Dose	5670	—	0.8
PTV 54/72 Gy	Min DVH	5670	95	0.8
Spinal cord + 3 mm	Max DVH	3000	50	0.2
Spinal cord + 3 mm	Max Dose	3300	—	0.6
Rt Parotid + 3 mm (minus PTV)	Max DVH	2000	50	0.2
Rt Parotid + 3 mm (minus PTV)	Max DVH	2600	30	0.2
Lt Parotid + 3 mm (minus PTV)	Max DVH	2000	50	0.2
Lt Parotid + 3 mm (minus PTV)	Max DVH	2600	30	0.2
Skin (minus PTV)	Max Dose	4900	—	1.5

DOSE DISTRIBUTIONS AND DOSE-VOLUME HISTOGRAMS

The endpoints used to evaluate and compare radiation therapy plans are the dose distribution across images that show the anatomy of interest and dose-volume histograms of targets and important normal structures. Space does not permit a display of all of the dose distributions that we review when evaluating an IMRT plan. Figure 1 shows representative dose-distributions in the coronal plane for Initial (A), Boost (B), and Composit (C) plans. Note that in the Initial IMRT plan (Fig. 1A), there is relatively little separation between the 49.5 and 54 Gy isodose lines, which indicates that a large portion of the standard-risk Planning Target Volume (PTV) receives the dose that we prescribe to the high-risk PTV. To limit the dose to tissues outside the high-risk PTV, we use a separate IMRT plan (Fig. 1B) to "Boost" the high-risk PTV to the final prescription dose (63 or 72 Gy). As shown in the Composit plan (Fig. 1C), the use of two separate IMRT plans results in a dose distribution where the 63 or 72 Gy isodose line conforms to the high-risk PTV.

Figure 2 shows dose-volume histograms (DVHs) for the Initial (A), Boost (B), and Composit (C) plans. In most patients, we expand the Clinical Target Volumes and

Table 5. Optimization Objectives for IMRT Plan #2 (Boost).

| Optimization objectives for IMRT plan #2 (boost) | | | | |
Region of Interest	Type	Target cGy	% Volume	Weight
PTV 54/72 Gy	Uniform Dose	1890	—	1.0
PTV 54/72 Gy	Min DVH	1890	95	1.0
Spinal cord + 3 mm	Max DVH	500	50	0.2
Spinal cord + 3 mm	Max Dose	1000	—	0.6
Rt Parotid + 3 mm (minus PTV)	Max DVH	700	50	0.2
Rt Parotid + 3 mm (minus PTV)	Max DVH	850	20	0.2
Lt Parotid + 3 mm (minus PTV)	Max DVH	700	50	0.2
Lt Parotid + 3 mm (minus PTV)	Max DVH	850	30	0.2
Skin (minus PTV)	Max Dose	1800	—	1.5

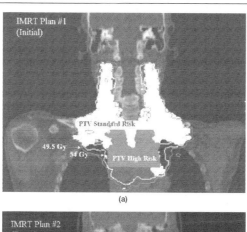

(a)

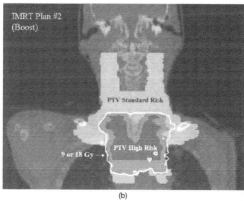

(b)

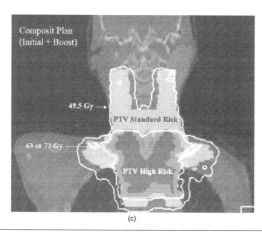

(c)

Figure 1. Coronal images showing the isodose distribution with the Initial (A), Boost (B), and Composit (C) IMRT plans.

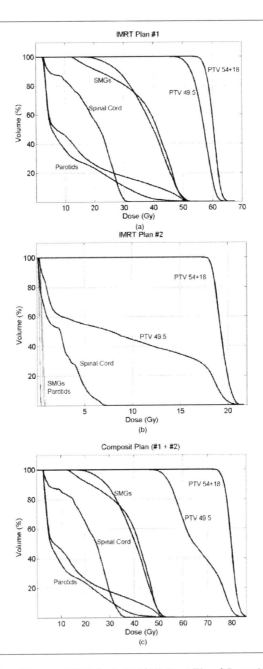

Figure 2. Dose–volume histograms (DVHs) for the Initial (A), Boost (B), and Composit (C) IMRT plans in a patient with a stage T4aN1b papillary carcinoma with positive nodes confined to the low level III, level IV and level VI regions.

normal structure volumes by 3 mm in all directions to account for setup uncertainty and organ motion. In other words, The Planning Target Volume (PTV) = the Clinical Target Volume + 3 mm and the Planning Organ at Risk Volume (PRV) = the Organ at Risk Volume + 3 mm.

We evaluate IMRT plans with the DVHs for the Planning Target Volumes and Planning Organ at Risk Volumes. Our target coverage goal is that at least 95% of the PTV receives the prescription dose and that 99% of the PTV receives at least 93% of the prescription dose. Our main tissue sparing goals are that the mean dose to at least one parotid PRV is ≤ 26 Gy and the dose to 0.1 cc of the spinal cord PRV is ≤ 50 Gy. Figure 2 demonstrates that we have met these goals.

9.7. DRAWING TARGET VOLUMES FOR INTENSITY MODULATED RADIATION THERAPY FOR THYROID CANCER

ROBERT J. AMDUR, MD, JONATHAN GANG LI, PhD, SIYONG KIM, PhD, CHIRAY LIU, PhD, WILLIAM M. MENDENHALL, MD, AND ERNEST L. MAZZAFERRI, MD, MACP

There are no standardized guidelines for drawing target contours for radiotherapy for thyroid cancer. The purpose of this chapter is to review the normal anatomic relationships that guide target definition and to present the contour atlas that we use to plan radiotherapy.

THE THYROID WRAPS AROUND THE INFERIOR HALF OF THE LARYNX

It is not possible to irradiate the thyroid bed without delivering the prescription dose to most of the larynx. Figure 1A is an anterior view of the relationship of the thyroid to the larynx. Figure 1B is a digitally reconstructed radiograph (DRR) that we created by contouring the thyroid gland, bottom of the cricoid cartilage, true vocal cords, and hyoid bone on axial images of a contrast-enhanced CT scan of a patient with normal anatomy. The important thing to notice from Fig. 1A and 1B is that the upper poles of the lateral lobes of the thyroid gland extend to the level of the undersurface of the true vocal cords. This means that the thyroid overlies the inferior half of the larynx.

Figure 1C shows why it is not possible to spare the posterior portion of the larynx when irradiating a patient with thyroid cancer. The lateral lobes of the thyroid wrap around the inferior half of the larynx and superior portion of the trachea. The posterior extent of the superior tip of the lateral lobe of the thyroid is at level of the arytenoids.

The variable extent and location of the pyramidal lobe of the thyroid further increases the uncertainty of target definition and serves to expand the superior extent of the target volume. In most of our plans, the majority of the larynx receives the dose that we prescribe to the high-risk target volume (63 or 72 Gy).

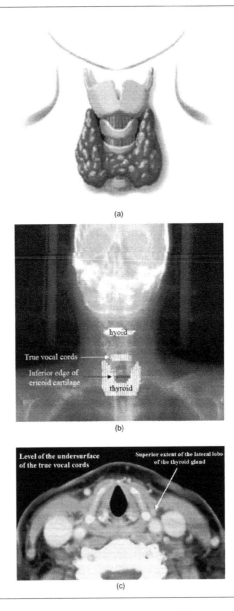

(a)

(b)

(c)

Figure 1. Artist illustration (A) of the relationship of the thyroid to the larynx on anterior view [Reproduced with permission from Forest Pharmecuticals, amourthyroid.com, 2005], Digitally Reconstructed Radiograph (DRR) after contouring the hyoid bone, thyroid gland, true vocal cords, and inferior edge of the cricoid cartilage on axial CT images of a person with normal anatomy (B), and axial contrast-enhanced CT image at the level of the undersurface of the true vocal cords (C). These figures show why most of the larynx receives the dose that we prescribe to the thyroid bed.

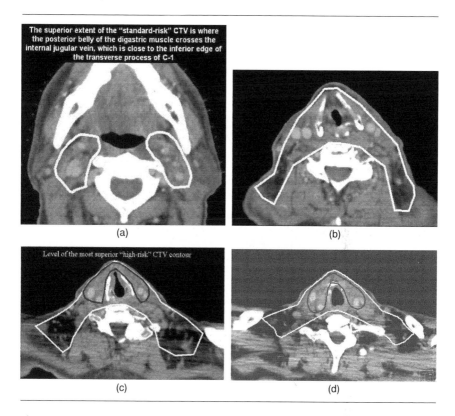

Figure 2. CTV contours for radiotherapy following thyroidectomy and neck dissection for stage T4aN1b papillary carcinoma with positive nodes confined to levels III–IV and VI. The white line defines the standard-risk CTV and the black (inner) line defines the high-risk CTV. In the absence of positive nodes in level II, the superior extent of the standard-risk CTV is at the level where the posterior belly of the digastric muscle crosses the jugular vein (A). At the level of the thyroid notch the standard-risk CTV covers the level V space bilaterally and the entire larynx (B). The most superior extent of the high-risk CTV is at the level of the undersurface of the true vocal cords (C). The inferior extent of the high-risk CTV is at the level of the arch of the aorta (F). The inferior extent of the standard-risk CTV is at the level of the carina (G).

GUIDELINES FOR CONTOURING TARGET VOLUMES

Figure 2 presents seven axial images from a CT scan that we used to plan IMRT in a patient with a T4aN1b papillary carcinoma with positive nodes confined to the low level III, level IV and level VI regions. We use the contours in Fig. 2 as a reference atlas that helps to simplify the contouring process and to standardize target volume definition among the different physicians in our group.

References at the end of this chapter review the boundaries of nodal stations based on CT scan anatomy and show examples of Clinical Target Volume (CTV) contours.

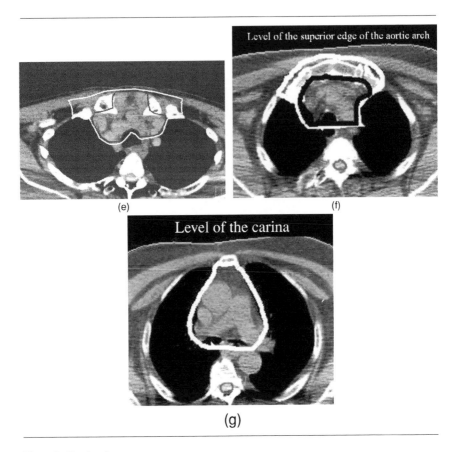

Figure 2. Continued.

In the absence of adenopathy in level II, we place the most superior standard-risk CTV contour at the level where the posterior belly of the digastric muscle crosses the jugular vein. In terms of bony anatomy, this usually corresponds to the level of the caudal edge of the transverse process of the first cervical vertebra. Excluding the most superior few centimeters of the level II nodes from the target volume makes it possible to keep the mean dose to the parotid below 26 Gy. However, when there is level II adenopathy we extend the "standard-risk" CTV on the side of the involved nodes to the jugular foramen.

As shown in Fig. 2B–D, we include the entire larynx in the "standard-risk" CTV. With our planning system, excluding the superior and central portions of the larynx from the CTV does not decrease larynx dose to a meaningful degree. With better software, it may be possible to achieve better dose distributions around the larynx but larynx motion will likely require PTV expansions that will make it difficult to exclude major portions of the larynx from the high-dose volume.

In Fig. 2C, the most superior "high-risk" CTV contour is at the level of the under-surface of the true vocal cords. We are reluctant to move this boundary more inferiorly in a patient with indications for external beam radiotherapy.

In Fig. 2F, the most inferior high-risk CTV contour is at the level of the arch of the aorta but should be extended more inferiorly in patients with level VII adenopathy. In Figure 2G, the inferior extent of the standard-risk CTV is at the level of the carina.

9.8. POTENTIAL TOXICITY OF EXTERNAL BEAM RADIOTHERAPY FOR THYROID CANCER

ROBERT J. AMDUR, MD, WILLIAM M. MENDENHALL, MD, AND
ERNEST L. MAZZAFERRI, MD, MACP

External Beam Radiotherapy (EBRT) for thyroid cancer causes acute side-effects and carries the risk of severe, permanent damage to normal tissues. The purpose of this chapter is to explain the problems patients may develop during and after EBRT in a way that helps both clinicians and patients evaluate the risk/benefit profile of EBRT in specific situations and to manage reactions to EBRT when they occur. The information in this chapter applies to EBRT with curative intent. The dose schedules that we use to palliate incurable disease are less toxic.

Data on the incidence of specific complications from EBRT for thyroid cancer are scarce. To inform patients and make decisions about giving EBRT we extrapolate from studies of patients with nonthyroidal malignancies. The incidence values that we present in this chapter are a combination of our interpretation of published studies on EBRT for thyroid and nonthyroid tumors as well as our unpublished experience over the past few decades.

SIDE-EFFECTS VERSUS COMPLICATIONS

Radiobiologists classify radiation effects on normal tissues as either acute side-effects or late complications. A detailed explanation of the rationale for this subdivision is beyond the scope of this chapter. Briefly, an acute side-effect results from radiation damage to rapidly dividing tissues such as the mucosa of upper aerodigestive tract, hair follicles, and epidermis while a late complication is the result of irreversible damage to cells that sustain long-term tissue integrity. In most situations, late radiation complications are due to damage to capillary endothelial cells, connective tissue fibroblasts, or neuroglial cells.

Table 1. Acute Side-Effects of External Beam Radiotherapy for Thyroid Cancer.

Acute side-effect*	Incidence
Overall acute side-effect incidence	Mild: 100% Moderate: 75% Severe: 2% Fatal: rare
Pharyngitis/Esophagitis	Requiring narcotics: 100% Requiring IV fluids as an outpatient: 20% Requiring a percutaneous feeding tube: 5%
Laryngitis	Causing discomfort and hoarseness: 75%
Skin reaction	Producing mild-moderate discomfort: 100% Ulceration requiring wound care: 1%
Nausea	Requiring antiemetics: 20%
Taste disturbance	Effecting eating habits: 100%
A disturbance, such as stress, dehydration, electrolyte imbalance, or infection, leading to myocardial infarction, stroke, pneumonia or other serious, but not fatal, problems	2%
Toxicity leading to a fatal event	rare

* Acute side-effects usually begin ~3 weeks after starting radiotherapy and usually resolve within 2 months of completing radiotherapy.

Table 2. Potential Late Complications of External Beam Radiotherapy for Thyroid Cancer.

Late complication*	Incidence (estimated life-time risk)
Overall complication risk	Moderate: 10% Severe: 2% Fatal: rare
Dry mouth	Mild-moderate: 50% Severe: 10%
Laryngeal edema	Effecting speech or swallowing: 25% Requiring tracheostomy tube: 2%
Laryngeal necrosis	Requiring laryngectomy: 1%
Esophageal or pharyngeal dysfunction	Requiring a special diet: 10% Requiring percutaneous feeding tube: 2%
Recurrent laryngeal nerve injury	Rare
Brachial plexopathy	Causing mild-moderate pain or weakness: 2% Causing severe pain or a useless extremity: rare
Carotid artery occlusion	~5%(risk from radiotherapy is unclear)
Spinal cord myelopathy	Rare
Pathologic fracture of clavicle or rib	Rare
Fibrosis of soft tissues of the neck	Causing mild-moderate discomfort: 15% Causing severe discomfort: 2%
Persistent skin ulceration	Rare
Hypoparathyroidism from EBRT	Rare
A radiation-induced second malignancy	Rare (more likely in patients who live for decades after radiotherapy)

* A late complication is a problem that develops or persists for more than 6 months after the completion of radiotherapy and is usually a permanent, or chronically recurring, problem.

Examples of late radiation complications are soft tissue fibrosis, esophageal stricture, persistent mucosal or skin ulceration, bone necrosis, and neuropathy.

RADIATION INDUCED SECOND MALIGNANCY

A special type of late complication from radiation therapy is a radiation-induced malignancy. Multiple papers document second malignancies following EBRT for thyroid cancer. The reference list at the end of this chapter contains articles that review the second malignancy issue in general and others that describe specific cases of second malignancies following radiation therapy for thyroid cancer.

PART 10. REFERENCE INFORMATION FOR PHYSICIANS AND PATIENTS

10.1. RESOURCE WEBSITES

ROBERT J. AMDUR, MD AND ERNEST L. MAZZAFERRI, MD, MACP

The purpose of this chapter is to list the major public-access websites that have information about thyroid cancer. Access to these websites is free and does not require pre-registration or organizational membership. In general the information is high-quality and up-to-date. Some of these websites are oriented to physicians while others are oriented to patients. All provide an enormous amount of information that will be useful to patients or health professionals who want to learn more about the topics that we discuss in this book.

NCCN MANAGEMENT GUIDELINES

http://www.nccn.org/professionals/physician_gls/PDF/thyroid.pdf

The National Comprehensive Cancer Network (NCCN) consists of the institutions that receive Comprehensive Cancer Center funding from the National Cancer Institute. The NCCN convenes a group of experts to draw up guidelines for management of each type of cancer. The thyroid cancer guidelines are updated frequently (most recently in year 2004). Some of the recommendations that we make in this book differ from those of the NCCN guidelines.

NATIONAL CANCER INSTITUTE PDQ SUMMARY ON THYROID CANCER

http://www.nci.nih.gov/cancerinfo/pdq/treatment/thyroid/patient/
http://www.nci.nih.gov/cancertopics/pdq/treatment/thyroid/HealthProfessional

The National Cancer Institute PDQ website gives patients and health professionals a concise summary of the current thinking on the treatment of specific cancer situations.

The information is available in two different formats. One format is for patients and the other is for health professionals.

NATION CANCER INSTITUTE "WHAT YOU NEED TO KNOW ABOUT THYROID CANCER"

http://www.cancer.gov/cancerinfo/wyntk/thyroid
This website explains all aspects of thyroid cancer diagnosis and management. The target audience for this website is patients and their families.

AMERICAN CANCER SOCIETY

http://www.cancer.org/docroot/CRI/content/CRI_2_4_1X_What_is_thyroid_cancer_43.asp
The American Cancer Society website is another source of educational information about the diagnosis and treatment of thyroid cancer. The information on this website is applicable to patients and health professionals.

THYROID CANCER SURVIVORS ASSOCIATION

http://www.thyca.org/
The Thyroid Cancer Survivors Association is a national organization that organizes a wide range of activities to help patients with thyroid cancer. The organization's web site gives patients educational information about all aspects of their disease, low-iodine diet menus, support group meetings, research findings and other useful services.

INDEX

Made in the USA
Lexington, KY
17 July 2010